A NEW SHORT TEXTBOOK OF

PSYCHIATRY

NEW SHORT TEXTBOOK SERIES

A NEW SHORT TEXTBOOK OF
PSYCHIATRY

LINFORD REES
CBE, DSc, MD, FRCP, FRCPsych(Hon),
FACPsych(Hon), LlD(Hon), DPM

Emeritus Professor of Psychiatry, University of London
Consulting Physician, St Bartholomew's Hospital
Governor of the Medical College of St Bartholomew's Hospital
Past President of the British Medical Association
Past President of the Royal College of Psychiatrists

HODDER AND STOUGHTON
LONDON   SYDNEY   AUCKLAND   TORONTO

To Catherine

British Library Cataloguing in Publication Data
Rees, Linford
   A new short textbook of psychiatry.—[New. ed.]
   1. Psychiatry
   I. Title   II. Rees, Linford. Short textbook of psychiatry
   616.89   RC454

ISBN 0 340 40543 0

First published as *A Short Textbook of Psychiatry* 1967
First published as *A New Short Textbook of Psychiatry* 1988

Typeset by Butler & Tanner Ltd
Printed in Great Britain
for Hodder and Stoughton Educational,
a division of Hodder and Stoughton Ltd,
Mill Road, Dunton Green, Sevenoaks, Kent TN13 2YD,
by Butler & Tanner Ltd, Frome and London.

Contents

Preface

The New Short Textbook of Psychiatry constitutes a major revision of earlier editions of the Short Textbook of Psychiatry and contains a great deal of new information and the addition of new chapters.

The first part, entitled Psychology as Applied to Medicine, now includes new chapters of clinical relevance and importance including Eating and Its Disorders, Sexuality, Sleeping and Associated Syndromes and the psychophysiology of Pain.

Part II has a new section on advanced technology in the diagnosis of psychiatric disorders and new chapters on Epidemiology, Social and Transcultural Psychiatry, Forensic Psychiatry and Legal Aspects, and Miscellaneous Disorders. Recommendations for further reading have been extended and been brought up to date.

1

Definitions and Scope of Psychiatry

Psychiatry is the branch of medicine which deals with the recognition, treatment and prevention of mental abnormalities and disorders. It deals with illnesses which predominantly affect a person's mental life and behaviour, i.e. his feelings, his thinking, his behaviour and social relationships.

The field of psychiatry is diverse and extensive. There are special branches dealing with children (child psychiatry) and old age (psychogeriatrics). Forensic psychiatry deals with medico-legal aspects. Social psychiatry includes all environmental factors, including epidemiology.

Psychiatric ill health is of great social importance. Nearly half of all the hospital beds in England and Wales are for mentally ill and mentally handicapped patients.

The most conservative surveys of general practice reveal that between 15 and 25 per cent of all patients seen by the general practitioner have a psychiatric illness or have important psychological features.

The prevalence of psychiatric illness as a cause of morbidity, loss of work and incapacity is revealed by Ministry of Pensions and National Insurance statistics. Similarly, the extent to which psychiatric illness is responsible for illness and discharge from the Armed Forces and is a cause of breakdown in University and other students, further testify to its importance.

A **psychiatrist** is a physician who has been trained and has had experience in the diagnosis and treatment of psychiatric illness. Postgraduate training extends over 5–8 years, during which time higher qualifications in general medicine as well as specialist qualifications in psychiatry are usually obtained.

A **psychotherapist** is a person with special training in psychotherapy. A psychoanalyst is a psychotherapist who is trained in the method of Freud.

The term **psychosomatic** means the influence of psychological factors in the production of physical disorders.

The term **somatopsychic** refers to the effect of a physical disease or disability on the person's mental state and behaviour.

Psychology is concerned with the study of mental life and behaviour. It stands in relationship to psychiatry in very much the same way as physiology does to general medicine.

A **psychologist** is not medically qualified and has a degree in psychology.

The clinical psychologist forms an integral part of the psychiatric team which comprises psychiatrist, psychologist, psychiatric social worker, nurses etc.

2

Historical Development of Modern Psychiatry

Psychiatry has been described as the oldest art in medicine and the newest science.

It is the oldest art because mental disorders were among the first types of illness to be recognized. The oldest prescription in existence is from ancient Egyptian medicine and calls for 'the exhibition of green stone as a fumigation against hysteria'.

Ancient medicine, both Egyptian and Greek, considered all disease to be caused by evil spirits or demons and similar concepts continued in Europe with regard to mental disorders throughout the middle ages.

Hippocrates (460–377 BC) replaced demoniacal concepts of disease by a theory and practice of medicine based on observation and natural causes. Hippocrates regarded mental illnesses in much the same light as he did physical illnesses. He considered that mentally ill patients needed to be investigated to discover the causes of the illness in order that these should be dealt with as effectively as possible.

The theories of disease causation of Hippocrates and Galen regarded disease to be due to a disturbance in the body of the distribution of the four humours—black bile, yellow bile, blood and phlegm. We still pay reference to these humoral theories by the everyday use of the terms melancholia, choleric, sanguine, and phlegmatic.

Despite the enlightened teachings of Hippocrates and Galen, beliefs that mental illnesses were due to possession by demons persisted throughout the middle ages and were responsible for cruelty to the mentally ill, who were flogged and ill-treated in order to drive out demons and evil spirits. Witch hunting occurred on a large scale in the fifteenth century and many supposed witches were put to death because they were believed to be possessed by evil spirits.

Three bright lights shone in the darkness of this period. One was a hospital which existed in the sixth century at Mount Cassino in Italy, which provided humane care for mentally ill patients, and later other hospitals which, similarly, treated mentally ill patients with understanding and humane care were founded in Lyons in the sixth century and Paris in the seventh century.

Development of Modern Trends in Psychiatric Care and Treatment

It will be convenient to consider the development of modern trends in psychiatric care under the following headings:

1 hospital care, including social and legal aspects
2 the development of psychological methods of treatment
3 the development of the organic or biological approach to psychiatric illness
4 the development of drug treatment in psychiatry.

1 Hospital Care, Social and Legal Aspects of Psychiatric Care

One of the most important dates in the history of psychiatry is 1795, which marks the inauguration of the humane treatment of the mentally ill by Pinel in Paris.

Pinel gave patients increased liberty and provided them with work and activities in the hospital. Previously, they had been restrained and sometimes chained and were noisy, destructive and disturbed but, when freed and given work to do, their behaviour dramatically improved and an air of tranquillity prevailed throughout the hospital.

This important social reform was continued by Rush in America and by Connolly and Tuke in England and these pioneers are the real founders of modern social psychiatry.

The work of Tuke in York and Connolly in Hanwell, Middlesex, not only started the movement for more humane treatment for the mentally ill in this country but also influenced public opinion to regard mentally disordered people as being ill and not criminals or possessed by devils, and that society had a duty to provide medical treatment as well as providing humane care.

In Britain a large number of mental hospitals were built during the nineteenth century. In 1890 the Lunacy Act was passed, which imposed on local authorities the duty of providing mental hospital accommodation. The Act made Certification and a Judicial Order a prerequisite for admission to public mental hospitals.

The effect of this was that people with early or mild degrees of mental illness were excluded from treatment, as Certification was only invoked when the behaviour or the medical condition of the person made admission to hospital imperative.

The Maudsley Hospital, by a special Act of Parliament, was allowed to admit patients on a voluntary basis in the early nineteen twenties. Subsequently, in 1930 the Mental Treatment Act enabled all mental hospitals to take voluntary patients.

This Act had far-reaching consequences; patients now sought admission at a much earlier stage of the illness, with the result that recovery and discharge rates improved. There was also a rapid development of outpatient clinic services to enable patients to be seen prior to admission and to be followed up after discharge.

The most striking change in social and legal provisions for psychiatric illness in this country was the Mental Health Act of 1959 which, in many ways, constituted a revolutionary change in psychiatric care. The Act abolished Certification and also did away with the distinction, from the legal viewpoint, between mental and general hospitals. Patients can now be admitted informally to psychiatric hospitals, just as they can to general hospitals. Compulsory admission, when necessary for observation or treatment, is not a judicial procedure but based on medical recommendations. This Act lays much greater emphasis on the care of a patient in the community, with increased opportunities for treatment of psychiatric illnesses at outpatient clinics, day hospitals and in the patient's home. The Mental Health Act 1983 provides more safeguards for detained patients and protection of staff.

The Department of Health and Social Security proposes closing down many of the older mental hospitals and establishing large psychiatric units at general hospitals which will serve specific catchment areas.

2   The Development of Psychological Methods and Treatment

Paracelsus, in the fifteenth century, put forward the view that health and illness were controlled by astral bodies such as the stars and the moon. The term lunacy is a relic of these theories which allege that mentally ill people are affected by the moon.

From this developed the concept of animal magnetism and Mesmer believed that ill health was due to a disturbance in the body of a fluid which was called animal magnetism.

Patients treated on the basis of the animal magnetism theory often went into a trancelike state, which was in fact identical with what we now know to be hypnosis. Hypnosis was later used by Charcot and others therapeutically. Charcot believed that hypnosis and suggestion were the keys to psychiatric treatment.

Freud started using hypnosis to treat psychiatric patients but later dispensed with it, as he found it was unnecessary and often created undesirable dependence on the part of the patient. He replaced it by his method of free association. This became the foundation of psychoanalysis, which proved to have far-reaching influences on thinking and attitudes as well as providing a method of treatment for certain psychiatric disorders, and laid the basis of modern dynamic psychiatry.

3 The Organic or Biological Approach

The organic or biological trend paid due attention to physical factors in mental illness and initiated somatic treatment methods, starting in the eighteenth century with Morgagni who held the view that mental illness was an organic disease. This concept was refined by various other neuropsychiatrists, laying the foundation for a biological, constitutional and organic type of psychiatry.

This led to a number of important treatments; in 1917 Wagner von Jauregg introduced malarial therapy for general paresis and later, Klaesi introduced prolonged narcosis therapy, Sakel introduced insulin coma therapy and Meduna cardiazol convulsive therapy. Moniz introduced prefrontal lobotomy in 1936 and in 1938 Cerletti and Bini introduced electroconvulsive therapy.

4 The Development of Drug Treatment

Herbal remedies and concoctions were used for the treatment of mental disorder by Hippocrates and were described by Burton in his Anatomy of Melancholy. Chloral hydrate was introduced into medicine in 1869 and Fisher synthesized the first barbiturate in 1903.

The drug treatment of mental illness has developed with remarkable rapidity during the past few decades. New drugs with potent actions on the higher functions of the central nervous system (**psychotropic drugs**) have been discovered, which have transformed psychiatric treatment.

The field of study of these drugs is termed **psychopharmacology**, which is one of the most rapidly developing areas of psychiatry (see Chapter 39).

Conclusions

The history of progress in medicine generally during the past two hundred years shows that the pattern of progress develops from clinical descriptions of symptoms and signs of the disease, description of morbid anatomy and the possibility of treatment and prevention, depending on the discovery of the relevant causal factors and the extent to which these could be modified by medical intervention.

This mode of progress has applied in psychiatry, but advances here also involve social, administrative and legal aspects culminating in the Mental Health Act of 1959 and the plans for transforming community and hospital care for the mentally ill and mentally handicapped.

Further Reading

Zilboorg, G. (1941) *A History of Medical Psychology.* Norton, New York.

Leigh, D. H. (1961) *The Historical Development of British Psychiatry. Vol I 18th and 19th Centuries.* Pergamon Press, Oxford.

Hunter, R. A. and MacAlpine, I. (1963) *Three Hundred Years of Psychiatry 1535–1860.* Oxford University Press, London.

Ackernecht, E. H. (1969) *A Short History of Psychiatry.* 2nd edn. Hafner, New York.

Jones, K. (1972) *A History of the Mental Health Services.* Routledge & Kegan Paul, London.

PART

I

Psychology as Applied to Medicine

3

'Milieu Interieur'

'La Fixite du Milieu Interieur est la Condition de la vie Libre'

Every organism has two environments, namely an external environment to which it must adjust and an internal environment ('milieu interieur') which for health, growth and well-being must be maintained relatively constant within narrow limits.

Claude Bernard propounded his now famous dictum that 'the condition for a free life is the constancy of the internal environment'.

Any variation in the internal environment, beyond certain permissible narrow ranges, causes a disturbance of well-being and abnormality of functioning in the organism and invariably the first functions to suffer with any change in the internal environment are the highest functions of the central nervous system.

Cannon introduced the term 'homeostasis' to refer to the maintenance of a steady state within the organism.

The internal environment refers to the body fluids which bathe the cells of the organism. It is a product of the organism and controlled by it and is the medium for the transfer of oxygen, foodstuffs and waste products.

Homeostasis is a tendency to restore or maintain a steady state or relative constancy of the composition of the body. The concept involves the persistence of an observable steady state with minor changes, thresholds of normality above and below this range of variation, information which is often a sensory input reporting changes in the steady state, and effector processes for restoring the steady state. The mechanisms may be biochemical or physiological, sometimes referred to as static homeostasis, or complex learned behaviour referred to as dynamic homeostasis.

Homeostasis involves:

1 obtaining from the external environment oxygen, food and water
2 eliminating waste products
3 maintaining temperature and the manifold physicochemical properties of the internal environment relatively constant
4 appropriate periods of activity, rest and sleep.

Mechanisms Involved in Achieving Homeostasis

Homeostasis is achieved by:

1 regulatory mechanisms occurring within the body
2 alterations in behaviour of the organism as a whole.

Internal Regulatory Mechanisms

These vary in complexity:

1 The simplest are the chemical buffer systems within the body fluids. These bring about automatic changes which serve to control slight variations in chemical composition; e.g. in acidity or alkalinity of the internal environment, buffering systems instantly make available bicarbonate or hydrogen ions, to restore neutrality and maintain a constant pH.
2 At the cellular level homeostasis is achieved by enzymatic balance; e.g. an excess of substrate will stimulate the production of the enzyme, whereas an excess of enzyme will result in a decrease in

enzyme production. This is a feedback mechanism which serves to control enzyme balance.

3 Mechanisms of metabolic storage and release; e.g. the constancy of the blood glucose level must be maintained within certain limits and this is regulated by the pancreatic hormones which control the transport of glucose for utilization by the tissue or for storage as readily available liver glycogen.

In hypoglycaemia, glycogen in the liver is broken down into glucose, tissue proteins may be converted to sugar, and the tissue utilization of glucose is lowered by a decrease of insulin secretion.

For emergencies, other mechanisms come into operation; hypoglycaemia causes a release of adrenalin which causes a rapid breakdown of tissue glycogen to glucose. It also stimulates the release of ACTH from the anterior pituitary which, in turn, stimulates the release of cortisol from the adrenal cortex, causing the breakdown of protein to glucose.

The fundamental importance of maintaining the blood glucose level for survival and well-being is illustrated by its not relying upon a single mechanism but on several which subserve the same purpose.

4 The autonomic nervous system plays an important part in internal mechanisms involved in homeostasis.

The sympathetico-adrenomedullary system, by release of catecholamines, serves to mobilize the organism for activity to be able to deal with threats. The parasympathetic nervous system, on the other hand, is concerned with restitution, repair and procreation.

The central nervous system and the autonomic nervous system form a unit which is integrated to subserve the functional unity of the individual.

The central nervous system also governs the organism's behaviour and, through the cerebral cortex, the limbic system, the reticular system and the hypothalamus, also influences neuroendocrine mechanisms in a variety of ways including the secretion of a series of releasing hormones which influence specific hormonal release by the anterior pituitary. The anterior lobe of the pituitary secretes trophic hormones which stimulate the thyroid, adrenal cortex, sex glands, etc. These glands in turn produce hormones which inhibit the activity of the anterior lobe of the pituitary, thus constituting a self-regulating mechanism.

Chapter 11 describes how the autonomic nervous system and the adrenal gland play a role in dealing with the effects of stress and maintaining homeostasis.

Some effects of changes in the internal environment

1 **Acidity and Alkalinity.** A slight shift towards acidity of the blood results in drowsiness or, if greater, leads to coma and possibly death. A shift towards greater alkalinity causes tetany, twitchings and fits.

2 **Oxygen.** When there is a fall in oxygen level in the blood the brain is the first to suffer. The cells of the grey matter of the cortex will die if deprived of oxygen for more than five minutes, whereas the cells of the medulla oblongata can survive up to thirty minutes' deprivation of oxygen. The oxygen needs of the brain as a whole are great and it has been estimated that during a state of bodily rest one quarter of the oxygen needs of the body are utilized by the brain.

J B S Haldane, during an experiment, stayed in a chamber in which the concentration of oxygen was gradually reduced. Haldane wished to determine the onset of colour changes in his face and lips and had a hand mirror with him for the purpose. After being in the chamber for some time he picked up the mirror and kept peering at the back instead of the mirrored surface, not realizing the absurdity of his action. This is a striking illustration of how lack of oxygen can impair judgment without the individual realizing it. With further reduction in oxygen pressure an impairment of recent memory and a tendency to impulsive and irrational behaviour develops. This can be an important hazard in air crews if their oxygen supply is decreased.

Exposure to high oxygen pressure will give rise to oxygen poisoning shown by faintness, fall in blood pressure and convulsions.

The body will only function properly if its oxygen content is kept within narrow limits.

3 **Water.** Hydration is a state of excessive water content of the body, as found in congestive heart failure and certain forms of nephritis or in any process causing retention of sodium.

Hydration may be deliberately produced by giving a person large quantities of water to drink and at the same time administering vasopressin, an antidiuretic. Hydration causes general malaise and can cause convulsions. The latter occur more readily in epileptic subjects.

Dehydration resulting from any cause also causes malaise and, if continued, death, for example in cholera.

4 **Blood Sugar.** With a progressive fall in blood sugar level, as will happen after a large dose of insulin, a series of changes in function and behaviour can be observed. These changes have been studied in detail during the treatment of schizophrenia by insulin coma treatment and the treatment of certain neuroses by modified insulin (subcoma) treatment.

With slight falls in blood sugar the subject feels weaker and relaxed. As hypoglycaemia deepens he becomes confused and later his response to stimuli diminishes and he becomes soporose. Eventually consciousness is lost and purposive responses cease. If the level of blood sugar continues to fall, we can observe a progressive loss of function starting with the higher levels; the cerebral cortex, then the basal ganglia, then the midbrain and finally the medulla. Medullary function maintains the vital functions of breathing and circulation and further increase in hypoglycaemia will cause loss of medullary function resulting in death.

Sugar is of supreme importance in the body economy as the brain can use oxygen and function in its presence and if deprived of sugar, ceases to function.

Homeostasis by Behaviour of the Organism as a Whole

For example, when the body is deprived of food the level of sugar in the blood is prevented from falling by mobilizing reserves, e.g. conversion of liver glycogen to sugar. This permits the continuation of normal functioning of cells, tissues and organs.

Further lack of food will also induce feelings of hunger which cause the organism to seek food to satisfy it. Interesting animal experiments have been carried out which indicate that the behaviour of an animal may be determined by homeostatic needs.

Rats in which the adrenal cortex was removed differed from intact rats, in that they tended to seek salty foods for which they developed a special appetite. This change of appetite and behaviour enabled the sodium needs of the rat to be maintained and the rats did not die. If no salty food was provided, death ensued. If the adrenal cortex is implanted in adrenalectomized rats, their appetite for salt diminishes and returns to normal.

In animals with parathyroid glands removed there is excess urinary calcium loss and lowered blood calcium. Such animals develop an increased appetite for calcium.

Similarly, animals with posterior lobe of the pituitary removed pass large quantities of urine. These animals develop an appetite for water and drink large quantities to maintain the normal water content of the body. If such animals are deprived of water, they die much more quickly than those with an intact posterior pituitary lobe.

A further interesting experiment consisted of allowing rats freedom to select from 15 purified substances including fat, protein and carbohydrate. These rats grew as well as those given a carefully balanced diet.

A study carried out on children revealed that when they were given free access to a variety of natural foods, they chose a well balanced diet resulting in normal growth and development. This finding may surprise many people and it seems that faulty parental guidance and the effect of advertising may be responsible for faulty dietary choice.

Thus, appetite and behaviour develop according to physiological needs in order to maintain homeostasis. There seems, therefore, to be some scientific support for the old saying 'a little of what you fancy does you good'.

Conclusions

Nature has provided the human being with a variety of mechanisms and processes which serve to keep the internal environment relatively constant, and that the behaviour of the organism may be determined by homeostatic needs. Man's ascent on the evolutionary scale was dependent on acquiring efficient homeostatic mechanisms. With any change that occurs in the composition of the internal environment the first to suffer is the brain, and the recent advances in knowledge give the strongest support to Claude Bernard's dictum that proper and healthy functioning is dependent on the constancy of the internal environment.

Disease in the final analysis is a disturbance of homeostasis.

Further Reading

Cannon, W. B. (1953) *Bodily Changes in Pain, Hunger, Fear and Rage.* Branford Co, New York.

Bernard, C. (1965) *An Introduction to the Study of Experimental Medicine.* Macmillan, New York.

Best, C. H. and Taylor, N. B. (1980) *The Living Body,* 5th edn. Chapman & Hall, London.

Brown T. S. and Wallace, P. M. (1980) *Physiological Psychology.* Academic Press, London.

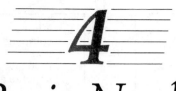

Basic Needs

The Role of Innate and Environmental Influences

An instinct is a disposition to perform a certain pattern of action without previous training. It refers to comparatively complex patterns of behaviour which are largely innate, in the sense of being genetic and unlearned, present in all members of at least one sex of the species and aroused by perception of certain objects or stimuli. Instinctive activity is endogenously controlled, i.e. once set in motion is not dependent on peripheral stimuli.

Instincts in clear cut form are not seen in the human and, when instincts are in operation, they are often largely masked by learning and cultural influences. Instincts can be seen most clearly in lower animals, particularly in insects.

The term drive is preferred by many to the word instinct but has a wider connotation as it covers all the various form of impulsion to activity. The term drive does not necessarily imply innateness; it is the resultant of the processes of heredity, maturation and environment.

A drive is a state of disequilibrium of the organism, set up from within or from without, which profoundly influences or directs the course of response and leads or tends to lead, as shown in Figure 4.1, to a state of equilibrium.

The following are the primary drives:

1 hunger and food-seeking
2 thirst and water-seeking
3 maintenance of body temperature
4 eliminative functions of micturition and defaecation
5 rest after prolonged exertion
6 activity after prolonged rest
7 sex and parental activities.

Contributions from Ethology

The study of the nature of instinctive behaviour in the human has not proved fruitful and, in recent years, considerable knowledge regarding the nature of innate patterns of behaviour has emerged from the field of ethology.

The term ethology is derived from the Greek 'ethos', meaning custom or habit, and is a new field of knowledge and enquiry based on the behaviour of animals studied with scientific rigour. The development of this field is associated mainly with the names of K Lorenz and N Tinbergen.

Observations of behaviour are made in the field rather than under laboratory conditions and ethology is concerned with their systematic interpretation.

Innate behaviour has figured prominently in the studies of ethologists, who favour the view that an instinct is not a complex reflex system but is a hierarchy of directed activities motivated from within and susceptible to priming and release at different levels by appropriate stimuli.

An instinct is a hierarchically organized nervous mechanism, which is susceptible to certain priming, releasing and directing impulses of internal as well as external origin, and which responds to these impulses by co-ordinated movements that contribute to the maintenance of the individual and the species.

The term hierarchic organization means that each part of the behaviour pattern is mediated by a discrete structure and that, in normal behaviour, these fragments are integrated into patterns by other

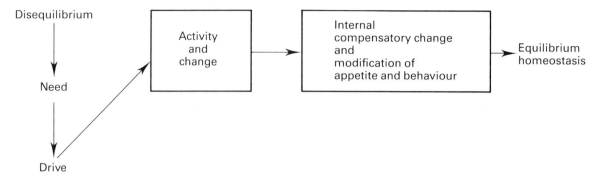

Figure 4.1

mechanisms which co-ordinate the activities of various structures. For example, the consummatory thrusts of the act of coitus are mediated by the sacral segment of the spinal cord, yet the entire body is involved in coitus.

Priming impulses are clearly distinguished from releasing impulses. Priming impulses, by their effects, build up a potential to act which is triggered off by the releasing impulses. Among the priming influences are:

1 endocrines, which facilitate certain patterns of behaviour
2 tissue needs
3 intrinsic activities of the central nervous system.

Instinctive activity is set into motion by specific stimuli which are referred to as **sign stimuli**. Animals, despite the complex pattern of stimuli available at a particular time, respond only to the sign stimulus. This specific response is probably genetically determined.

The male stickleback will fight another male stickleback intruding into his territory. Detailed experiments using different models resembling sticklebacks revealed that the sign stimulus is the red belly of the male stickleback. Any source of the colour red can act as this sign stimulus, e.g. a red vehicle passing the window of the room containing sticklebacks under observation by Lorenz, whereupon the males immediately went into attacking behaviour.

The sign stimulus acts upon an **innate releasing mechanism** (IRM). A special type of innate releasing mechanism is **imprinting**. Imprinting is a process observed in some birds and fish whereby the young acquire the image which will subsequently come to serve as a releaser of filial or sexual behaviour, as a result of confrontation occurring soon after hatching.

Imprinting is a mechanism involving the immediate response to the first sign stimulus experienced, with a rapid or immediate learning of such a response. Tinbergen was able to illustrate this mechanism with a newly hatched gosling, by presenting himself to it as the first available large moving object and allowing the gosling to follow him. Thereafter, the gosling always followed him.

Ethological studies have thrown interesting light on mechanisms which may be relevant in human behaviour, particularly the development of abnormal or disorganized behaviour.

Behaviour in Conflict Situations

Sometimes animals encounter situations in which conflicting tendencies occur. For example, the territorial song bird will attack a male of the same species within its territory and, when the latter is off the territory, it flees. When the boundary of the territory is reached, the tendency to attack and the tendency to flee become similar in degree and then the bird may show alternating attack and escape behaviour, i.e. **ambivalent behaviour**.

In the presence of two conflicting drives, e.g. either to attack or to escape, or when confronted with two contrasting sign stimuli or when instinctive drives are frustrated or thwarted, the animal may show a number of forms of **derived activities**:

1 A bird will stop feeding when it sees a flying predator and immediately flees to cover. This may become an established pattern by a process of avoidance conditioning.

Masserman, in his experiments on experimental neurosis in cats, found that they would not feed in the situations in which they had been frightened, even though they were on the point of starvation.

2 Intention movements appropriate to only one of the conflicting drives. For example, a bird might repeatedly carry out a fraction of the movements involved in attack and this fractionation of behaviour may become a fixed pattern of behaviour by learning.

For example, elephants in close confinement show an unhappy rocking, which is derived from intention movements of locomotion.

3 **Compromise behaviour:** the animal shows aspects of two types of behaviour which, in themselves, are incompatible but nevertheless share some components:
a) there may be **alternation** between attack and flight;
b) the animal may show **ambivalent posturing,** showing some aspects of attack and some aspects of retreat.

4 **Redirection activities:** for example, the female black-headed gull elicits both sexual and aggressive behaviour from her mate who may redirect his aggressive behaviour on to a passer-by.

5 **Displacement activities:** this is when an animal, whilst showing behaviour belonging to one function or group of activities, suddenly shifts to behaviour more usually characteristic of a quite different context, e.g. fighting starlings may suddenly start to preen their feathers in the middle of a fight.

Displacement activity occurs when the animal is subjected to conflicting tendencies or when the animal is thwarted and the excess drive thus created sparks over into the displacement activity.

Sexual Inversion

This is another example of apparently irrelevant behaviour but can be understood in terms of priorities. Behaviour of lower priority appears when patterns of high priority are temporarily impossible.

Inversion of sexual behaviour in birds can be understood on the assumption that sexual arousal in either sex involves an increased tendency to show both male and female patterns, although the male pattern is normally of a higher priority in males and vice versa. If the behaviour of the characteristic type is thwarted, the other may be shown.

Reflexes

Instincts have been compared with reflexes and at one time were regarded as a chain of reflexes. There are, however, some important differences between reflexes and instincts. A reflex may be defined as a response of a muscle or gland to a stimulus applied to a sense organ and traversing the path of a reflex arc.

Thus the contraction of the pupil to light is a reflex contraction of the muscle of the iris, brought about by the light stimulus traversing the reflex arc consisting of nerves travelling down the optic nerve and relaying in the midbrain to motor nerves which cause contraction of the pupil.

Instinctive Behaviour in the Human Being

Instincts, by definition, have certain characteristic features:

1 they are present in all members of at least one sex of the species
2 relative perfection (i.e. biologically adequate) at the first performance
3 although they can be modified and postponed, there is relative invariability
4 they are adaptive and subserve the needs of the individual or race.

In human beings the importance of instincts is not at all clear.

McDougall described 18 instincts which were varied, ranging from such actions as breathing, coughing and excretion, which are usually classified as reflexes, to such forms of behaviour as flight, curiosity, pugnacity, self-abasement and self-assertion, parental care, reproduction, acquisition, construction and so on. According to McDougall, these instincts were associated with specific emotions, e.g. flight associated with fear, repression with disgust, pugnacity and aggression with anger etc. Considerable controversy has taken place regarding the validity of McDougall's description of instincts.

Table 4.1

Reflex	Instinct
Reaction of part of the organism. The operation of a reflex is not conscious.	Reaction of whole organism. The operation of an instinct involves consciousness (e.g. perception of the object and emotional accompaniment).
The response is immediate. The response has absolute priority.	The response can be postponed. The response can be varied and modified.

Environmental Influences

In the McDougall list it is difficult to pick out what is innate and what may be determined by learning, social or cultural factors.

Thus Margaret Meade found that even such fundamental drives as maternal and sex behaviour may be largely culturally determined. In her study of three tribes in New Guinea of similar racial composition, she observed considerable variation.

In one tribe, which is peaceful and docile, there is a minimum of distinction between men and women. Boys and girls play the same games which are co-operative and gentle. The father takes as much interest in the upbringing of the children as the mother and both parents give plenty of love and attention to the children.

In another tribe there are also similarities in temperament of the sexes, but both men and women are aggressive and violent. Children are given little affection and are resented and generally rejected.

In the third tribe the women are dominant, aggressive and do the important work. The men do the domestic tasks and are more submissive and do all the gossiping.

This shows the extent to which temperamental characteristics can be determined by the cultural and social factors.

Again, with regard to aggressive behaviour, it is known that many factors may be responsible; for example, certain parental attitudes may foster aggressive reactions in children. Certain relationships with the father may produce, in later life, aggressive attitudes to authority. In some unstable individuals, aggressive behaviour can be related to changes in the electrical activity of the brain which may be brought out by hypoglycaemia, over-breathing or hydration. Cultural patterns may also foster aggressive behaviour.

Further Reading

Meade, M. (1949) *Male and Female.* Morrow, New York.

Tinbergen, N. (1951) *A Study of Instinct.* Clarendon Press, London.

Lorenz, K. (1952) *King Solomon's Ring.* Methuen, London.

Tinbergen, N. (1972) *The Animal in its World: Exploration of an Ethologist.* Harvard University Press, Cambridge, Mass.

Hinde, R. A. (1974) *Biological Bases of Human Social Behaviour.* McGraw Hill, London.

McGurk, H. (1975) *Growing and Changing.* Methuen, London.

McGuire, M. P. and Fairbanks, L. A. (1977) *Ethological Psychiatry.* Grune & Stratton, New York.

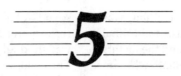

Development During Infancy and Childhood

The Needs of Infants

Infancy may be arbitrarily defined as the period extending from birth until the end of the second year.

Before birth, the infant is completely dependent on the mother for all its needs, e.g. food, oxygen and warmth.

The newborn infant, despite its physical separation from the mother and the establishment of independent respiratory and circulatory functioning, remains dependent on the mother for important physiological and psychological needs.

The newborn infant has the basic need to maintain homeostasis in order to permit growth and development. This is achieved, inter alia, by obtaining oxygen, food and water and by eliminating waste products.

Other basic needs are periods of sleep, rest and activity and to receive appropriate sensory stimulation.

Oxygen

The birth cry is a reflex and serves to bring into action the infant's automatic adjustment to postnatal respiration. During the first few months of life, prolonged crying may be due to lack of oxygen and the principle of letting a baby cry it out does not apply at this early age. It will be seen later that mothering and sucking activity have an important bearing on the proper establishment of breathing functions.

Feeding

The second basic need of the infant is intake of food. The mechanism of feeding in early infancy is sucking and it is only in recent years that proper recognition has been given to the physiological and psychological importance of sucking.

Sucking, which is usually regarded as an automatic and readymade function, is not always found in adequately functioning form in a newly born child. In addition to its primary purpose of feeding, sucking has other functions which are important in development:

1 Sucking brings a better blood supply to the face, thus aiding the development of facial structures
2 Sucking makes breathing deeper and more regular
3 The process of sucking is associated with various kinds of sensory stimulation:
    (a) touch sensations from the mouth
    (b) touch and pressure sensations from the body surface
    (c) proprioceptive impulses from muscles and joints
    (d) auditory and visual stimuli from the mother.
    All these stimuli impinge on the child's consciousness during sucking activity and form the very beginnings of consciousness.
4 Sucking is a source of pleasure to the infant. The mouth is one of the early erogenous (pleasure-producing) zones in the body. Oral pleasure continues into adult life, hence the popularity of smoking and kissing.

Studies of a group of babies allowed unrestricted

sucking revealed that in this group breathing was deeper and more regular, digestion, gastro-intestinal and eliminative functions were better and the infants were more relaxed and contented. Infants who, on the other hand, had restriction or frustration of sucking activity tended to show two distinctive types of reaction. One group was restless, tense and crying a great deal, and the other tended to be inert, atonic and rather stuporous, with a high incidence of gastro-intestinal disturbances. Babies allowed complete freedom regarding sucking only rarely exceeded two to five hours a day in sucking activity and were usually free from thumb sucking later. Sucking activity spontaneously wanes during the fourth month when oral activity is supplemented by biting and vocalization.

It is clear that adequate sucking activity is a very important need in the first few months of life.

Sensory Stimulation

It is not sufficiently realized that an adequate amount of sensory stimulation is essential for normal healthy development of the child. The process of mothering provides the type and degree of sensory stimulation needed by the infant. Mothering really consists of the sum total of the various acts by which a normal mother consistently shows her love for the child and thus, instinctively, stimulates its emotional development. Inadequate mothering can have serious effects on the child. Ribble found that in a group of babies that had not received adequate mothering, two main kinds of response tended to develop:

1 a negativistic response
2 an aggressive type of behaviour.

The negativistic reaction consisted of restlessness, restiveness and hyperextension of the trunk. Other infants showed another reaction to inadequate mothering, the skin becoming paler and losing its normal turgor, breathing becoming irregular and gastro-intestinal disturbances occurring. Vomiting and diarrhoea gave rise to dehydration. The treatment of this condition consists of giving saline to restore body fluids, and bodily massage to provide sensory stimulation.

The infant's first satisfaction, that obtained by sucking, is derived from his mother and the instant attachment to the mother grows as satisfaction is obtained by sensory stimulation and soothing sounds of the mother's voice. The importance of sensory stimulation in invoking emotional responses was strikingly shown in the story of the 'wolf child'. The child, which had apparently been abandoned in the wilds of India, was reared by wolves. When found by a missionary, the child walked on all fours, emitted unintelligible sounds and showed no social responses. The first sign of affection occurred when the missionary's wife began to massage the child.

Kinaesthetic stimulation is also required by infants and the old methods of rocking a child in a mother's arms or cradle supplies this need. It has been found that the children receiving inadequate mothering tend to develop head rolling and body rolling which, as it were, tend to compensate for the lack of rocking.

Thus, mothering provides an adequate source of sensory sensations of the right kind and degree, and it helps functional integration and emotional and general development.

Eliminative Functions

In the exercise of the eliminative functions of urination and defaecation, the infant is no respecter of time or person. Nowadays there is a tendency to start the child's toilet training very early, even during the first few months of life. The tenth month is early enough to start toilet training, and any attempt to start before this is merely the establishment of conditioned response which often breaks down at the end of the first year.

Toilet training should not be started before the infant can sit up securely and not before he is able to give some sign of his urge to defaecate. Furthermore, toilet training should not be started before he has a strong positive and emotional attachment to someone. Toilet training, in effect, constitutes a frustration of natural impulses and it is important that it should be carried out without emotional tension. Often mothers are so concerned with cleanliness and regularity of bowel action that toilet training may be enforced too early or too harshly. It must be remembered that training must be based on love and security, and the less anxiety and tension focused on eliminative functions the better it will be for the child and the more normal and regular will his elimination functions be.

The Effects of Loss of Maternal Care

Dependency is a central feature of infancy. During the first months of life the mother should supply the infant's needs as an individual and not merely act as provider of food and comfort. All feelings of security in fact are vested in his mother. The child of 18 months to 2 years is fiercely possessive, selfish and utterly intolerant of frustration. When a child of 18–24 months of age who has previously had a normal relationship with his mother and has not been separated from her for more than a few hours, is then brought up in an impersonal environment, he usually progresses through three phases of emotional responses—protest, despair and denial.

Protest

Lasts for a few hours to eight days. He is anxious that he has lost his mother and is confused by the unfamiliar surroundings. He will cry loudly, shake his cot and throw himself about and look urgently towards any sight or sound which might be his missing mother.

Despair

He may cry monotonously and intermittently. He is withdrawn and apathetic. He is quiet but in a state of mourning. This is often mistakenly taken to indicate reduced distress.

Denial

If a substitute mother is available he reacts with a denial for the need of mothering by his own mother. The second type is denial of all need for mothering. He becomes more and more self-centred, transferring his desires and feelings from people on to material things such as sweets, toys and food. These are dependable satisfactions.

In hospital these reactions can be avoided or minimized by extended visiting and allowing mothers to help in the care of their children.

Summary of General Principles

We may now formulate certain psychological rules on upbringing in infancy:

1 The baby should have a long and uninterrupted period of consistent and adequate mothering. If the mother is not available, it should preferably be given by one person
2 Freedom of sucking activity is a necessity during the first few months of life
3 The child's stage of development should determine the age of weaning and toilet training:
   (a) weaning should be initiated gradually when the child supplements sucking by biting and vocalization and then is able to grasp and carry things to its mouth
   (b) toilet training should not be started before the infant can sit up alone and can indicate his needs
4 The infant must be given time to learn and accept one thing at a time as he progresses from infancy to childhood
5 One must provide consistent and healthy emotional satisfaction
6 Consistent security lays the foundation for the transformation of the energies of the primitive impulses into activities which satisfy the child, are acceptable to others and achieve better emotional, intellectual, social and ethical development.

Forms of Behaviour during Infancy and Childhood

The behaviour of the infant falls into four groups of activity: motor behaviour, speech, emotional and social.

Motor Behaviour

The following are useful guides:

1 month—should attempt to lift head when held against the shoulder.
2 months—can hold head erect for few moments.
4 months—can hold head steady when carried.
6 months—sits up momentarily without support.
9 months—can sit without support.
1 year—can walk with help; can lower himself from standing position.
15 months—standing and walking.
18 months—climbs stairs and gets on to chair.
2 years—runs and builds a pile of 6 blocks.
$2\frac{1}{2}$ years—builds 7–8 blocks and goes down stairs alone.

Linguistic and Speech Behaviour

2 months—attends to speaking voice.
6 months—syllables.
9 months—'Da-da'.
1 year—knows about two words.
15 months—four words.
18 months—six words; can point to eyes, nose.
2 years—can name objects.

Emotional Behaviour

Emotional reactions are shown to satisfaction or frustration of instinctive drives.

In the first few months emotional disturbance is shown by increased muscular tension. Oxygen lack may be the first stimulus to produce anxiety but later hunger becomes the most frequent cause.

The infant's awareness of the outside world develops during the 3rd–6th months when specific emotional reactions to the mother begin to appear.

During infancy, pleasurable emotional reactions occur while defaecating. The achievement of bowel control at about 18 months coincides with greater play activities which help to canalise emotional and instinctive energies.

Social Behaviour

Although the infant is mainly biological and governed by bodily needs (for instance, for care and protection) he has to participate in social interaction to obtain satisfaction of these needs. The infant is not born into a vacuum but into a world in which persons, customs and other environmental influences are brought to bear on him at a very early age.

The first social influence is that of the mother, without whose provision of nourishment, care and protection the infant would not survive. This dependence of the infant on the mother for primary needs is essential for survival and is the basis on which love, sympathy and co-operation are built.

In the early months of infancy there is no appreciation of what is self and non-self. The idea of self is only gradually built up and it is only during the second year and later that the child develops a clear knowledge of himself as an entity. This is probably first noticed when the child finds that certain things, e.g. his limbs, can be moved when he wishes, whereas objects in the environment do not respond in this way.

Development During Childhood

The period of childhood extends from infancy until puberty. All schools of psychological thought agree that the period of infancy and childhood are of paramount importance in determining and patterning future character development and behaviour.

The human being, compared with other animals, has a long period of dependency. Many actions which are spontaneous in animals have to be acquired gradually in the human, e.g. walking. The child has to learn a variety of performances which in adult life become habitual, e.g. dressing, personal care and hygiene, talking, control of desires and emotions in a socially acceptable way.

During growth and development the child has to adjust and adapt himself to the needs of the surrounding environment. The adjustments required become increasingly complex and he has gradually to learn a greater degree of independence.

There are two main sets of factors determining behaviour and personality:

1 the individual with his inborn and learned needs which demand satisfaction
2 the environment, both physical and social-cultural (i.e. persons, groups and traditions), to which the individual must adapt.

Three phases of social development can be described in infancy and childhood:

1 elementary
2 domestic
3 community

Elementary Socialization

The period of elementary socialization extends from birth until 18 months to two years. During this stage, the infant is governed by physiological needs and urges. The satisfaction of these needs is provided by the mother.

During the first two years, growth and development are proceeding which permit of greater degrees of adaptation. The infant develops greater physiological integration and is developing his sensory capacities of sight, hearing and perception in general. Motor skill and co-ordination improve. The period is characterized by marked dependency on the mother for psychological and physiological needs which are inextricably intermixed.

Domestic Socialization

The family is the unit of society. The newborn infant is a result of inherited qualities and pre-natal growth, and it is upon this that society in the form of mother, father and other persons begin to influence its patterns of life and behaviour.

As we have seen, the primary needs of the child for nutrition and bodily care and protection are satisfied by the mother. Later the child is trained to exercise control over eliminative functions and sleeping and eating. The modification of primary needs to meet the requirements of the family is the first process in training.

The satisfaction of physiological needs gives rise to a pleasurable state. The child tends to seek stimuli which are pleasurable and to avoid those unpleasant or painful. This pleasure-seeking (hedonistic) tendency has to be modified and controlled to meet the needs of other people. The child has from an early age to conform to conditions and rules laid down for him by older and more experienced persons. The child demands satisfaction of his needs but has to find means which are acceptable to others. This in fact is the process of education and training.

Security

One of the most important needs for satisfactory development in children is a feeling of emotional security.

The child must feel safe and secure in his relationships, firstly with his mother and later with father and other members of the family. A feeling of security develops from interaction between the child and his parents or others participating in his upbringing. A feeling of security will depend on:

1 love and affection
2 approval
3 consistency in relationships

Love and affection

Love and affection to the child are as important for his development as food and other bodily needs. This fundamental truth has only been sufficiently stressed in comparatively recent times. The child deprived of love is stunted in his personality development. Affection must be genuine and direct and not given in the form of tokens such as presents.

Approval

Everyone likes to feel that he or she is acceptable and approved of by others. It is important for the child to feel that he is liked as a person not so much for what he does or achieves but for what he is.

Consistency

Consistency in all matters and relationships helps the child to form a stable attitude to life and enables him to develop standards and rules of behaviour which help him in reaching decisions and appropriate behaviour.

Consistency is important in:

1 love and affection
2 approval
3 training
4 praise, reward and punishment

Consistency in love and affection is important for feelings of security. If the mother lavishes affection one day and the next day has a different attitude because she may be feeling off colour, it does not give the child an opportunity for forming stable attitudes or habits. In the case of praise and punishment, consistency is of the utmost importance. It is important for the child to know why he is being punished and that it is because of the act itself and not because he himself is rejected. If punishment is given because the parent is in a bad mood or suffering from a hangover the child becomes bewildered and is prevented from establishing stable rules of conduct and behaviour.

For proper and healthy personality development the child must be loved, accepted and approved by the parents in a consistent manner. Certain parent-child attitudes have undesirable effects on the child and militate against his normal personality development. Examples are attitudes of rejection, over-protection and perfectionism.

Rejection

Parental attitudes of rejection to a child may vary in degree and also in the way in which they are manifested. A parent may have this attitude to a child for the following reasons:

1 The child may be unwanted. The parents may have enough children and rejection is on economic or selfish grounds.

   The child may be unwanted for other reasons:
   (a) some parents are unwilling to accept responsibility of rearing a child because it might interfere with their freedom and their pleasure.
   (b) sometimes the child may be wanted for a special motive, e.g. to try to cement an unhappy marriage. If the advent of the child fails to achieve this it may then on this account be rejected.
2 Fear that the child might inherit some undesirable mental or physical condition.
3 Because the child is a product of an unhappy marriage.

A parental attitude of rejection may show itself directly by neglect or excessive punishment. The parents may not be aware of their underlying attitude of rejection but show it by refusing to give the child affection or by demanding high standards of behaviour and achievement. This perfectionistic attitude accepts him only if he is perfect, giving him affection and approval only when he achieves the high standards set in behaviour, industry and obedience. Affection is only given when he reaches the high standards set for him, and not for the person he is.

Another manifestation of rejection is over-protection. Here the parents over-compensate for a feeling of rejection by over-solicitude and, by doing so, try to expiate their guilt.

Overprotection

Overprotection may be due to causes other than rejection:

1 It may be a manifestation of the mother's temperament. She may be over-anxious and have an apprehensive and anxious attitude to life in general. She seeks out potential dangers. She sees dangers lurking round every corner from which she feels she must protect her child. She fears

germs and may give excessive medicines, may clothe him excessively, etc.
2 If the parents have previously lost children through illness or accident, they may fear that something may happen to the child and for this reason overprotect him because he has now become very precious. An only child may be overprotected for similar reasons.
3 The parent may be suffering from her own emotional problem which makes her anxious; this results in over-anxiety for the child and consequently overprotection.

The overprotected child is usually timid and apprehensive and usually more childish than his years. His natural development has been hindered by 'smother love' instead of aided by mother love.

Perfectionism

Here the parent only gives approval when the child attains high standards in behaviour, achievement, cleanliness and obedience. He is not accepted for what he is but only for what he achieves. These attitudes are invariably frustrating and conducive to emotional insecurity.

Development of Speech, Language and Thinking

Speech has three main functions: (1) Representation, i.e. to convey meaning, (2) Expression of the individual's needs, desires and ideas and (3) Appeal, that is to attempt to control other people's behaviour.

The birth cry is the first use of the respiratory mechanism involved in speech and is of physiological rather than psychological importance.

The earliest vocalizations are reflex and have no meaning.

The infant responds to the sound of the voice between 2–3 months. During and after the third month cooing and babbling occur and the child expresses pleasure in this way. After the sixth month the child will imitate sounds and echo-babbling increasingly develops. By the end of the first year the infant knows two or three words such as mama, dada and bye-bye.

The above may be regarded as a preliminary to

speech and the first period of speech development is between 12–18 months. The first words are really sentences of one word; the child saying 'ball' may mean 'give the ball to me'. At this stage there is no understanding of grammar.

From 18–24 months the infant gradually becomes aware of the object of speech, i.e. that everything has a name. His will to master it increases and he asks questions about the names of things and his vocabulary shows a sudden increase. He first learns nouns, then verbs and lastly adjectives and adverbs.

From 2–2½ years he learns the finer shades of ideas by modifying words and his vocabulary is now between 300–400 words.

After the age of 2½, the vocabulary rapidly grows and he has about 900 words at 3 years, 1500 words at 4 years, 2000 at 5 and 2500 at 6 years.

Speech development falls into the following stages:

1 preliminary—during the first year.
2 true speech, from 1–5 years, in which words as symbols of objects, acts, situations, qualities and relations are learned in a manner more or less acceptable to the particular society or group to which the child belongs.

Development of Thinking

Words become linked with objects, relations, qualities etc. and are, in fact, symbols for them.

Meaning has two features:

1 denotation, i.e. the properties and qualities of the object perceived or conceived in time and space
2 connotation, i.e. the suggested and implied ideas and feelings attached to a word.

The following are the stages in thought development in children.

1 **Physiognomic or syncretic stage,** in which the child gives animate or human physiognomic qualities to inanimate objects. If he falls on the floor, he may kick the floor for coming up to meet him; if he jams his finger in the door, he may say the door has bitten him. He may play with a broomstick and refer to it as a horse.

Thinking at this level is asocial and is used merely to express the child's needs. It is egocentric and unreal.

2 **Concrete thinking** is realistic and literal. Each object or situation is regarded only as to its individual qualities. It is the main mode of thinking up until the age of 7 years. Thinking may remain at this level in mental defectives or may revert to this level in patients with organic brain disease.

The word chair to a child of 6 years will usually mean a particular chair he is familiar with and will not conjure up an idea of a class of objects with certain common features which would bring them into the generic meaning of the word chair.

In concrete thinking things may be regarded as the same because of some common feature; thus, if Daddy has a blue car, the child will refer to all blue cars as Daddy's because they have the same colour.

An individual who is only able to think at this level will not be able to see the deeper meanings of proverbs, e.g. if asked what 'a new broom sweeps clean' means, he is likely to tell you that a new broom will sweep cleaner than an old one.

3 **Conceptual or abstract thinking** gradually develops after the age of 7 years and is characteristic of the educated adult.

Conceptual thinking is an active process which involves the voluntary assumption of a mental set and the ability to shift one aspect of the situation to another and make a choice. Various aspects of the situation have to be kept in mind and the whole has to be split up into parts and common qualities abstracted. It involves active intellectual exercise and involves planning ahead intentionally and thinking symbolically.

A concept represents a reorganization of various aspects of perceptual experience, in which some element or feature at a verbal level comes to stand for the whole experience.

It involves finding both similarities and differences in the larger field of concrete experiences with specific objects or persons. Thus, a child comes into contact with chairs, tables, sideboards, etc. and eventually will be able to classify such objects under the term furniture. The word green will come to stand for a variety of shades of the colour. Similarly, honesty, justice, etc. will come to mean general attributes of everyday conduct.

Conceptual thinking is the highest level of thinking and it enables us to use concepts (ideas)

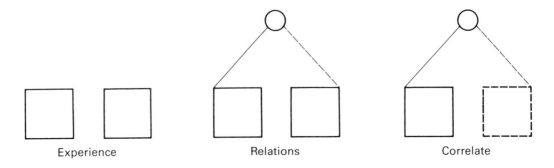

Figure 5.1   *The development of a new idea. The continuous lines denote occurrence and dotted lines tendency.*

instead of concrete situations and may allow us to form conclusions without resort to direct experience or trial.

The development of new knowledge depends on certain processes. Firstly we experience certain things, e.g. colour or odour and then we tend to perceive various relations, that one red is like another or one odour more pleasant than another. Having noticed relationships between things, the knowledge of an object and a relationship can give rise to a new idea.

The operation of these processes can yield entirely new ideas by the eduction of correlates. Sometimes new ideas are elaborated subconsciously. We may have been grappling with a problem for a long time and we 'sleep on it' and it may happen that when we wake up in the morning the solution appears, we may even wake up at night with the answer we have been seeking.

Thus, subconsciously a sorting out of the relationships has been occurring, resulting in the discovery of the solution. This process is referred to as **subconscious elaboration**.

Helmholtz, the famous physicist, when confronted with a problem used to read as much as he could about the various aspects of it and he used to find that, although deliberate effort would not produce the answer, the answer would come into his mind during moments of relaxation, e.g. whilst in the bath or going on a country walk.

Darwin used to keep a series of envelopes in his pocket to jot down the various ideas that used to come into his mind at odd times.

The perception of relations and the eduction of correlates is a high level of thinking and obeys the laws of Logic.

Further Reading

Bowlby, J. (1952) *Maternal Care and Mental Health*. World Health Monograph series No. 2

Lewis, S. (1954) *Deprived Children: The Mersham Experiment, a Social and Clinical Study*. Oxford University Press, Oxford.

Harlow, H. F. and Foss, B. M. (eds) (1961) *Determinants of Human Behaviour*. Methuen, London.

Bowlby, J. (1969) *Attachment and Loss Vol. 1*. Hogarth Press, London.

Laufer, M. (1975) *Adolescent Disturbance and Breakdown*. Penguin, Harmondsworth.

McGurk, H. (1975) *Growing and Changing*. Methuen, London.

Sandstrom, C. I. (1977) *The Psychology of Childhood and Adolescence*. Penguin, Harmondsworth.

Tanner, J. M. (1978) *Education and Physical Growth: Implications of the Study of Children's Growth for Educational Theory and Practice*, 2nd edn. Hodder and Stoughton, Sevenoaks; *Foetus in Man: Physical Growth from Conception to Maturity*. Open Books, London.

Bowlby, J. (1979) *The Making and Breaking of Affectional Bonds*. Tavistock, London.

Coleman, J. C. (ed) (1979) *The School Years*. Methuen, London.

Rutter, M. (1979) *Changing Youth in a Changing Society: Patterns of Adolescent Development and Disorder*. Nuffield Provincial Hospitals Trust, London.

Coleman, J. C. (1980) *The Nature of Adolescence*. Methuen, London.

Kagan, J. (1980) *The Growth of the Child*. Methuen, London.

Bee, H. (1981) *The Developing Child*, 3rd edn. Harper & Row, Washington.

Rutter, M. (1981) *Maternal Deprivation Reassessed*, 2nd edn. Penguin, Harmondsworth.

Weiner, I. B. (1982) *Child and Adolescent Psychopathology*. John Wiley, Chichester.

6

Growth and Maturity

Adolescence

Adolescence is the period of transition from puberty to adult life. Roughly speaking, it extends from 13 years to 21 years in girls and from 15 years to 21 years in boys. Adolescence is a period of profound changes in physical, psychological and social spheres.

The individual has to adjust to manifold changes. In the majority of people the period is passed through uneventfully, but in others it may be a period of instability and adjustment difficulties.

Physical Changes

During the early years of adolescence growth is greatly accelerated. This adolescent growth spurt results in increase in height and weight.

Growth occurs at varying rates in different parts of the body. Growth of the long bones of the extremities is marked. In boys the chest becomes deeper and broader and in girls the figure becomes more rounded, the hips broaden and the breasts increase in size. Concurrently with skeletal growth, bodily muscularity increases in size and strength.

Puberty is the period in which the individual becomes capable of fulfilling reproductive functions. In girls it is marked by the appearance of the menses, the age of which shows considerable individual variation with an average of about 13 years. Girls, on average, reach puberty $1\frac{1}{2}$–2 years ahead of boys. Glandular changes occur and most of the endocrine glands increase in size and in particular the ovaries and testes.

Thus the accelerated general growth and differential growth rates, the complex glandular changes, the maturation of reproductive organs and functions and the development of secondary sexual characteristics make the adolescent period a time of marked physical change.

Psychological Changes

Intellectual growth proceeds steadily during childhood and in the majority of people maximum mental capacity is reached by middle adolescence. In individuals of low intelligence the maximum capacity may have been reached earlier and in some individuals of superior mental capacity intelligence may continue to grow throughout the adolescent period.

Following the achievement of maximum intellectual level, further mental enrichment occurs by the acquisition of knowledge, study and experience. Interests grow and spread over wider spheres including vocational, recreational, intellectual and social.

Emotional Changes

The physiological changes at puberty result in reinforcement of heterosexual drives and of strivings for independence and personal responsibility. The physiological changes stimulate sex drives and the adolescent normally develops greater interest in the opposite sex. Frequent associations occur and falling in and out of love is common in adolescence. These experiences help the individual to decide on the sort of person he really likes.

During adolescence the individual has to wean himself from the family and acquire a greater degree of independence and responsibility. This may evoke in some individuals feelings of insecurity and anxiety.

Parents may not like the emotional changes that often accompany the striving for independence. Previously the individual might have been docile and co-operative and may now become resistant, irritable and disobedient.

Identity Crises

The marked physical, physiological and psychological changes of adolescence, the development of sexual awareness and the reactions to these changes by family and society threaten the continuity of self and ego identity. These conflicts are the bases of identity crises in adolescence, the resolution of which is of paramount importance in successful adjustment. The chief characteristics of the normal adolescent are hope, ambition, being affectionate and desire for social contact. He tends to feel anger, disappointment and other emotions more acutely. In some individuals serious maladjustment may develop during adolescence such as delinquency, neurosis, psychosis, marked emotional instability etc. The tendency to maladjustment will be determined by the individual's constitution and personality, his upbringing, the nature of parental influences and the unfavourable environmental influences he has had to contend with in the past and in the present.

During adolescence the individual gains a keener appreciation of the needs of society, develops standards in moral, ethical and religious matters and, in short, develops his philosophy of life.

Maturity

Maturity refers to the full development of the individual's capacities and potentialities. This is, of necessity, a relative matter as we have to take into account the great range of individual variations in what may be termed maturity of personality in its manifold aspects. Furthermore, the concept and definition of maturity has to be related to social and cultural standards.

Physical and physiological maturity are the easiest to define. Physical maturity is reached when skeletal and bodily growth reaches its maximum. Similarly, physiological maturity can be readily defined. Emotional maturity, on the other hand, is a more complex matter requiring a more detailed assessment.

A person may show mature behaviour in certain situations, e.g. at work, but may show emotional instability in his home and marital life.

The concept of emotional maturity denotes a stable, satisfactory adjustment to life in its various spheres. Such adjustment is achieved when the individual is able to control his selfish interests to meet the needs of society and other people. The main processes involved in the achievement of emotional maturity are as follows:

1 The achievement of independence and self-reliance.
2 The diversion of biological urges and emotional outlets into socially accepted outlets.
3 The person must have a clear appreciation of reality and, whilst having imagination, should not distort reality unduly by fantasy or fanciful thinking.
4 The individual has to achieve a balance between giving and receiving.
5 He must be relatively free from undue egoism and excessive competitiveness.
6 Aggression and hostility must be controlled. Only the strong can be gentle and hostility is a sign of weakness.
7 Goals must be reasonable and within the person's opportunities and capacities.
8 The individual should have reasonable appreciation of his assets and handicaps, in work, play and leisure.
9 He must show flexibility and adaptability to meet the demands of new situations.
10 Pleasure needs of the moment must be considered and fulfilled in relation to future needs.
11 The development of conscience as a guide and to further development. Excessive conscience training in childhood will give rise to anxious and inhibited adults. Inadequate training in this respect will give rise to impulsive and childish behaviour.

Thus, the achievement of emotional maturity involves overcoming the dependency and egocentricity of childhood and controlling desires and impulses to meet the needs and wishes of other people with the aim of increasing personal and social good. Ideally, the mature person should:

1 Be independent and self-reliant with little need to return to childish attitudes or patterns of behaviour.
2 Have his desires and interests reasonably controlled to meet other people's needs and wishes. He should be able to give as well as receive.

3 Be co-operative and live and let live.
4 Have minimum hostility and aggression to himself or others but this should be fully available for defence and constructive activity when needed.
5 Be in relative harmony with his conscience.
6 Realize his assets and handicaps and their relevance or influence on work, play and rest.
7 Have good habits of work, sleep, eating and leisure.
8 Have goals that are reasonable and within his capabilities.
9 Have a clear grasp of reality and, whilst having imagination, it should be checked by reality.
10 Have needs that are acceptable and modifiable in relationship to reasonable ethical ideas.
11 Be able to control his needs.
12 Behave in a relatively predictable way.

Involution and Senescence

Later in adult life there occurs a gradual falling off of various capacities, e.g. visual acuity, learning and reasoning. The gradual loss of physical and mental capacity becomes more marked during the fifth decade and after.

The period of decrease in various physical and mental capacities is referred to as the **involutional period**. Roughly speaking, it extends from 45–60 in women and 50–65 in men.

Following this period and merging with it is the period of **senescence** which is characterized by an increased impairment in mental and physical capacity, a narrowing of interests and increasing rigidity in personality and outlook.

The term **senility** refers to a pathological state in which the above processes become very marked and new changes supervene which interfere with the person's happiness, behaviour and adjustment.

Senescence, therefore, is the normal process of growing old and senility refers to the abnormal mental states which sometimes supervene towards the close of life.

The study of the causes and medical treatment of ill health associated with old age is called **geriatrics**. The study of the processes of ageing in health and disease is called **gerontology**, from which geriatrics derives its knowledge and guidance. Gerontology is to geriatrics what physiology and pathology are to medicine.

Senility occurs when impairment of physical and mental capacity becomes excessive and when initiative, the ability to form well considered opinions and sustained effort fail and social maladjustment results. Patients become less concerned with external events, become increasingly egotistical and their emotional life becomes impoverished.

Memory, which is the keystone of mental life, becomes impaired—especially memory for recent events—whereas memories of the past which are well established can be recalled vividly. The past, therefore, for the elderly patient is often more realistic, important and significant than the present. The failure in remembering recent events causes failure of appreciation of current events which may cause the elderly person to be suspicious of his surroundings.

Previous emotional conflicts which were successfully kept under control during adult life may now appear. The elderly person tends to be anxious, depressed, to have anxious forebodings for the future and is restless, particularly at night.

The tendency for senescence to develop into senility will depend on a number of factors. It will partly depend on heredity and constitution as senility has a familial tendency. The person's physical health will also have a bearing, such as the degree of arteriosclerosis and kidney function impairment etc., which may reduce the ability of the elderly person to adjust to stressful situations. The person's way of life and his personality and previous level of adjustment will also affect his ability to maintain a satisfactory adjustment during senescence.

Retirement

The individual's reaction to and method of dealing with retirement has an important bearing on mental health. If the individual feels that he is finished and is incapable of further useful work or activity then he will tend to become morose, apathetic or depressed. If he feels that he is now superfluous and unimportant this will exaggerate feelings of inadequacy and inferiority. If he now enters into a scale of relative inactivity in place of his regular routine of work and leisure, he will lack adequate outlets for his constructive and creative urges.

Reaction to retirement in the above ways will tend to lead to inefficiency and maladjustment. The person should therefore continue to engage in work,

Table 6.1 Comparison of phases of human development			
Physiological and physical aspects			
Childhood	*Maturity*	*Senescence*	*Senility*
Anabolism	Anabolism = Catabolism	Catabolism	Catabolism
Organs developing	Fully developed	Organs lose in efficiency	Pathological degenerative changes
Homeostasis— unstable at first	Homeostasis stabilized	Homeostasis within narrow limits	Homeostasis impaired
Physiological integration becoming more perfect	Integration well established	Integration less secure	Loss of integration
Increase of physical capacity	Full development of physical powers	Decline of physical powers	Decline with pathological changes
Increase of mental capacity	Mental capacity maintained or slowly rises	Increasing decline in mental capacity	Pathological loss of mental capacity
Increasing development of independence	Independent	Increasing dependence	
Flexibility	Flexibility diminishing	Rigidity increases	Rigidity
Interests increasing	Interests continue	Interests diminish	Interests limited

hobbies and activities which will give a good outlet for his creative energies and give him feelings of confidence and the satisfaction of achievement. He should maintain and broaden his interests, take an active part in current affairs and express his opinions on them in discussions with his friends. He should, by taking a greater interest in others, try to counteract any tendencies to increasing egocentricity.

Medical and Nursing Care of the Elderly Patient

A knowledge of the psychological and physical changes in old age will greatly help in the understanding and treatment of elderly patients. Due allowance for the patient's handicaps must be made. The elderly person has a special need for affection and attention but requires to be treated as an adult. Patience and a sense of humour are important. The elderly patient must not be expected to remember instructions as well as younger people. All efforts should be made to increase the person's confidence and self-esteem. He should not be expected to do things beyond his capacity. He should be encouraged to talk and to describe events about his younger days. Interest in current things should be fostered. He should be allowed to do simple tasks and persuaded to complete them even if he may be slow and clumsy.

The keynote of nursing and medical care from the psychological point of view is to make due allowance for handicaps, being patient, encouraging, good humoured and treating the person as an interesting adult, doing everything possible to encourage confidence and self-esteem and trying to maintain and widen the patient's interests.

Further Reading

Saul, L.M. (1960) *Emotional Maturity*. Lippincott, Philadelphia.

Bower, T.G.R. (1979) *Human Development*. Freeman, San Francisco.

Arie, T. (1985) *Recent Advances in Psychogeriatrics*. Churchill Livingstone, Edinburgh.

7

Intelligence and Ability

Intelligence has been variously defined as all-round general ability, the capacity to benefit from experience, the ability to see relationships and utilize such knowledge in future thought and action.

It is difficult to obtain a definition which will cover the manifold aspects of intelligence. It is generally agreed that general intelligence is the innate potentiality of the individual which determines how educable he is in any direction. A person's innate intelligence determines the maximum level that he can achieve, although other factors will influence what is actually achieved. It is necessary to distinguish between ability and capacity; ability refers to achievement and capacity to potential.

For many years there has been considerable controversy regarding the essential components of intelligence. Spearman carried out a wide variety of tests of ability in a random sample of the population. The tests included performance ability, verbal and non-verbal intellectual ability. The results in all the tests were intercorrelated; then, by means of the statistical procedure of factor analysis, it was found that there was a general factor which influenced all tests. This was called the general factor of intelligence or 'g'.

In addition to general intelligence there are specific factors such as verbal ability, numerical ability, spatial ability, perceptive ability, inductive reasoning, ability to remember, etc. These are relatively independent but not fully so.

General intelligence can be measured, at least fairly efficiently if not with complete accuracy, by standardized tests such as those devised by Burt, Thomson, Raven and others. The scores obtained on such tests in samples from the whole population reveal that it is distributed along the 'normal frequency (Gaussian) curve'. This means that there will only be a comparatively small number of people with the very highest ranges of intelligence, a larger proportion above the average and below the average and there will be a small proportion with very low intelligence. At the lower end of the IQ distribution curve there is a small hump in the frequency curve which represents those persons suffering from special types of mental subnormality.

Although the actual success achieved by a person will depend on other aspects of personality, particularly industry, persistence and willpower, in general it is possible to relate intelligence level to vocational categories as follows:

Highest professional and administrative	IQ	150+	(0.1% of adults)
Lower professional and technical	IQ	130–150	(2.2%)
Clerical and highly skilled	IQ	115–130	(14%)
Skilled and ordinary commercial	IQ	100–115	(34%)
Semi-skilled and poorest commercial	IQ	85–100	(34%)
Unskilled and coarse manual labour	IQ	70–85	(14%)
Casual labour	IQ	50–70	(2.2%)
Institutional mentally subnormal patients	IQ	50–	(0.1%)

During the growth of the individual child, intelligence becomes progressively more and more specialized, more and more comprehensive and differentiates into a hierarchy of cognitive abilities— sensory, perceptual, associative and relational. The basic quality common to all these is referred to as intelligence.

Binet (1857–1911) held the view that intellectual backwardness was not a result of lack of education but of some basic handicap arising from defect of or damage to the central nervous system. Binet considered that intelligence in the normal person and the capacity to acquire knowledge were dependent not on education but mainly on some inherited endowment.

In 1904 he was requested by the authorities of Paris to devise a method of identifying, at the earliest possible stage, children who were unlikely to be able to cope with normal schooling. Binet was anxious to differentiate between ability and capacity and he applied to all age groups a large variety of tests, which were believed to involve intelligent behaviour and to be independent of what had been taught. From the results he was able to devise an age scale. The test scores, when related to performance of the normal population, provided a measure of the individual's mental age.

The intelligence quotient (IQ) is the ratio formed by dividing mental age by chronological age and multiplying the result by 100 as follows:

$$IQ = \frac{\text{Mental age}}{\text{Chronological age}} \times 100$$

Intelligence—How Much Innate and How Much Acquired?

Orphans and foster children, who are not brought up by their own parents, nevertheless continue to show some correlation in intelligence with their true parents. Also, many intelligent individuals come from a poor background and, on the other hand, professional parents sometimes have a very dull child whose educational and vocational achievements remain low, despite the best upbringing and intellectual stimulation that they can provide. These differences between child and parents are to be expected on a genetic basis and are difficult to account for by the influence of environmental factors.

Studies on identical twins reared apart and non-identical twins reared together show very clearly that both intelligence and tests of educational attainment are affected by heredity and environment but the relative effects of the factors are markedly differ-

ent. Intelligence test scores depend very heavily on heredity and attainment test scores more heavily on environment.

In the case of children, it is important to have suitable environmental stimulation in order that intellectual capacity may develop to its maximum. Similarly, thinking processes also need stimulation and exercise provided by the home and school environment.

Hebb makes the useful distinction between what he calls Intelligence A and Intelligence B. Intelligence A is the innate potentiality which we can never observe or measure since from birth there is no interaction with environmental stimulation. Intelligence B is the intelligence we actually observe and try to measure. It is the all-round capacity to comprehend, to learn new habits and skills, to grasp relations and to build up and use abstract concepts.

According to Burt, 80% of intelligence is determined by genetic factors and only 20% by environmental differences within a homogeneous cultural group.

In addition to the genetic contribution to intelligence, environmental factors are important in order to enable the person's innate capacity to develop to the optimum. A person's intellectual capacity is built up gradually as a result of his interaction with the environment.

The intelligence we measure is, therefore, a product of the innate potentiality and its interaction with environmental influences.

Measurement of Intelligence by Tests

Intelligence tests may be classified in various ways, e.g. group tests, individual tests, paper and pencil tests, oral tests, verbal and non-verbal tests, perceptual tests and performance tests.

Verbal

1 **Binet type of test** consisting of questions arranged in mental ages corresponding to the ages of children who could pass them. The test has been revised by Burt, Terman and Merrill and restandardized to provide British norms. The results of the test are expressed as mental age from which one can easily calculate the Intelligence Quotient.

   The disadvantages of the Binet scale are that it

is not very satisfactory for adults, both on account of the fact that the questions appear childish to the adult and also because of the small number of items for the higher mental age groups. Furthermore, the tests are heavily loaded with tests of educational achievement.

2 **Spearman's Approach.** Spearman declared in 1904 that all branches of intellectual activity have in common one fundamental function or group of functions, whereas the remaining or specific elements seem in every case to be different from that in all the others. The common factor he called 'g' and the specific factor 's', specific for each test.

The following are the kinds of tests used to measure 'g': analogies, inferences, classifications, synonyms and antonyms.

3 **The Weschler tests** are for individual administration and consist of a series of tests for adults, the Weschler Adult Intelligence Scale (WAIS), with six verbal and five non-verbal tests.

In addition to a total test IQ, two separate subtotal IQs can be calculated, one for verbal subtests and one for performance subtests.

A special scale for children is available, called Weschler Intelligence Scale for Children (WISC), for subjects under the age of sixteen years.

4 **Raven's Mill Hill** vocabulary test is used as a verbal complement to the non-verbal perceptual Raven's matrices test.

5 **Kent Oral** consists of a short battery of tests and can be given to both adults and children.

Non-Verbal Tests

1 **Sleight's Non-verbal Intelligence Test** for ages 6–10 years. The series of ten tests consist of pictures and drawings for substitution, classification or series continuation.

2 **Raven's Progressive Matrices** consist of five sets of twelve designs of matrices. The tests are progressively more difficult, both in the series of matrices comprising a set and in the series of sets. The matrix contains a missing piece and the testee has to select the correct one from a number of designs underneath, so that the analogy between the designs is completed. The analogy may be similarity, opposition or addition.

Performance Tests

The following are some performance tests of intelligence in common use.

1 **Koh's Blocks.** The test consists of 16 coloured inch cubes. All the cubes are printed in the same way—white, yellow, blue, red, red and white diagonally divided and yellow and blue diagonally divided. The subject has to construct designs with the blocks, according to given patterns of increasing difficulty. The result is usually expressed as MA (Mental Age) and IQ.

2 **Knox Cube Test** consists of five 1-inch cubes painted black. Four of the cubes are placed in front of the subject about 2 inches apart. The fifth is used by the examiner and subject for tapping. The examiner taps out a pattern of movements or taps with his cube on the four placed cubes, then hands the cube to the subject who has to repeat the movement or pattern. Twelve patterns of increasing complexity are used.

3 **Domino Test.** This, like the previous test, is a test of memory span like the memory span for digits.

4 **Size and Weight Test** consists of arranging in order of size, five cubes, five others being used for demonstration purposes, and arranging five blocks of wood in order of weight, five brass weights being used for demonstration.

5 **Manikin and Profile Test** consists of noting the subject's ability to rebuild a manikin or reconstruct the profile of a face from component pieces.

6 **Form Boards** are of various types and consist of fitting pieces correctly into spaces of a board. Examples—Pintner's, Seguin, Goddard, Minnesota.

7 **Cube Construction Test** consists of reconstructing a cube from a number of component pieces.

8 **Picture Completion Tests,** e.g. Healy's, are self-explanatory.

9 **Carl Hollow Square Test** consists of fitting pieces of wood of varying sizes, shapes and bevel into a hollow square space in a block of wood. The pieces are arranged in a series of increasing difficulty and the results are scored on the time taken and the number of trials to achieve success.

10 **Maze Tests**—Porteus and others.

Advantages of performance tests

1 Can be used on illiterates, foreigners, deaf mutes and those with speech difficulties.
2 Measure ability to deal with concrete problems and practical usefulness in addition to 'g'.
3 Less determined by education than verbal tests.

Disadvantages

1 Usually take a long time to do.
2 The norms of many are inadequately based, especially for different cultures.

Assessing a New Intelligence Test

The assessment of the value of a new intelligence test is made by applying certain criteria.

1 **Reliability.** This term refers to the constancy of results given by a group at different times. Obviously if the same group gave divergent results on different occasions, some other factor would be influencing the results in addition to the trait one wishes to measure. The reliability is calculated by correlating the results of the test given to the same group at different times. The degree of correlation indicates the retest reliability.
2 **Validity.** The term validity refers to the degree to which a test measures what it sets out to measure.
   Validity may be determined by:
   (a) External criteria, e.g. correlating the results of the test on a sample, with gradings made by teachers or others on the same sample.
   (b) Internal criteria. If one applies various intelligence tests to a goup of people and calculates the intercorrelations between the tests, one will be able to ascertain how closely they agree with each other, as it is assumed that there must be a common factor.
      In the above experiment one would expect to find significant correlations, as the tests are all supposed to measure intelligence. Spearman found that a general factor of 'g', as it is called, is present which accounts for the correlation between the tests. The presence of such a factor can be elicited by the statistical technique of factorial analysis, which will also tell us how much each test correlates with this general factor 'g' or, in other words, how much the test is saturated with 'g'.
      This gives us a method of determining validity. If the test is devised to measure general intelligence, its validity is indicated by its saturation with 'g'.
3 **Norms and Standardization.** Norms for the general population should be available and expressed in terms of Mean, Standard Deviation or Percentile Ranks, and the norms should also be standardized for age and sex.
4 **Objectivity.** The less subjective the interpretation required for a test, the more reliable and valid it is likely to be. The scoring of the test should be objective, so that results by different markers will be comparable.
5 **Practicability.** The test should be easily given and scored and the results graded without difficulty.
6 **The Items.** The number of items in the test should be large enough to allow a sufficient range of variation.
7 The test results should not be greatly influenced by knowledge and education as opposed to native intelligence.

Further Reading

Richardson, K. and Spears, D. (eds) (1972) *Race, Culture and Intelligence*. Penguin, Harmondsworth.
Vernon, P. E. (1972) *Intelligence and Cultural Environment*, 2nd edn. Methuen, London.
Jensen, A. R. (1976) *Educability and Group Differences*. Methuen, London.
Vernon, P. E. (1979) *The Structure of Human Abilities*. Greenwood Press, London.

8

Learning and Remembering

Learning is probably the most important field of psychology. Most of our behaviour is learned. In fact, all the behaviour which characterizes the civilized person and that which distinguishes a particular person as a member of a race, a religion or a social group is learned.

It should also be noted that man learns reactions of guilt feelings, fear and anxiety and many symptoms found in psychiatric illness.

Essentially, learning is the modification of behaviour by experience as a result of interaction of the individual with his environment.

Instincts and reflexes are unlearned forms of response to stimuli.

The learning process may be described as establishing new connections between sensory organs and effector organs. The form that learning takes varies in complexity from simple conditioned reflex responses, as when children learn to avoid fire, to very complex acts and processes whereby a scientist constructs a theory.

All forms of learning, from the simplest to the most complex, have important common factors—drive, response and reinforcement.

Drive

The term **drive** refers to the force which impels the subject to act or respond. Any stimulus which impels action is a drive. The intensity of the drive usually increases according to the strength of the stimulus.

Primary drives

Primary drives are stimuli fundamentally important in determining motivation. Examples are pain, thirst, hunger, fatigue, cold and sexual stimuli.

The strength of primary drives, as a rule, increases with deprivation.

Secondary drives

Socio-cultural influences provide secondary (learned) drives. These are based on unlearned drives and are important in human behaviour, in processes of social adjustment and also in achievement.

Cues denote stimuli which determine when the response to a drive actually takes place; for example, when the motorist applies his brakes on seeing the traffic lights change from green to amber. A cue can be any stimulus which is sufficiently distinctive.

Response

A response to a drive must occur before it can be learned. Some responses do not become learned, whereas others do. The factors which determine whether or not a response is learned are:

1 frequency of occurrence of response
2 whether a reward is associated with response.

Among the various possible responses to a drive and cue, the particular response rewarded is the one most likely to be learned. If the correct response is achieved the first time and rewarded, learning is greatly facilitated and automatically takes place.

Trial and Error Learning

Animal studies have thrown light on the various types of learning. The method usually employed is to place the animal (dog, cat, rat, etc.) in a maze, puzzle box or some other obstacle between the animal and the satisfaction of some need, e.g. hunger.

When a dog, for example, is placed in a cage with food outside, he first of all makes various attempts to get out and eventually might touch the latch which opens the door of the cage. If the experiment is repeated over and over again, the successful action is reached earlier, until eventually the correct action is carried out without errors.

This is an example of trial and error learning. It is learning by parts of a whole until the successful response becomes stamped in by practice. The golfer learns the proper stance, the correct way of holding the club and the follow through, etc. Many of the preliminary efforts are in the nature of trial and error but, in the human being, observation of someone else carrying out the skilled movement and training in the various actions greatly shortens the period of learning, as compared with trial and error methods alone. The golfer practises the strokes and actions until they all become co-ordinated and the stroke sends the ball with the desired force in the desired direction.

Conditioned Responses

One of the simplest forms of learning is by the establishment of conditioned reactions. We owe much of the knowledge of conditioned reflexes to the Russian physiologist, Pavlov. Pavlov made intensive use of the reflex secretion of saliva in dogs for his studies on conditioned reflexes.

The secretion of saliva in response to eating food is an innate reflex, is therefore unlearned and is present in all members of the species. Pavlov found that if a bell was rung at the same time as the dog was given food to eat, and if this was repeated over and over again, eventually the ringing of the bell alone produced a secretion of saliva. In other words, a new reflex had been established by the conditions of the experiment. This new reflex of salivary secretion in response to the ringing of a bell produced by the experiment is called a conditioned reflex.

The establishment of conditioned reflexes is one of the simplest and earliest forms of learning. The process of conditioning may be illustrated as follows:

Unconditioned stimulus (eating food)	→Unconditioned response →Secretion of saliva
Unconditioned stimulus and conditioned stimulus (sound of bell)	→Secretion of saliva
Conditioned stimulus alone (sound of bell)	→Conditioned response →Secretion of saliva

The watering of our mouths when we are hungry in response to the smell of food or the sight of a well-laden table is a typical example of a conditioned response. Another example is the baby's sucking movements of the lips when he sees the feeding bottle. Some conditioned responses are negative, such as a child who avoids fire after being burned.

Conditioning makes us seek pleasurable activities or objects and avoid unpleasant activities or situations. Habits to Pavlov were a series of conditioned reflexes, the arousing of one reflex serving to stimulate the next. Although some simple habits may be conditioned reflexes, many habits are more complex and not based on reflexes.

Conditioning is probably most important in the early years of life. Some phobias (fears of certain objects, things or situations) may be the result of conditioning, for example, a fear of being in enclosed spaces may have arisen from a frightening experience in early life of being locked up in a cupboard as a punishment for some misdemeanour.

Verbal Learning

Verbal learning refers to learning in which language predominates. Learning to speak is based on attempts to imitate and also on trial and error activity. Verbal skills are to some extent motor as the mechanism of articulate speech is involved and motor skills in man may also have verbal components.

Configuration in Learning

We know from personal experience that all learning is not achieved by trial and error. For example, in solving a mechanical puzzle we make a number of trials without success and then suddenly the solution becomes apparent and the successful action is carried out forthwith. This becomes possible when insight into the solution of the puzzle occurs, i.e. when the parts of the problem are seen as a whole. When we learn a melody we learn it as a whole and it may be recalled entirely even after only a few bars are played. The melody is retained even if all the notes are changed, as happens when it is played in a different key. In other words, we appreciate the parts as having a certain relationship to each other, i.e. belonging to either.

In an experiment in which an animal was placed before two open boxes illuminated by lights of different brightness, one being twice as bright as the other, it was trained to go into the more brightly lit box. Later the brightness was changed but the ratio of brightness was maintained. The animal continued to go to the brighter box indicating that the animal reacts to the total situation, in particular the relationships between the stimuli rather than the stimulus itself.

An experiment by Kohler which has now become classical, was that of a chimpanzee named Sultan who was put in a cage outside which food was placed beyond his reach. Two sticks were placed in front of Sultan; neither stick was long enough to reach the food by itself but they were so constructed that they could be fitted into each other like the pieces of a fishing rod. Sultan tried reaching the banana with his hand, then with each stick separately without success. He then played with the sticks inside the cage and quite suddenly found that they fitted each other. He then immediately, without further trial and error, used the conjoined sticks to bring in the banana.

This method of learning is learning by insight. Insight appears when the various aspects of the situation are seen as a whole, each part having a definite relationship to the other. In other words, sultan had learned the appropriate action to reach his goal. The correct action, being the last one carried out before the next trial, would be more likely to be remembered as it was the most recent. This is the **law of recency**.

Another thing which tends to ensure that the correct action is the one that is learned is the fact that it enables achievement of the desired effect, i.e. getting out of the cage and obtaining the food. This is expressed in the **law of effect**, which states that an action resulting in reward is the more readily learned than an action not resulting in reward or associated with discomfort or punishment, which will tend not to be repeated.

Motivation in Learning

We have noted that rewards influence learning. In animals, drives arising from basic physiological needs relating to food and sex, etc. are the strongest motives in learning. The strength of motivation will depend on the state of the organism and, in general, the stronger the motivation the more efficient the learning.

Factors Influencing Learning

A study of the factors influencing learning is of great practical as well as theoretical interest:

1 exercise
2 effect
3 reward
4 incentive

Exercise

The **law of exercise** is pithily expressed in the saying 'practice makes perfect'. The more often we repeat an action or a response to a situation or stimulus, the more firmly and strongly will such an action or response be established. This applies to conditioned reflexes which require a certain number of repetitions before the conditioned reflex becomes established.

All learning activities from multiplication tables to serving effectively in tennis depend on practice. Genius has been said to be 90% perspiration and 10% inspiration.

Rewards are better than punishment but a combination of both is better than either alone.

Competition stimulates learning providing it is not extreme, when it may interfere with it.

Whole versus Part Learning

The question of whether it is better to learn material in parts or as a whole is continually put forward. Children tend to learn better by part, whereas adults and more intelligent children learn better by whole. If the material is long it may be necessary to break it down in order to learn it.

Distribution of Learning

It is found that learning is more effective if distributed over a period. Thus, learning to serve in tennis would be less effective if done in a three-hour period during a day than if the same time were spread over three successive days.

It has been found that learning a new material tends to inhibit or interfere with material learned previously, especially if very similar; this effect is called retroactive inhibition and is one of the disadvantages of cramming.

Over-learning

In order to achieve skills and knowledge which will be retained and made available most efficiently, it is desirable to practise for a longer period than is necessary to learn the action. This is called over-learning and it is found that over-learned material is retained and remembered for the longest time.

Over-learning is clearly seen in the learning of multiplication tables by children. Soldiers in training also have to over-learn various things so that they will be able to carry them out in unfavourable circumstances.

Memory

Memory involves three processes:

1 registration
2 retention
3 recall

Registration

Registration is the imprinting of an experience in the mind. Registration will be influenced by the factors governing perception. The more lucid the perception, the better the registration. It will, therefore, be affected by attention and we have noted that the most clearly perceived objects are those in the focus of attention. Concentration and focusing our attention on the task to be learned will greatly influence the quality of registration.

Attention may be interfered with by fatigue, anxiety and preoccupation. Concentration of attention will also be influenced by interest, motives, mental set, etc. Interest and motive will determine how concentration will be applied and how long

sustained. Mental set and attitude will determine what things in particular are registered.

Students often complain that they cannot concentrate. It is usually found that the difficulty in concentration is due to lack of interest or preoccupation with some personal worries. When the worry regarding the problem is resolved, the student is able to study quite easily and concentrate well because these worries no longer distract attention.

Similarly, people in love often have difficulty in concentrating because their minds tend to wander to the beloved person more than the particular work in hand.

Retention

There are marked differences between short term memory and long term memory. Short term memory, involving seconds or minutes, is much more easily disturbed during the period immediately following learning. The nature of the memory trace remains unknown.

Recently it has been suggested that storage of information may involve changes in the structure of RNA molecules within the neurones. However, it is also assumed that storage involves either changes in synaptical resistance or the creation of reverberating activity within neural loops.

Memory is more readily disturbed within a few seconds of learning and is more difficult to disturb after more than an hour has elapsed.

Persons show considerable differences in their power of retention. Some people are able to retain almost everything—their minds are like sealing wax on which impressions make a permanent and clear imprint—whereas in others the mind reacts like jelly which, when touched, wobbles but is left with no permanent impression.

Intimately related to retention is the opposite process of forgetting. One of the best studies on the processes of forgetting was carried out by Ebbinghaus. He learned a list of nonsense syllables until he could repeat them correctly. Then he tried to repeat them at intervals of time. It was found that 50% was lost by the first hour, 66% by twenty-four hours and 80% by the end of a month.

Relearning, however, was achieved much more quickly. The reason nonsense syllables were chosen for the study was because they had no association with anything else, enabling the process of retention and forgetting to be studied more simply. Nevertheless, it was soon found that even with nonsense syllables people tried to form associations, e.g. some people saw associations between the syllables wed and nag.

In normal life, however, we learn meaningful material and it has been shown that we retain material that is well understood much better than poorly understood facts. In order to improve our ability to retain learned material, we must try to form as many bonds of association as possible. Many schemes for memory training depend on the principle of developing as many associations as possible with material that is being learned.

Retention, of course, will also depend a great deal on how effectively registration is carried out. If the person concentrates well and is interested in the task, retention will be improved. Similarly, practice, repetition and recitation will improve retention.

Recall

The process of recall, or remembering an experience, is quite an active process and is far from being a photographic reproduction of the experience.

The experiments of Bartlett have shown that we tend to remember the main outlines as a frame of reference and that we fill in details and often distort things in the process. In forming the frame of reference, people will tend to select different things from their own experience and, in recalling it, will distort it. For example, the parlour game in which people form a ring and something is whispered into the next person's ear and the message has to be passed from one person to the next all round the circle. The message coming out at the other end is usually totally different from the one going in. The message is continually changed as it is passed on from one person to the other. There is a story of a message sent from the front line—'The General is going to advance, please send reinforcements.' By the time it got to headquarters it read 'The General is going to a dance, please send three and four pence.'

When people are asked to remember stories at intervals, they also tend to distort the material in various ways such as:

1 rationalization
2 conventionalization
3 omissions
4 displacements

Rationalization is the tendency to make the material understandable, reasonable or meaningful. Conventionalization is the tendency to bring the material within usual or commonplace limits. Omissions are frequently made and material is frequently displaced.

The distortion of material in this way has an important bearing on the validity of the testimony of witnesses in Courts of Law and explains why even well intentioned and sincere witnesses are sometimes quite inaccurate and misleading, even though they do not realize it. This is also why it is desirable for policemen or other people reporting on accidents or events to observe accurately and to commit to paper their observations without delay. The longer the delay, the more likely is distortion to occur.

This also has an important bearing on the writing of medical and other notes. Clinical observations should be recorded immediately and not entered later, when the processes described above may lead to distortion of the material so as to make it fit into some preconceived idea.

Other factors also operate in remembering—thus, we tend to remember pleasant experiences easily, whereas unpleasant or painful experiences tend to be forgotten. This is why, when we look back on our lives, they often appear much more rosy than they actually were.

People often forget to do things that they do not really want to do—this explains the high frequency with which people forget their dentist's appointments, forget to pay back debts or to return borrowed books.

How to Improve Efficiency in Study and Learning

Some of the most important factors in study and learning are **interest, motivation** and **incentive**. Motivation refers to a drive from within, whereas incentive refers to the external stimulus.

There is probably an optimum level of anxiety to promote learning. Too much anxiety impairs performance, whereas the person who 'never has a care in the world' is probably operating below his best level.

Planning of Work

The most difficult part of any task is the beginning. One has to overcome inertia to make a start and, in all forms of work, a warming up period is necessary to get accustomed to the task and reach optimum output. Interruptions tend to cause loss of efficiency because the warming up process has to be repeated.

It is important to tackle work when one is fresh and to tackle it with vigour. It is better to work for suitable periods—say one to two hours—with intensity and then to take a break before starting again. Attempts to work hour after hour throughout the day or night lead to boredom and fatigue.

Interest, once it develops, tends to continue on its own momentum; this is an example of the operation of the law of autonomous functions. Fatigue can, to some extent, be relieved by changing the task but eventually, general fatigue develops to an extent that change no longer gives relief. It is important to have adequate sleep and periods of recreation in order to maintain alertness and freshness.

Efficiency in the Initial Act of Learning

It is important to work with intensity and concentration so that registration is clear and accurate. Attention and concentration determine the success of registration. Interest, motivations and incentives will stimulate application to work, acuity of attention and concentration and, also, the amount of effort put into the task.

Improvement after the Initial Act of Learning

Revision shortly after learning a particular task is a good thing, followed by revision at intervals. Recall, repetition and recitation are the keynotes for consolidating what is learned.

A student should develop as many associations as possible with the learned material, both by discussion with fellow students and by further reading. It is desirable to learn in meaningful wholes and as much as one can at a time. It is also desirable to have a basic book to serve as a frame of reference, to which further material and additional associations can be added by reading, discussion and experience.

One of the best ways of imprinting learned material is by committing it to writing. Bacon said ... 'Reading maketh a full man, conference a ready man and writing an exact man.'

Cramming has disadvantages as it does not give the opportunity to develop adequate associations and it may inhibit recall of material previously learned by the process of retroactive inhibition.

Plan of Work

In planning one's work it is necessary to allow sufficient time for learning and revision. It is essential that the newly learned material has a chance to become linked up with the knowledge one already possesses.

It is also important to give learned material time to be assimilated, as there is evidence that mental activity proceeds below the level of consciousness. Scientists and others have often found that, having been perplexed by a problem for long periods without success by conscious deliberation, they have reached the answer during periods of relaxation—for example, when lying in the bath or going for a walk in the country. This process is termed subconscious elaboration of ideas.

Further Reading

Burt, C. (1949) *Handbook of Tests.* Staples Press, London.

Eysenck, H. J. (1953) *Uses and Abuses of Psychology.* Penguin, Harmondsworth.

Skinner, B. F. (1953) *Science and Human Behaviour.* Macmillan, New York.

Hunter, I. M. (1958) *Memory Facts and Fallacies.* Penguin, Harmondsworth.

Eysenck, H. J. (1962) *Know Your Own IQ.* Penguin, Harmondsworth.

Hebb, D. O. (1972) *Textbook of Psychology*. W. B. Saunders, Philadelphia.

Mowbray, R. M. *et al.* (1979) *Psychology in Relation to Medicine*. Churchill Livingstone, Edinburgh.

Vernon, P. E. (1979) *The Structure of Human Abilities*. Greenwood Press, London.

Hill, W. F. (1980) *Learning*, 3rd edn. Methuen, London.

Davey, G. (ed) (1981) *Applications of Conditioning Theory*. Methuen, London.

9

Perception

Perception is the process whereby a meaning is given to a sensation produced by sensory stimulation.

Perceiving involves both the awareness and the recognition of meaningful sensory stimuli. It is an active process whereby present experience is related to past experience and given a meaning.

Perception involves a two way process of organism-environment interaction. This interaction is an active process throughout life and it is believed that perceptual mechanisms are slowly established by initial learning in childhood but that, later, the established mechanism permits more rapid learning in new situations.

Properties of the Stimuli

Perception depends on sensory data, both from the environment and from within the body. An interesting example is provided of the role of internal stimuli when a person wears an inverting prism; everything appears upside down at first but, after a period of about eight days, the world becomes normally oriented.

The process of perception is often a response to change in the environment. For example, at the surface of the earth there is a pressure of 15 lb on each square inch of our bodies and yet we feel nothing; but if 15 lb *more* pressure were applied to one square inch we would perceive it acutely.

Perceiving is selective. At any given moment hundreds of stimuli are impinging on our sense organs; the organism has to select the particular one to which he will attend.

Objective Factors in Perception

The sense organs and the brain together organize a number of stimuli into a larger unit to which the organism may respond in a simple fashion.

The grouping together of stimuli by the brain is based on a number of principles:

1 Similarity

```
        A                        B
 . o . o . o             . . . . . .
 . o . o . o             o o o o o o
 . o . o . o             . . . . . .
 . o . o . o             o o o o o o
 . o . o . o             . . . . . .
 . o . o . o             o o o o o o
```

In A we perceive the dots and circles running vertically and in B horizontally. This is because stimuli which are similar tend to be grouped together.

2 Promixity. In the following series;   OO   O
we see the near circles as a pair.

3 Closure. The following 8 lines (A) appear as separate units with little tendency to be grouped:

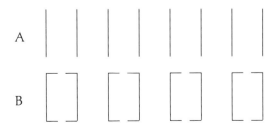

If a short line is added to the ends of the lines as in B, we see them as 4 pairs of incomplete rectangles.

4 Symmetry

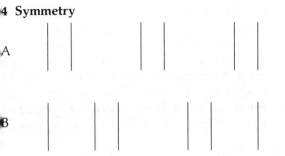

In A, proximity makes us group the lines into pairs. In B the end lines are paired, not because of proximity but because of symmetry.

The mind likes to group stimuli into wholes—a tendency seen by the principle of closure.

5 Good continuation

Fig. 9.1 is seen as a curved line and a line with two right angle bends, although proximity would tend to link a with b, or c with d.

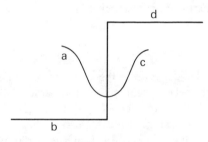

Figure 9.1

This principle was made use of in camouflage of factories, aeroplanes etc. during the Second World War. The 'good continuity' of the outline was broken up in the camouflaging process by wavy lines and coloured patches, thus tending to make the object merge with the surrounding land when seen from the air.

We tend to perceive any change and we select stimuli which tend to be grouped into a simple pattern or unit.

Subjective Factors in Perception

The actual object, thing or stimulus perceived is influenced by the attention of the subject. Attention will be attracted by the intensity of the stimulus, e.g. a very loud noise, the nature, location, colour, movement, repetition or unusualness of the stimulating conditions.

Subjective factors influencing attention and perception include:

1 needs
2 interests
3 desires
4 attitude and mental set
5 mood

Need

When we are hungry we will pay particular attention to things related to food.

Interests

We do not all necessarily see or perceive the same things. Thus, if a geologist, artist and botanist went for a walk together and were asked to describe the walk afterwards, the respective accounts would probably differ considerably and to such an extent that one might think they had been on different walks. The geologist would describe the conformation of the land, the type of rocks seen etc., the botanist would pay particular attention to the plants, trees and flowers seen, whereas the artist would notice features of beauty or artistic interest.

Mental Set

Mental set, such as expectation and anticipation, can influence perception. For example, when we are meeting someone from a train, as we scan the crowds along the platform, we commonly mistake people in the distance for the person we are waiting for.

Mood

Our moods also influence our outlook and perception. When we are sad things tend to appear black and unpromising and when we are happy the same things take on a different and more pleasing appearance.

There is much truth in the old saying 'we see things not as they are but as we are'.

Anomalies of Perception

Illusions

An illusion is a misinterpretation of a stimulus. There are four types of illusion.

1 **Optical illusions.** Experienced by everyone, irrespective of emotional state. These include the Muller–Lyer and Danzio illusions, as seen from the diagrams, where one of the lines looks longer due to the position of the neighbouring lines. In the Muller–Lyer illusion the diverging end lines make the line look longer and in the Danzio illusion the converging lines are typical perspective lines, giving a depth effect and setting the scale for size accordingly.

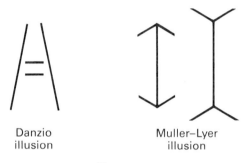

Danzio
illusion

Muller–Lyer
illusion

Figure 9.2

2 **Illusions due to lack of attention and concentration.** We have noted that many subjective factors can influence what is perceived. In reading we quickly scan the written word and, if not sufficiently attentive, we may make a mistake. We overlook misprints and interpret the meaning according to the general context.

   Some illusions in delirium, subdelirium and dementia are of this type. The way in which a person recalls the experience may also distort the reported perception.

3 **Emotionally determined illusions.** Whilst walking home in the countryside in the dark, many people have experienced the misinterpretation of shadows, trees and other objects as human figures or animals.

   In depressive states with feelings of guilt and the conviction that punishment is rightly coming, various stimuli may be misinterpreted as the police coming for one.

   Illusions of this kind are usually fleeting and

understood in terms of the prevailing mood at the time.

4 **Pareidolia.** This form of illusion arises from ill-formed stimuli such as the flames in the fire, clouds in the sky, patterns on curtains, patchy walls etc. Emotions do not come into this type and the person knows it is not real but a product of imaginatory activity.

Hallucinations

Hallucinations are the experiencing of a perception with more or less sensory vividness in the absence of the relevant stimulus. They are false perceptions which are not distortions of real perceptions and may occur along with normal perceptions.

Hallucinations vary in complexity, from simple sounds or flashes of light to complex and highly differentiated perceptions.

They may occur in a setting of clear consciousness as in schizophrenia or in clouded consciousness as in delirium and confusional states.

Observer Error

Clinical skill depends on the ability to perceive similarities between members of the same class and differences from members of a different class. In the wards we must perceive features indicative of a particular illness and how it significantly differs from the normal and even from other persons with the same illness.

These similarities and differences are perceived via the sense organs. We have noted the variety of factors which can influence what is perceived. Even carrying out straightforward readings such as that of a burette are found to be influenced by expectations. The observer unwittingly moved his head up or down to get the preferred result, whether this was derived from a previous estimation or from knowledge of the expected result.

Similarly, in reading X-rays a wide variation was found, even among highly qualified physicians.

Errors will be minimized by:

1 Knowledge of what there is to see. In detecting signs of disease a knowledge of what is to be found will make its discovery more likely.
2 Concentration and alertness which will facilitate accurate perception.

3 Avoiding prejudging the case, as we may over-look features which do not fit in and only perceive those which support our preconceived idea of the disorder.
4 Improved methods of records and measurement which will also minimize the likelihood of error.

The physician should be familiar with all the above factors which influence accuracy of perception if he is to improve and perfect his clinical skill.

Body Image

The body image, or body schema, is the plastic tridimensional perception of the body at the fringe of consciousness.

The image we have of our body is not provided in ready-made form but is gradually built up during childhood. By the age of 9 months the child is able to distinguish himself from the environment but it is not until the age of 2 years that he learns to appreciate himself as a unit. The body image is gradually built up out of various perceptive elements viz. proprioceptive, vestibular, visual, superficial and deep sensibility. The orifices of the body are the first clearly demarcated limits of the body image.

Play is an important factor to form the body image. It is unlikely that the body image is fully developed until the age of 8 years.

The three cardinal factors which contribute to the formation of the body image are visual factors, tactile impulses and proprioceptive stimuli. All are usually important but none is essential; a blind person will have his own type of body image which will be determined by tactile and proprioceptive impulses.

In patients who have lost a limb, all three factors are excluded, i.e. there is no limb to be seen and the proprioceptive and tactile stimuli no longer ascend from the periphery yet, despite this, a phantom sensation of the limb persists, thus keeping the integrity of the body image.

Pathological Changes of the Body Image

Any type of pain or discomfort is liable to cause the affected part to loom largely in the body schema. Patients suffering from Buerger's disease complained that the affected leg felt bigger and heavier compared with the good one.

Some patients, after anaesthesia or during toxic infective states or at the point of going off to sleep, experience disturbances of the body image, various parts appearing larger, smaller or otherwise changed in size or shape.

Sometimes the body image may be projected outwards, the so-called somatic doubling. The projected body image may be similar or different in size and characteristics from the person's normal body image. This can occur during narcosis or in states of fatigue, with hypnosis and in states of intoxication.

Disturbances in body image can also occur in neurological disorders, particularly lesions of the parietal lobe, especially the left side. One such disorder characterized by finger agnosia, acalculia and agraphia is known as Gerstman's syndrome.

An allied condition to somatic doubling is when the patient has the mental impression that he is not alone, but does not have an actual hallucination. This occurs in states of exhaustion, hunger, thirst or loneliness; it has been described by Antarctic explorers, shipwrecked sailors and by climbers marooned on the Alps.

Vestibular disturbances can also affect the body image and produce distortions of part of the body image or may cause somatic doubling.

Disturbances of the body image also occur with states of sensory deprivation and with drugs such as phencyclidine (Sernyl), which produce effects similar to sensory deprivation, and also with hallucinogenic drugs such as mescalin or lysergic acid.

The Effects of Prolonged Sensory and Perceptual Deprivation

The central nervous system is bombarded by stimuli from visual, auditory, tactile, kinaesthetic and other sensory modalities. Great interest has been devoted in recent years to the study of the effects of reduction in environmental stimulation. Professor Hebb was the first to investigate the matter thoroughly, as he wished to understand the mechanisms underlying brain-washing and the lapses of attention which occur under monotonous environmental conditions. The results of his researches were startling. The subjects who were paid to do nothing except to lie in a cubicle and wear translucent goggles became hallucinated, deluded and had distortions of the body image; they became emotionally disturbed.

There are two main forms of reduction of sensory and environmental stimulation:

1 **Sensory deprivation,** in which the sensory input from the outside world is as low as possible, using dark, soundproof rooms and keeping the subject by himself and lying quietly. Ear plugs or ear muffs are used and communication between subject and experimenter is minimal.
2 **Perceptual deprivation** attempts to reduce the patterning and organization of sensory import while maintaining the level of input nearly normal.

In perceptual deprivation the subject lies in a cot in a cubicle with translucent goggles, which permit diffuse light to enter the eyes but eliminate all pattern vision. A masking sound (white noise) is piped into both ears. White noise is produced by mixing together tones with frequencies from the whole range of audibility, in equal amounts.

The effects of sensory deprivation

1 Affective changes include panic, fear and anxiety, depression and irritability.
2 Changes in perception: the room appears to alter in size and contour. Pronounced negative 'after' images occur.
3 Changes in perceptual motor skills, a significant decline in rotary perceptibility and also gross motor skill, e.g. a rail-walking test was adversely affected, especially after 72 hours of sensory deprivation.
4 Time is usually over-estimated by half an hour to three hours.
5 Changes in level of consciousness. In all the lengthy periods of deprivation, subjects pass varying periods in sleep.
6 Level of attention. Inability to concentrate is frequent.
7 Cognitive efficiency. Abstract thinking, distortion of thinking, diminished or lost concentration, lack of clarity in thinking, difficulty in organizing thoughts.
8 Disturbance of body image.
9 Imagery. Auditory phenomena like voices, visual phenomena from daydreams to hallucinatory experiences, kinaesthetic, tactile, gustatory and olfactory images occur.
10 Some experimenters have found sensitivity feelings of a rather paranoid character.
11 Somatic complaints, complaints of weakness etc.

These effects sometimes last for over 24 hours after the completion of the experiment. Gross visual disturbances usually disappear quickly.

The reticular activating system, situated at the crossroads of input and output systems, is able to sample and monitor all such activities. If the reticular system normally is deprived of its sensory input, it meets an unfamiliar situation. It is believed that this change accounts for the manifestations of sensory deprivation. The adaptive capacity of the normal brain depends on sensory input to maintain its reality-adapted activity.

Interference with input allows function to continue, but it tends to become increasingly out of phase. It is interesting that phencyclidine, a drug which interferes with sensory input if given under conditions of sensory deprivation, does not result in its somatic and psychological sequelae.

Further Reading

Hebb, D. O. (1958) *A Textbook of Psychology.* W. B. Saunders, London.

Gregory, R. L. (1977) *Eye and Brain: The Psychology of Seeing.* Weidenfeld & Nicholson, London.

Wilding, J. M. (1983) *Perception: From Sense to Object.* Hutchinson, London.

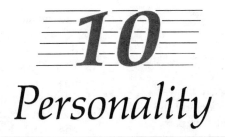

Personality

The term personality is frequently used to refer to certain qualities possessed by some people which influence or impress others. This notion of personality is incomplete and superficial.

In psychology the term personality has a wider meaning and refers to the sum total of a person's psychological and physical characteristics which make him a unique person. The term embraces his behavioural tendencies, his intellectual qualities and his emotional disposition.

Character

The term character refers to an evaluation of personality, according to some standard whether moral, ethical, religious, social, etc. In describing the person as good, dishonest or wicked we are describing his character.

Temperament

The term temperament refers to the emotional aspects of personality, namely the person's enduring emotional disposition. For example, a person may be anxious, pessimistic or cheerful in temperament.

Two fundamental concepts have operated in the description of personality in the past, namely concepts of types and concepts of traits. A trait of personality is defined as the observed constellation of individual action tendencies. A type may be defined as a group of correlated traits.

Throughout the ages man has tended to classify his fellow beings into types. In the time of Hippocrates and Galen four temperaments were described corresponding to the four humours—blood, black bile, yellow bile and phlegm—and we still use terms derived from this concept, e.g. sanguine, phlegmatic, etc.

Very many classifications of personality type have been proposed in modern times, e.g. introvert and extravert types of Jung and the schizothymic and cyclothymic types of Kretschmer.

Whichever typological classification is used, we find no evidence of separate and disparate personality types. Instead there is a continuous gradation from one extreme to its antithesis at the other extreme distributed along the normal frequency curve. For example, with regard to introversion and extraversion the majority of persons are midway between the two extreme types. As Pope succinctly put it ... 'Virtuous and vicious all men must be, few in the extreme but all in a degree.'

Determinants of Personality

Personality is the product of the interaction of genetic constitutional (intrinsic) factors and the environmental (extrinsic) factors.

Among the **intrinsic** factors are:

1 genotype
2 genotypic milieu
3 constitution comprising physical, physiological and biochemical aspects
4 endocrine influences
5 growth and maturation processes

Extrinsic factors include:

1 parental and family influences
2 social cultural factors
3 life experiences
4 physical or mental handicaps, reaction to illness

Genetic Factors

Genetic studies in animals and humans have shown that certain emotional and autonomic characteristics are inherited.

The closer similarity in personality between siblings than between unrelated persons and the high correlation found in identical twins in personality attributes testify the importance of heredity. Furthermore, identical twins who have been brought up apart still show a close similarity in personality even when brought up by parent figures of markedly different personality.

The distribution of most measurable personality traits is along the normal frequency curve and this indicates a polygenic mode of inheritance.

Constitution

Constitution denotes the sum total of an individual's morphological, physiological and psychological characteristics determined mainly by heredity.

Physical constitution

That there is a relationship between mental and moral qualities and physical attributes has been held from ancient times.

Various types of physique are held to be correlated with personality. In Shakespeare we find 'let me have men about me that are fat, sleek headed men and such as sleep at nights'. An old proverb says 'Fat and Merry, Lean and Sad.'

Kretschmer (1921) described the following types of body build:

1 asthenic or leptosomatic, characterized by being narrow in relation to length with narrow, shallow thorax with narrow subcostal angle. The limbs are long and the neck slender with a prominent Adam's apple. The very marked asthenic person tends to disappear when he turns sideways.
2 the pyknic type is characterized by large body cavities, relatively short limbs and large subcostal angle with rounded head and short, fat neck.
3 the athletic type has wide shoulders and narrow hips with well developed bones and muscles.

The leptosomatic and athletic types tend to be associated with shyness, reclusiveness and self-centredness.

The pyknic build is associated with an outgoing, frank, sociable and extraverted personality with a tendency for recurrent changes in mood, varying from depression to elation.

In recent times a number of newer techniques for classifying physique have become available. Sheldon in the USA, from a series of standardized photographs, concluded that there were three main components determining the variations in physique which he termed **endomorphy, mesomorphy** and **ectomorphy,** as he believed that they consisted of structures derived from the three primary germinal

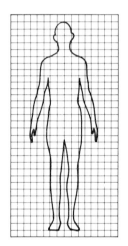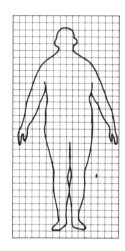

Fig. 10.1 *Some correlates of physical type.*

layers. Each of these components was rated on a 7-point scale; a person rated as a 711 would be an extreme endomorph and would preponderate in breadth and circumferential measurements compared with length, whereas a 117 would be an extreme ectomorph and would preponderate in length compared with breadth. This system has been criticized because the available data enables the correlations to be explained in terms of two factors instead of three.

The method of factor analysis has proved fruitful in the study of physique. This consists of taking a random sample of physical measurements, intercorrelating them and then carrying out an analysis to elicit the factors responsible for the correlations. Two factors are usually extracted; (1) A general factor of body size and (2) a factor of physical type, with persons at one extreme being narrow and preponderating in length and at the other extreme broad and of relatively short length.

The distribution of these types, according to the authors using the Rees-Eysenck index derived from the results of factorial analysis, was along the normal frequency distribution curve using as arbitrary points of demarcation one standard deviation above and below the mean, giving three ranges of physique designated the **leptomorph**, the **mesomorph** and the **eurymorph.**

The correlations which have been reported between various physical types, personality and various diseases are given in Table 10.1.

When the thyroid functions inadequately we get the apathy and inertia found in myxoedema, the person is slow and lacking in energy and inactive and he finds everything too much trouble. His skin is dry and his hair tends to fall out.

Oversecretion of the cortex of the adrenal gland tends to produce masculinizing effects. Women tend to grow beards and to have husky voices. Male hormones produced by the adrenal cortex and the testes are responsible for the external secondary sexual characteristics and some of the masculine traits of personality. It is interesting to note that birds, when living in a group, have a certain peck

Table 10.1			
	Author	*Linear*	*Lateral*
Typology	Hippocrates	habitus phthisicus	habitus apoplecticus
	Beneke	habitus scrofulous-phthisical	rachito-carcinomatous
	Italian School	microsplanchnic	macrosplanchnic
	Kretschmer	leptosomatic	pyknic
	Rees and Eysenck	leptomorph	eurymorph
	Sheldon	ectomorph	endomorph
Personality characteristics		introvert	extravert
		schizothymic	cyclothymic (syntonic)
		inhibition, anxiety and depressive tendencies	sociability and cheerful emotions
		form reactions in tests	colour reactions
		more persevering	less persevering
		quicker tempo	slower tempo
		autonomic instability	greater autonomic stability
Neurosis		anxiety and reactive depression	hysteria
Psychosis		schizophrenia	manic depressive psychosis
Physical disease		duodenal ulcer	gall bladder disease in women
		cardiac neurosis (effort syndrome)	coronary disease
		pulmonary tuberculosis	arterial disease

Endocrine glands

The role of endocrine glands in determining personality has been a subject of much interesting speculation and research. Certain facts are clear. For example, overactivity of the thyroid gland makes the person overactive, restless, tense and anxious; personal tempo is increased, there is a general alertness and a quick response to stimuli.

order. The highest pecks all those below it and so on. If a bird low in the peck order scale is given male sex hormone, it soon gets to the top of the scale and pecks other birds who previously pecked it.

Similarly, female sex hormones influence mood and interests. When the oestrogen level in the blood is high women tend to be more active and restless, whereas high progesterone level is associated with a calmer and more receptive attitude.

We may conclude by saying that, whereas endocrine glands can have an influence on our mental life, emotions and behaviour, the main effects of hormones become apparent when marked deviations from the normal occur. Providing there is a constancy in the internal environment with regard to hormones, endocrines cannot be regarded as one of the more important determinants of personality.

Environmental Factors

In the factors determining personality we can include:

1 family influences and early experiences
2 school and community influences
3 personal experiences
4 illnesses, accidents and disabilities
5 social and cultural forces

Family influences

We have already seen how important the mother and other members of the family are in determining the child's behaviour reactions. It is commonly said that the first five years of life are the most important in moulding future personality and character. Normally, personality development in children requires:

1 adequate affection and love
2 security
3 consistency in relationships
4 proper balance between stimulus and outlet

If the family unit is happy and stable and the child is accepted, loved and brought up with consistency, he will have favourable conditions for his personality development and his future adjustment to society will be helped.

Overprotection tends to give rise to timidity and delay in emotional development. Rejection produces a variety of reactions from apathy to resentment and aggression.

Maladjustment and delinquency are sometimes traceable to faulty homes and parental attitude. Similarly, attitude to brothers and sisters, jealousy and undue rivalry can influence the personality of the child.

School and community influences

These affect, by education and interpersonal relationships, the development of character.

Personal experiences

Experiences in early life can play an important role in determining personality. If the child is deprived of his mother or a satisfactory substitute at an early age, or has not the advantage of a stable family background, he will be at a great disadvantage in personality growth and development.

The reaction of the child to illness or disability may be important. If the child has had to spend any period in bed or in hospital during his childhood and was mismanaged at this time, he may develop an invalid attitude which may affect his adjustment in life and predispose to breakdown under stress.

Reaction to disability

The person's reaction to a disability varies; some reactions are favourable, others are not salutary.

A person can react to a disability such as paralysis of one or more limbs in the following possible ways:

1 He can accept the disability and try to compensate for his deficiencies in a way which helps his happiness and adjustment. This method is the most satisfactory.
2 He may use his disability to avoid taking his proper role in life and to avoid responsibility. He succumbs to the disability and uses it as an excuse for his shortcomings or failures.
3 He may overcompensate for his disability in an undesirable way such as becoming unduly aggressive, competitive or hostile, or by becoming spiteful and trying to elevate himself by running other people down. He may become sly, spiteful and jealous and become morbid in his personality in this way.

Social cultural influences

These play a very important part in determining the characteristics of a race or nation and, to a lesser extent, individual personality differences. The importance of cultural influences in determining personality is strongly borne out by the studies of Ruth Benedict and Margaret Meade.

Assessment of Personality

Personality can be assessed by:

1 subjective methods
2 objective methods

Subjective methods include interview by one person or by a panel, as in Officer Selection procedure in the Forces.

Objective methods utilize various tests such as:

1 Questionnaires containing items relating to various aspects of temperament and personality. Examples of well standardized tests are Eysenck's EP Questionnaire and Cattel's Personality Factor Questionnaire.
2 Projection tests. An example of a projection test is the ink blot test of Rorschach. This consists of a series of black or coloured ink blots. The ink blots are a plastic medium which the individual alters according to his personality pattern. People react differently to the shape, colour, details, shading etc. Extensive research has now enabled a detailed personality assessment to be made from the person's response.

The Thematic Apperception Test (TAT) consists of a series of pictures with people and objects in ambiguous situations. The person is asked to describe how he thinks the situation in the picture was reached, i.e. what events led up to the situation in the picture, and what he thinks will be the outcome.

Some Clinical Personality Types

The following are varieties of personality type or traits which are important in clinical practice. They are not mutually exclusive as one person may show a number of traits, e.g. timidity, sensitivity and anxiety often go together.

General instability

Difficulties in adjustment at school, at home, at work, in marriage, with frequent succession of jobs and a tendency to impulsive behaviour without due regard to the consequences, are all manifestations of emotional immaturity and will be considered in more detail later when we deal with Psychopathic Personality.

Timid personality

This person shows subnormal assertiveness, is aware of feelings of anger or hostility but has difficulty in verbalizing these, even to the physician. This type of person, when he is assertive, experiences anxiety or guilt feelings and subsequently withdraws to his habitual pattern or for a time becomes excessively ingratiating, submissive, apologetic etc.

Sensitive personality

A tendency to take offence, even when none is intended, being easily hurt and tending to brood over hurts or insults.

Anxious personality

This person is always worrying unduly, even about trivial matters; he meets troubles half way and anticipates apprehensively problems and difficulties that lie ahead. He crosses his bridges before meeting them; he is tense, apprehensive, fearful regarding himself and everything else and constantly in need of reassurance.

Obsessional personality

This can vary in degree. Obsessional traits consist of meticulousness, over-conscientiousness, attention to detail, a resentment if plans are interfered with. Obsessional people are tidy, orderly, cannot stand anything out of place, are painstaking, persistent, rigid in habits.

Hysterical personality

This person craves attention, always wants to be in the limelight, tends to exaggerate, will manipulate people and situations in order to get the attention and affection craved for. They are excessively demanding and dominating people, their emotions tend to be superficial and they are, in general, unreliable.

Schizothymic (introverted) personality

A schizothymic person is shy, reserved, has difficulty in making social contacts and in communicating with others. He prefers to be solitary when in trouble, tends to be awkward, tense and rather inhibited.

Cyclothymic (extraverted) personality

These are outgoing people, express themselves freely, make social contacts easily, are warm, friendly. In the cyclothymic person, mood swings varying from mild depression to elation are common but sometimes their mood is equable; this is referred to as the syntonic personality.

Clinical Description of Personality

In describing a patient's personality, he should be described as a living person; with reference to his attitudes, conduct and general demeanour and, when significant, his attitude towards the life situation and his illness. The description should take into account his aspirations, goals and whether these are realistic, his drive and energy, special skills; his affective disposition, his interpersonal relationships, his attitude towards others, whether he is excessively dependent or tends to deny dependent needs, becoming emotionally detached, or whether he is actively aggressive and immature. His attitude to himself, what degree there is of self-absorption or egocentricity; what his views are of himself, the basis of his self-esteem and confidence and the specific areas of failure of self-esteem; his goals and actual achievements, to what degree do they coincide, to what degree is there a discrepancy. His capacity for rapport, his interests.

Further Reading

Vernon, P. E. (1969) *Personality Assessment: A Critical Survey*. Tavistock, London.

Eysenck, H. J. (ed) (1973) *Handbook of Abnormal Psychology*. Pitman, London.

Ewen, R. B. (1980) *Introduction to Theories of Personality*. Academic Press, London.

Fransella, F. (ed) (1981) *Personality*. Methuen, London.

11
Emotions and Stress

Definition

Emotions (affects) are more or less intense feelings with the following components:

1 affective (feeling) aspect
2 cognitive (knowing) aspect
3 behavioural changes
4 bodily concomitants
  (a) facial expression, posture and mobility
  (b) changes in neurohumoral functions and autonomic activity.

Watson, from his studies of infants, concluded that there were only three innate emotional reactions—fear, rage and love. Fear could be aroused by loud sounds or sudden removal of support, rage by hampering the infant's movements and love by gentle stroking or rocking.

Babies were found to have no inborn fear of snakes, rats etc and only developed fears of these objects by learning (conditioning). One of the babies studied by Watson played with a rat without fear; subsequently a loud noise was made when he was playing with the rat and the child showed the natural fear reaction to the noise. After the loud sound had been repeated a number of times in the presence of the rat the baby developed a fear reaction to the rat itself. The child subsequently showed fear reaction, not only to rats but to all furry objects.

Watson maintained that all emotions were derived by conditioning from the three primary emotions of love, fear and anger.

Physical Aspects of Emotions

It would indeed be difficult to imagine emotions without their physical accompaniments. A theory that emotions were the conscious appreciation of body changes was put forward in 1886 by William James in America and shortly afterwards by Lange, a Danish psychologist.

Common sense tells us that when in danger we feel afraid and then run, or we feel angry and then strike our opponent. This sequence is wrong, according to the James–Lange theory, who considered the proper sequence is that we run away and then feel afraid, and anger follows physical action. The James–Lange theory is not accepted nowadays and there is convincing evidence against it:

1 The physical concomitants of widely different emotional states are often similar.
2 There is not sufficient range of physical change to account for the variety of emotional experiences.
3 Sherrington was able to show that in dogs whose autonomic connections between head and body were severed and also whose spinal cord in the neck region was divided so that all forms of sensation between somatic tissues and viscera were cut off from the head region, all emotional reactions were manifest as in intact dogs.
4 The example of a patient with a cervical injury, which resulted in completely cutting off sensations from the body, who in fact felt all emotions as he used to previously.

Emotions, therefore, are not dependent on peripheral stimuli and in fact can be experienced in the absence of such stimuli.

Emotions are always the reactions of the total organism.

Stress

The term 'stress' in medicine and biology today is used in a number of different ways. It may refer to external forces or conditions experienced by the organism, or to the reaction of the organism to these. When applied to external forces the term stress is similar to its use in physics and applies to an external stimulus or force which is strain-producing, or potentially strain-producing, to the person to whom it is applied. Anything may be considered a stress if it threatens the biological integrity of the organism, whether directly by its physical or chemical properties or indirectly because of its symbolic meaning.

Selye uses the term 'a state of stress' to denote a specific syndrome occurring in the body in response to certain agents to which he refers as 'stressors'.

In medicine and psychiatry the term stress is usually used to denote various psychosocial situations which can produce disorganization of behaviour, including physical and mental illnesses.

A convenient definition of stress is any stimulus or change in the external or internal environment which disturbs homeostasis which, under certain conditions, can result in illness.

Adaptability and resistance to the effects of stressful stimuli are fundamental prerequisites for life and survival.

Stresses cannot be considered in isolation. We need to know what stimuli or situations are potentially stressful and we need to know the effect produced by such stresses on the organism and, finally, the pathways and mechanisms mediating the organism's response to stresses.

Pathways Mediating the Reactions of the Organism's Responses to Emotional Changes and Various Stresses

Three principal systems are involved:

1 the autonomic nervous system
2 the neuro-endocrine system
3 the neuromuscular system

The autonomic nervous system and the neuro-endocrine system are concerned with maintaining the relative constancy of the internal environment of the body (homeostasis) whereas the neuromuscular system is concerned with the organism's reactions to the external environment, including behaviour in its many facets. The co-ordination of these three systems in reaction to various stresses and emotional changes is complex and illustrates the psychosomatic unity of the organism, and these reactions are of vital importance to adaptation and survival.

The Autonomic Nervous System

The autonomic nervous system has two main divisions, the sympathetic and the parasympathetic, and both these divisions are controlled by higher centres at various levels in the brain.

The sympathetic nervous system arises from the thoracic and first three lumbar segments of the spinal cord, whereas the parasympathetic arises in its cranial part from the cranial nerves 3, 7, 9 and 10 and in its sacral part from the 2nd and 3rd sacral nerves.

The sympathetic and parasympathetic nervous systems are anatomically and physiologically distinct. The sympathetic nervous system is principally concerned with the mobilization of the organism's resources to deal with emergencies or threats. Most of the functions of the sympathetic nervous system deal with increasing alertness, reactivity and the efficiency of the organism to deal with a threat by action, whether it be by fight or flight. The parasympathetic nervous system, on the other hand, is concerned with repair and restitution; whereas the sympathetic nervous system tends to discharge and function en masse, as it were, the parasympathetic has a more discrete function supplying certain organs, glands, tissues and functions.

It is very important to remember that in certain emotional states both sympathetic and parasympathetic manifestations may appear, particularly when they serve the needs of the organism for survival; for example, during marked fear the bladder and bowel may be emptied, along with generalized sympathetic over-activity. This gets rid of unnecessary weight, thus increasing efficiency of activity to deal with emergencies.

With regard to effect on functions of individual organs and tissues, the sympathetic and parasympathetic systems tend to have antagonistic actions.

When we consider the role of emotions in the

etiology of various physical illnesses, both sympathetic and parasympathetic nervous systems will be seen to play an important role.

Neuro-endocrine Mechanisms

Adaptability and the development of resistance to the effects of stresses and noxic stimuli are prerequisites for life and survival. Such adaptation may involve specific defence reactions as exemplified by the development of specific antibodies to allergens, the mechanisms involved in adaptation to cold or to life at high altitudes and the hypertrophy of muscles which are subjected to prolonged heavy work.

Adaptation may also be non-specific, as described by Selye in the form of a general adaption syndrome.

The general adaptation syndrome

Selye of Montreal described a syndrome of adaptation to non-specific stresses which he referred to as the General Adaptation Syndrome (GAS for short). GAS has three stages: (1) the alarm reaction with two component phases of shock and countershock; (2) the stage of resistance and (3) the stage of exhaustion.

Alarm Reaction

The phase of shock is mediated by neural mechanisms involving the sympathetic nervous system stimulating the medulla of the adrenal gland. Similarly, higher centres stimulate the anterior and posterior lobes of the pituitary, which increase production of ACTH from the anterior lobe of the pituitary and a hormone controlling water balance from the posterior pituitary.

The phase of shock is followed by the phase of countershock in which the various changes occurring in shock are reversed.

Stage of Resistance

This is characterized by hypertrophy of the adrenal cortex, increased parasympathetic activity, increased secretion of glucocorticoids from the adrenal cortex, increased secretory activity of the thyroid and islets of Langerhans and, in general, increased protein anabolism.

Stage of Exhaustion

When exposure to the stressor is sufficiently prolonged and severe the adaptation which has been developed is no longer maintained and this leads to the changes which comprise the stage of exhaustion.

The Neuromuscular System

Under this heading we are considering the reactions of striated (voluntary) muscles. The reactions of unstriated muscles have already been dealt with under the autonomic nervous system.

In contrast to autonomic and neuro-endocrine mechanisms already considered, the reactions of the neuromuscular system are under voluntary control. The reactions in the voluntary muscular system to emotional changes and to psychosocial stresses, although capable of being influenced voluntarily nevertheless occur automatically, either affecting specific regions of the body or affecting the musculature as a whole. It is only comparatively recently that physicians have paid adequate recognition to the fact that tensions in voluntary muscles, supposedly entirely under voluntary control, are just as likely to be determined mainly by emotional factors, by the patient's personality and by his response to various stresses as are changes in the smooth musculature of the body which are controlled by the autonomic nervous system.

The biological functions of voluntary muscles are:

1 static, for maintenance of posture and for enclosing body cavities and therefore serving a protective function,
2 purposive relations with the environment as in aggression, defence and other purposeful activities. In these activities the muscles of the extremities are mainly involved,
3 local reactions such as the muscles involved in facial expression and chewing, swallowing, speech, breathing and those pelvic sphincters under voluntary control.

By measuring the action potentials from muscles of different parts of the body it has been possible to demonstrate that many bodily symptoms associated with emotional tension are, in fact, due to a sustained increased muscular tension in the muscles of these areas. A knowledge of this mechanism is extremely helpful in the understanding of the manifold symptoms of bodily pains and disabilities found in patients suffering from anxiety states and other psychiatric disorders.

The Co-ordination of Emotional Reactions

It is now known that the hypothalamus, the thalamus, the limbic system and the reticular system all have important functions in emotional life.

The hypothalamus controls both sympathetic functions which are concerned in mobilizing the body's resources for action and the parasympathetic which is concerned with restitution and repair.

In the limbic system, the amygdala complex is concerned with food intake, i.e. the preservation of the body, and the septal area with sexual and reproductive activities, i.e. the preservation of the species.

The reticular system integrates sensory input of various modalities and is concerned with wakefulness.

All these structures are interconnected in the form of reverberating circuits.

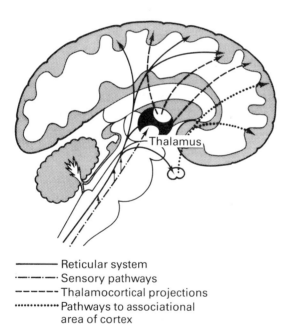

————— Reticular system
—·—·—· Sensory pathways
—————— Thalamocortical projections
················ Pathways to associational area of cortex

Figure 11.1

The famous circuit described by Papez is as follows:

Hippocampus → Hypothalamus
↑   ↓
Cortex → Thalamus

This circuit is concerned with reactions related to emotions attaining awareness.

The reticular system is connected to some of these structures as follows:

Reticular system → Hypothalamus
↓
Amygdala and septal area

By means of these circuits the functions of self preservation and species-preservation can enlist the hypothalamus in support of their functions. Similarly, these circuits linking the reticular system, hypothalamus, hippocampus, thalamus and cortex serve to mobilize the body resources in times of danger and stress.

Many of the potent psychotropic drugs used in treating various mental illnesses exert their main actions on these important structures.

Arousal

There are varying degrees of arousal, ranging from sleep and coma to stupor, drowsiness, alertness, over-alertness, excitement and extreme arousal as in panic and hypomania.

In normal healthy life there is a continuum between sleep, drowsiness, alertness and excitement to extreme arousal, as in panic. Increased sympathetic activity is associated with increasing arousal and higher frequencies in the electroencephalogram. The neural mechanism underlying arousal is mediated by the ascending reticular activating system (ARAS).

Drugs which increase arousal are the central nervous system stimulants such as amphetamines, cocaine and caffeine, whereas central nervous system depressants, such as alcohol, benzodiazepines and other tranquillo-sedatives, have the opposite effect.

There is an important relationship between arousal and performance which takes the form of an inverted U-curve, referred to as the Yerks Dodson Curve.

Increasing arousal may arise from external stimuli or inner driving forces, giving increasing productivity and performance until reaching an optimal level. If the arousal continues to increase, performance deteriorates. Workaholics tend to try to maintain arousal until fatigue and depression set in, sometimes with psychosomatic or stress related disorder.

Stress, Distress and Disease

Stress can be defined as stimulus or change in the external or internal environment of such a degree, in terms of strength or intensity or duration, as to tax the adaptive capacity of the organism to its limit, and which, in certain circumstances, can lead to a disorganization of behaviour or maladaption or a dysfunction which may lead to disease. What may constitute a stress may consist of physical stimuli, infections (bacterial, viral or fungal) or allergic reactions, or may refer to a whole series of stimuli or change in the social or psychological spheres of life.

Selye's (1950) definition of a stressor really is one which evokes the manifestation of a General Adaptation Syndrome. Thus this is a physiological response, and the effect of the stressor can be measured in terms of action on the hypothalamus, the adrenal cortex, the sympathetico-adrenomedullary system, and the secretion of different hormones. Physiological stressors differ from psychosocial stressors in that the power or force of the psychosocial stress will be determined not only by its inherent threat but also by the way in which the individual perceives and appraises the significance of the potentially challenging event, and what degree of threat he perceives as appertaining to the stimulus situation. When an event is perceived as being harmful or threatening a variety of coping mechanisms may be used as a defence. Reality may

be discounted by denial, which is a very common mode of dealing with distressing events, including illnesses like cancer, leukaemia and myocardial infarction. The degree of subjective distress may be modified by displacement, e.g. anxiety or hostility into smiling or laughter, into sleep, or into eating, drinking or smoking. Other coping mechanisms are rationalization and self-deception (which are merely manifestations of denial) and withdrawal from the stressful stimulus or situation. These coping mechanisms can ameliorate the experience of distress as well as its bodily concomitants.

Distress denotes an unpleasant emotional experience which may arise in response to environmental influences or to changes in some internal environment, or as a reaction to some disease or disability.

Disease is a notoriously difficult term to define, but for pragmatic purposes the term disease is used to denote disability arising from bodily or mental malfunction which imposes difficulties in coping with everyday work and responsibilities, interferes with well-being and produces distress.

This theme is shown in Fig. 11.2. We will consider

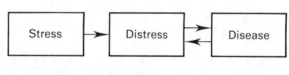

Figure 11.2

the ways in which stresses or stressors produce distress in the individual and in which, in certain circumstances, they may produce disease, which in turn can also cause distress by the threat of the illness itself, or the disability it causes.

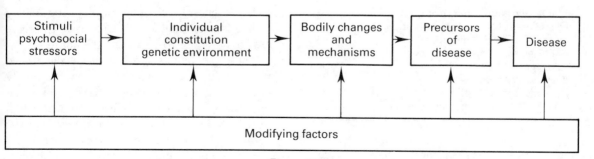

Figure 11.3

Figure 11.3 shows the sequence of events that may occur. The individual's response to such stimuli will be influenced by genetic-constitutional factors and by the environmental modification of his genetic make up.

Previous experiences, particularly in childhood, may also influence the susceptibility to respond to psychosocial stressors. These stimuli, acting on the individual, give rise to bodily changes involving hypothalamic-pituitary control of the adrenal and other endocrine glands and a variety of biochemical and physiological changes which may constitute the precursors of disease and these in turn, if they continue, lead to disease. These changes may be modified at all stages.

We have noted the effects of coping mechanisms. It is sometimes possible to modify the response of the individual by changing the internal environment, e.g. at the premenstrual phase. It is possible to modify the mechanisms involved in the precursors of disease by psychotropic drugs or psychological means to prevent the changes actually leading to disease.

Stress and Life Changes

Holmes and Rahe quantified life events giving point value to life changes that require adaptation. They found that there was a critical level at which too many of these events happening to one person

Table 11.1   Social Re-adjustment Scale

1	Death of spouse	100
2	Divorce	73
3	Marital separation from mate	65
4	Detention in jail or other institution	63
5	Death of a close family member	63
6	Major personal injury or illness	53
7	Marriage	50
8	Being sacked from work	47
9	Retirement from work	45
10	Changing to different type of work	36

during a one year time span, put that person at great risk of illness. Of those people who accumulated 300 points in one year 80% were at risk of illness in the near future, with 155 to 299 points 50% became ill in the near future. Of those with fewer than 150

stress points, 30% became ill shortly after the life events.

It has been found that situations relating to occupation, marriage and parenthood were the most likely to produce anxiety and depression. The life changes affected both sexes but women and poor and disadvantaged groups were more vulnerable. The change created significant strain when it was unexpected and when it not only involved adjustment to a loss, for example a job, but the need to adjust to a new status that involved further hardships and problems.

Loss of work constitutes a stress and may tax the adaptive capacity of the person to the maximum, particularly if it means marked loss of financial status, marked loss of prestige, or creates additional problems with the family.

Psychological Sequelae to the Event of Unemployment

Following the event of unemployment the individual goes through a series of psychological phases:

1 Initial response, as in bereavement, is one of shock and, depending on the circumstances, disbelief. During this phase the worker maintains a certain degree of optimism, regards his loss as only temporary and tends to look at his new situation as if it were a long deserved holiday. He will further stick to this idea if he has received considerable redundancy settlement. This is the time when the handyman comes to the fore and completes overdue jobs about the house.

2 The second phase is one in which the reality in all its harshness becomes inescapable. The holiday feeling is over, money is getting short and there are no more jobs to do around the house.

   The first attempts at job finding having been unsuccessful, the 'unemployed identity' slowly develops. The day is spent in forced and meaningless leisure and there is a feeling of inertia with its debilitating effect on personal self-esteem. The concept of time changes drastically, days will seem to fly past with nothing to distinguish them or to remember them by. People often lose interest in what day of the week it is, they feel exhausted and lacking in energy and most of the day is spent in bed. Tensions develop between members of the family: petty disagreements are likely to become full blown arguments. An adjustment during this period will depend on whether the ex-worker felt he was sacked unjustly or selectively, or on his ability to accept a low status job if these are the only ones available, and on the extent to which support is provided by the family.

3 The third and last phase is defined by Fagin as the 'unemployed state'. A new non-occupational identity has now been established with the necessary psychological adjustments. The anxiety and depression characteristics of the earlier phase life and the family and the individual settle down to the new standards and a different way of life. The job seeking is not done regularly and actively but in a haphazard, casual way, without any real hope of change. Social activities are curtailed, for emotional and financial reasons. At this stage there is a general feeling of inferiority, submissiveness and inability to provide sufficiently for himself or his family. This has been called the broken state.

The unemployed state as it continues in time has an indelible effect on the individual personality which will remain even in future situations of economic prosperity and full employment. There is statistical evidence to indicate that past periods of long unemployment increase the chances of losing future jobs through inability or redundancy.

Kasl and Cobb carried out an interesting prospective longitudinal inquiry on the effects on the health of employees when a firm closed down in Pakistan. Blood pressure recordings taken at monthly intervals revealed that blood pressure rose during the time that closure was anticipated, continued at this higher level for those remaining unemployed, only returning to normal levels upon, or a few months after, re-employment. The increased blood pressure readings were correlated closely with measures of depression, irritation and loss of self-esteem. Increased serum uric acid levels followed the same pattern as the blood pressure.

Entire families are likely to be affected by the consequences of unemployment by the wage earner. Jahoda studied the effects of unemployment on family life during the great recession years in a village in Austria. Families lost interest in events and were broken apart owing to forced and unwilling emigration. The women seemed to bear the greatest burden and assumed a central role in the family. Jones found similar disruption of the family in unemployment areas of the Welsh valleys.

The most vulnerable are the extreme age groups, the young and the old workers; the unskilled; the immigrants; the disabled and the executive class. The professional and managerial staff suffer dramatic psychological changes following redundancy as shown by Harley and Cooper and Tarrant.

Effects on morbidity and mortality

Harvey Brenner found an increase in deaths due to heart and kidney diseases, cirrhosis of the liver, homicides and higher rates of admissions to mental hospitals and prisons among the unemployed. Harvey Brenner, who is a leading research worker in the field, found in a number of studies a relationship between the state of economy and the state of an American subject's physical and mental health. He found that as unemployment increases, so do mental hospital admissions and the suicide rate. He found that it is not the people with a previous history of mental disorder and hospitalization who account for the increase in admissions. Studies in the United Kingdom from 1950–1956 also revealed that hospital admissions rise with unemployment. Women show a greater sensitivity to economic change and the two groups most at risk are women between 20–24 and men between 35–44. It is reported that the unemployed suffered much higher levels of anxiety, guilt, hostility, self-criticism, personal distress and were comparable to a group of mixed neurotic disorders. George Brown, in his survey of depressed women in South London, found that one of the factors that made them vulnerable to depression after certain life events was lack of employment outside the home.

Further Reading

Wolff, H. G., Wolf S. E. and Hare, C. C. (eds) (1950) *Life Stress and Bodily Disease*. Williams & Wilkins, Baltimore.

Wolff, H. G. (1953) *Stress and Disease*. C. C. Thomas, Springfield, Illinois.

Selye, H. (1957) *The Stress of Life*. Longman, Harlow.

Holmes, J. H. and Rahe, R. H. (1967) The social readjustment scale. *J. Psychosom*, **11**, 213–18.

Venables, P. H. and Christie, M. M. (eds) (1975) *Research in Psychophysiology*. Wiley, Chichester.

Barrett, J. E. (1978) *Stress and Mental Disorders*. Raven Press, New York.

Cooper, C. L. and Payne, R. L. (eds) (1978) *Stress at Work*. Wiley, Chichester.

Parkes, C. M. (1978) *Bereavement: Studies of Grief in Adult Life*. Penguin, Harmondsworth.

12
Sleep and Dreaming

Sleep is essential for health and for mental and physical well-being. Our knowledge of its nature is scanty—we do not even know why it is necessary for us to spend at least one third of our lives asleep.

Throughout the animal kingdom there are periodic sleep-wakefulness periods. During development the sleep-wakefulness relationship changes and in the adult more wakefulness is possible during the 24 hours, which approximates a fourfold increase on that of early childhood. The newborn child has two hours sleep for an hour of wakefulness, whereas the adult has half an hour's sleep for the same period.

Changes during the Period Immediately before Sleeping

Some people slip into sleep with great ease and rapidity, others more gradually and some experience unusual sensations. Jerking movements are common at the point of falling off to sleep and many people experience hypnagogic phenomena, such as fleeting visual or auditory hallucinations or changes in body image or feelings of floating in space.

Changes during Sleep

The most obvious change during sleep is generalized inertia and muscular relaxation. Not all muscles, however, relax; the eyeball exhibits rapid movements during dreams and at intervals limbs are moved and many changes of posture occur during the night. Sleepers usually change their position 25 to 40 times during the night, irrespective of the depth or shallowness of sleep. Blood flow through muscles is decreased but blood flow through the skin is increased. The skin is flushed and the sweat glands function freely. It is for these reasons that the body tends to lose heat quickly during sleep. Heart rate and blood pressure falls, breathing is slower, deeper and more regular. Relaxation of the jaw and throat muscles is responsible for snoring.

Levels of Depth of Sleep

Depth of sleep can be monitored by recordings of the electroencephalogram, eye movements, blood pressure, heartbeat etc. Recent work has shown that there are three to five distinct stages from the onset of sleep to very deep sleep. Dreaming occurs in the shallow levels of sleep.

The following stages usually take place: where one is falling asleep, thoughts become inconsequential, reveries or visual images pass through the mind. This is followed then by a more rapid passage into deep sleep reaching the deepest level of sleep for the entire night. This deep sleep period lasts half an hour. Then there is a gradual lightening of sleep, reaching the lightest state of sleep about 70 minutes after falling asleep. It is during this stage of light sleep that the first dreaming spell occurs and lasts about 10 minutes. This is followed by a deeper phase of sleep but not quite so deep as the first. This is followed during the third hour of sleep by a lighter phase with a second and more protracted spell of dreaming. The third spell of dreaming occurs in the fifth or sixth hour of sleep and lasts for 25 minutes. In the seventh hour there is another spell of light sleep and dreaming for another hour or so.

During recent years our knowledge of the physiology and biochemistry of sleep has greatly advanced, as has our understanding of the relationship between sleep and associated disorders, such as night terrors, nightmares, sleep walking, enuresis, sleep apnoea, narcolepsy and delirium tremens.

The following methods have helped the elucidation of the physiological and behavioural states occurring during sleep; the electroencephalogram (EEG), the electro-oculogram (EOG), and the electromyogram (EMG).

Sleep is indicated by the appearance of sleep spindles consisting of 12 to 14 Hz bursts of EEG activity which wax and wane within the space of a second or two. During deep sleep, slow waves also occur often with spindles superimposed. EEG recordings reveal that periods of light sleep alternating with deep sleep occur throughout the night as many as half-a-dozen times.

Sleep begins with the appearance of sleep spindles and there are no rapid eye movements and no dreaming. This is referred to as non-rapid eye movement sleep or NREM sleep, which is characterized by a slow regular heart and respiratory rate with blood pressure reaching its lowest level. Muscles retain a fairly high tone, maintaining the posture of the body which is demonstrated by high background activity in the EMG.

Thermal Regulations

Maintenance of a constant body temperature is one of the basic homeostatic functions. A temperature trough occurs during the first third of the sleep cycle. Alterations in endogenous body temperature cycle have been linked to sleep disorders, such as insomnia and hypersomnia.

Investigations have shown that NREM sleep is associated with a homeothermic condition whereas REM sleep is a poikilothermic state, reflecting ambient temperature.

The relationships between the circadian temperature cycle and the distribution of sleep stages provides an explanation for the jet-lag syndrome and its association with sleep disturbances.

Rapid Eye Movement (REM Sleep)

After about 90 minutes sleep, muscle tone becomes extremely low for a time, with an increase in heart and respiratory rates and periodic elevation of blood pressure. Brain oxygen consumption is increased during REM sleep. During this phase penile erections occur in men and an increase in vaginal temperature in women. REM sleep alternates with a more familiar orthodox sleep (NREM) and constitutes about 20%

of a total night's sleep. It used to be thought that dreaming occupied very few seconds and that some people did not dream at all, but this has been proved incorrect. It is now known that if you wake people up during REM sleep they report dreams. The periods of REM activity occur at roughly $1\frac{1}{2}$ hour intervals, so that usually at least four periods of dreaming activity occur, taking up one-fifth of the night's sleep.

Nightmares occur during REM sleep. Nightmares are frightening dreams which wake us up with ability to remember the content of the dream whereas night terrors (pavor nocturnus), which occur in children are quite different. The child sits up with a scream and does not respond to words of reassurance. They therefore are inaccessible and have amnesia for the episode. This also applies to sleep walking where the mind continues to be asleep and the body is active. Night terrors and sleep walking take place during deep orthodox NREM sleep. It would be, in fact, impossible for these disorders to happen during REM sleep because of the marked muscular hypotonia.

Narcolepsy

Narcolepsy is a condition in which the patient has uncontrollable episodes of sleep even at times when nobody else would; for example, walking in the street or when eating a meal. It is sometimes associated with hypnagogic hallucinations (visual or auditory sensations experienced whilst dropping off to sleep), sleep paralysis (being awake but unable to move one's limbs), cataplexy (collapsing to the ground powerless) and is precipitated by strong emotions such as laughter or anger.

Most people have their first period of REM sleep one to one and a half hours into orthodox sleep, but the patient with narcolepsy may begin the night with a burst of REM activity.

The Kleine–Levin syndrome occurs in male adolescents who suffer from prolonged periods of hypersomnia and on wakening feel extremely hungry and eat ravenously. The body temperature may be raised and extreme changes of mood are sometimes noticed.

Hypersomnic states such as narcolepsy and the Kleine–Levin syndrome may be treated with central nervous system stimulants like amphetamines or methylphenidate. Alternatively, tricyclic antidepressants such as clomipramine are helpful. Clomipramine is particularly helpful for cataplexy.

Cataplexy

Sleep paralysis occurs when the patient has the hypotonia of REM sleep, but is awake rather than dreaming.

Delirium Tremens

Delirium tremens occurs as part of a withdrawal syndrome to physical dependence on chloral, meprobamate, benzodiazepines, alcohol, barbiturates and related hypnotics which cause a suppression of REM sleep and when the medication is withdrawn, a marked REM rebound occurs with disorientation and fearful visions.

Sleep Prevention

Sleep prevention has been reported to be a useful method for the treatment of depression. The patient is kept awake all night for a number of nights during the week and this has been reported to relieve depression, but controlled studies are needed to evaluate its efficacy.

Sleep and Respiration

The study of sleep and respiratory function has proved fruitful in the understanding and management of common disorders such as chronic pulmonary obstruction. It has also revealed newly recognized pathological conditions occurring exclusively during sleep, e.g. sleep apnoeic syndrome.

Monitoring both air flow and inspiratory effort during sleep enabled three types of apnoeic events to be demonstrated:

1 The obstructive apnoea characterized by a cessation of air flow with a continuation of inspiratory effort.
2 The central apnoea characterized by a simultaneous cessation of inspiratory effort and air flow, and a simultaneous resumption of both.
3 A mixed apnoea which is characterized by an initial central apnoea, followed by an obstructive apnoea.

Chronic sleep deprivation, due to apnoeic events,

is the primary cause of excessive daytime sleepiness in such persons.

It has become increasingly evident that sleep evaluation is important for the full understanding of the pathogenesis of many forms of respiratory disorders.

Classification of Sleep and Arousal Disorders

Disorders of Initiating and Maintaining Sleep

These may be transient or persistent. They are mainly associated with affective disorders and other severe psychiatric illnesses, tolerance to or withdrawal from CNS depressants, use of CNS stimulants or chronic alcoholism. They may also be associated with sleep induced respiratory impairment, sleep apnoea, alveolar hypoventilation, or with sleep related restless legs (Ekbons disorder) or myoclonic jerks.

Excessive Somnolence

Excessive somnolence may be transient and situational. It can be persistent when associated with depression, schizophrenia, use of sedatives or alcohol, sleep induced respiratory impairment such as sleep apnoea, alveolar hypoventilation, sleep related restless legs (Ekbons disorder) or myoclonic jerks, narcolepsy and related disorders such as the Kleine–Levin syndrome, menstruation associated syndromes, disorders of the sleep-wake schedule such as the jet lag syndrome, work shift change, dysfunctions associated with sleep such as sleep walking, sleep terrors, sleep related enuresis, sleep related asthma or coronary insufficiency.

Sleep Deprivation

During recent years studies have been carried out on the mental and behavioural effects of depriving a person of sleep. A critical period of sleep deprivation is 100 to 120 hours, after which a characteristic abnormal mental state develops. This is preceded by a prodromal phase which develops during the first four or five days without sleep and is characterized by a progressive increase in drowsiness and by brief lapses of awareness (these are micro-sleeps which last only a few seconds).

There is an increasing tendency to stare; auditory sensations increase as the prodromal phase continues, with feelings of pressure bands on the head, tingling feelings in the skin, noises in the ears, a decrease in vigilance, a growing sense of fatigue, drowsiness and lack of interest.

On the fifth night a 'psychotic' syndrome develops with gross disturbances of reality testing which may persist for varying periods of time. Hallucinatory experiences become more prolonged and vivid, the person's facial expression is elongated and immobile, brows are furrowed and he has to make a great effort to keep his eyes open. There is intermittent clouding of consciousness and disorientation for time, then place and person. Paranoid ideas are common.

By night the picture resembles a delirious state. During the daytime the picture somewhat resembles paranoid schizophrenia.

When the person eventually sleeps he is usually likely to sleep for 12 to 15 hours and during this period dreaming occurs frequently and quickly, as if the person is catching up not only with his sleep but also his dreams.

Recent work in fact has demonstrated that a certain amount of dreaming each night is a necessity for health. When people were prevented from dreaming by being deliberately awakened at the commencement of their REM periods, it was found that there was a marked increase in percentage dream-time on subsequent nights of undisturbed sleep. It was also found that such dream-deprived subjects became unhappy and ill at ease.

Content and Meaning of Dreams

Freud was able to demonstrate that dreams had a manifest content which was derived from events of the preceding day or from the person's life which were not very revealing, but that there was also a latent content which could be revealed by getting the dreamer to free-associate to the manifest content of the dream.

A number of processes occur in dreams which are collectively referred to as dream-work. For example, condensation is common, e.g. parts of a number of people may be all condensed into one person.

Displacement is another mechanism; important or serious happenings may be made to appear trivial and vice versa.

Ideas are usually presented in a concrete form and usually in images, and often in the term of symbols. For example, dreaming about missing the bus may stand for letting an opportunity pass by.

There are some symbols which tend to be universal; for example, sharp, pointed objects like daggers, swords, steeples usually denote male sexuality, whereas caves, tunnels, jewel boxes refer to the female.

At the point of waking, dreams tend to be distorted in order to be made meaningful or worked up into a story; this is the process of secondary elaboration. If one intends analysing dreams it is important that the patient should have pencil and paper ready to jot down the dream as early as possible to avoid the distorting effect of secondary elaboration and to avoid the very rapid forgetting of dreams.

Further Reading

Hartmann, E. L. (1967) *The Biology of Dreaming.* C. C. Thomas, Springfield, Illinois.

Drucker-Colin, R. R. (ed) (1979) *Functions of Sleep.* Academic Press, London.

Oswald, I. (1980) *Sleep,* 4th edn. Pelican, Harmondsworth.

Christie, M. and Mellett, P. G. (1986) *Psychosomatic Approach: Contemporary Practice of Whole-person Care.* Wiley, Chichester.

13
Eating

Hunger and Satiety

Hunger is the subjective experience of sensations felt when one is deprived of food and results in behaviour which is relieved by the intake of food.

Satiety refers to the active suppression of interest in food and of feeding behaviour, rather than just the absence of hunger.

The available evidence indicates that there are rigid regulatory control mechanisms over body weight level and, by inference, eating behaviour. It has long been known that lesions of the hypothalamus can result in obesity. Lesions of a specific hypothalamic area, the ventromedial nucleus, are followed by hyperphagia and obesity.

Bilateral lesions of the lateral hypothalamic area result in aphagia and adipsia in animals. It has been suggested that these two brain centres mediate eating behaviours by reciprocally inhibiting each other. The lateral hypothalamic (LH) has predominant control and is regarded as the feeding centre of the brain, stimulation of this area eliciting ingestive behaviours. The ventromedial nucleus (VMH) has been traditionally regarded as the satiety centre. Bilateral symmetrical lesions in this nucleus produce hyperphagia and obesity.

Both chronic obese patients and VMH lesion rats eat fewer meals a day, eat more per meal, eat more rapidly than normal controls and are also less active.

Neurochemical factors can also be important; for example, administration of catecholamines, or their precursors, has marked effects in reducing food intake. This is due to a peripheral effect as these substances do not cross the blood brain barrier. Acting centrally, noradrenalin suppresses hunger and feeding activity, which can be blocked by beta blockers such as propranolol and also by chlorpromazine.

5-Hydroxytryptamine (5HT, serotinin) is believed to act centrally as an appetite stimulating agent. This is supported by the clinical findings that fenfluramine is an effective anorexic agent and that cyproheptadine increases appetite. Both act on 5HT metabolism in different ways.

The role of 5HT in eating behaviour is by no means clear. However, it appears that multiple neurochemical mechanisms exercise control over feeding and these include dopamine and other catecholamines and serotonin.

Glucostatic Mechanisms

Glucose metabolism is not only regulated by a complex series of endrocrine relationships but is also a regulator of fat synthesis and oxidation as well as protein synthesis and mobilization. Blood glucose stimulates insulin release from the pancreatic cells which, in turn, stimulates the uptake of glucose as well as free fatty acids and amino acids into peripheral tissues.

The carbohydrates are used for energy or stored as glycogen. The free fatty acids are converted to fat and stored in adipose tissue. Amino acids are incorporated into protein. When the blood glucose level falls adrenalin and glucagon are released from the adrenal gland and pancreas, producing increased blood glucose levels by inhibition of cellular uptake.

There is strong evidence that glucose receptors occur in the hypothalamus which control feeding.

Endocrines

In recent years considerable evidence has emerged that the gastrointestinal system is a powerful source of endocrines, which appear to play an important part in the regulation of carbohydrate metabolism, gastric acid secretion, pancreatic secretion, gall bladder function, gastrointestinal motility and blood flow. Some endocrines are found both in the gut and the brain and these include cholecystokinin (CCK), somatostatin, thyrotrophic releasing hormone and adrenocorticotrophin (ACTH). Somatostatin is involved in the fine tuning of insulin and glucagon secretion, inhibiting the release of both. It also inhibits gastrin release, acid secretion and delays gastric emptying.

Vasoactive intestinal peptide (VIP) is found both in the gut and the brain, is a potent vasodilator, stimulates insulin as well as inhibiting gastric acid secretion, increases glycogenesis and pancreatic secretion of water and bicarbonate.

Of the gastrointestinal hormones identified so far, CCK appears to be most closely implicated in satiety regulation. A major stimulus for its release is the presence of fat in the lumen of the gut.

Psychological Factors in Hunger and Satiety

In addition to the physiological and biochemical processes already discussed, there are many psychosocial factors which help to regulate our eating behaviour and may override physiological factors. These include conditioning, learned differentiation of inner states, sensitivity to external stimuli, cognition and education as well as cultural factors regarding food intake and body size. The variety of stimuli relating to eating, such as smell, taste, texture and touch of food, together with pharyngeal and gastrointestinal sensations and stimuli relating to places where eating occurs, can lead to sensations of hunger by a process of conditioning.

It has been pointed out that people with obesity or anorexia nervosa never properly develop the ability to differentiate hunger and satiety from other internal tensions and never have a sense of mastery or control over their bodies. Many people misuse the eating function and eat in response to a variety of psychological states, such as boredom, anxiety and depression. Cognitive factors can also be important in determining what and when we eat. Changes

have occurred in eating habits based on beliefs that high cholesterol is conducive to heart disease and also the alleged relationship between the fat content of food and longevity.

Obesity is largely a lower social class disorder whereas anorexia nervosa and bulimia nervosa are highly correlated with the upper and middle classes.

Western society tends to value leanness and this is conducive to the development of dieting and ultimately to the risk of developing anorexia nervosa and bulimia nervosa.

Obesity

Obesity is a major health hazard in modern society. It is a perplexing disorder without agreement regarding causation or treatment.

Overweight can be defined as a deviation greater than 20% above the desirable weight for age and height obtained from norms established by insurance companies.

Nowadays, however, body mass index (BMI) is a preferred method for measuring obesity. The index relates to weight and height according to the formula

$$\frac{Wt(Kg)}{H^2(m)}$$

This index enables a grading of obesity to be made; mild—BMI of 20 to 30, moderate—30 to 40 and severe—40 plus.

The causation of obesity is complex and can best be understood in terms of interrelationships between cultural and physical aspects of the external environment. The behavioural act of eating is, both quantitively and qualitatively, the process of ingestion and assimilation of foods and the storage and utilization of energy. Brain mechanisms are involved in the control system and subjective states, such as attributions and cognitions, which may be relevant. There are direct relationships between metabolism and eating behaviour. Food consumption increases energy expenditure and heat production. This is referred to as diet-induced thermogenesis and is clearly an adaptive response. Reducing food intake does not simply deny calories to the body but leads to an adjustment in metabolism and, again, the lowering of metabolic rate is an adaptive response to food restriction.

The relationship between eating and metabolism, in particular oxygen consumption, is a fundamental link in the interaction of systems relevant to obesity. It has been shown that an obese person will tend to eat meals infrequently. A similar pattern has been shown in experimental animals, who, when allowed to, choose to eat as much as they wish from a variety of tasty foods, with an increase in weight leading to a decrease in the frequency of meals. This indicates that infrequent meals in human obese subjects is not necessarily a consequence of social-cultural pressures.

Obesity is a disorder which does not fit into the traditional medical model of illness involving a link between a possible cause and a cluster of symptoms or disorder. Neither can obesity be explained purely on psychological terms. It can only be understood as a disorder standing on the boundary between the internal environment and its physiology and biochemistry, and the external environment with its various stimuli.

Restricting calorie intake would be effective if all of the parts of the relevant systems remained stable. However, a number of changes occur, such as lowering of the metabolic rate and also psychological changes, such as the development of restraint, the occurrence of periodic hypoglycaemia and the development of cravings due to the avoidance of certain nutrients. It should also be remembered that benzodiazepines and many antidepressants tend to increase appetite.

Treatment of obesity must be multimodal, comprising:

1 Dietary restriction which must be accompanied by programmed physical activity to augment and to increase metabolic rate and to counteract any suppression of metabolic rate.
2 Promotion of coping abilities to help to deal with situations involving increased vulnerability for the patient.
3 Psychological methods of treatment—the two main methods are psychotherapy and behaviour therapy. A large scale collaborative study by psychoanalysts in the United States revealed that obese people derive considerable benefits from this treatment, including alleviation of the usually intractable problem of body image disparagement. There is also significant weight loss which people can maintain as effectively as those treated by other methods.

Behaviour therapy involving self-monitoring stimulus control, slowing of rate of eating, self-reinforcement, cognitive restructure, contingency contracting and exercise management also has proved effective. The low drop-out rate and the availability of treatment from less highly trained therapists has made this the treatment of choice for mild obesity and moderate obesity, with better results than those achieved by pharmacotherapy.

Anorexia Nervosa

Anorexia nervosa is a disorder which is almost confined to young women, but occasionally occurs in older women and much less frequently in men.

The term 'anorexia' is a misnomer. Initially, there is a deliberate restriction of eating, particularly of carbohydrates and fatty foods and usually the patient will take minimum quantities of the most slimming foods and will secretly dispose of food or vomit it afterwards or hide it in various places. The patient will pick at her food and eat mainly salads and other slimming foods.

There is an intense fear of becoming obese which does not diminish as weight loss continues, even where there is weight loss amounting to at least 25% of the original body weight.

The patient usually has a disturbance of body image perception and perceives herself to be much fatter than she is or to have wide hips, a large bottom and large breasts, even when emaciated. Loss of appetite usually only occurs after severe emaciation.

Anorexic patients are preoccupied with food and will collect recipes and prepare elaborate meals for others, but refuse to eat themselves. One patient had severe weight loss and looked like a skeleton. Her husband was a very large and obese man of 114 kilograms and her two sons were 95 kilograms and 88 kilograms respectively. The most remarkable thing was that the family dog was by far the fattest one in the area.

Anorexic patients are usually active and energetic. Sometimes a growth of fine downy hair appears over the body which is similar to that found in other types of intense starvation.

Amenorrhoea is characteristic, weight loss usually occurring before or simultaneously with the onset of amenorrhoea. Menstruation is unlikely to return until the patient is about 80% of normal weight, but the majority will not start menstruating until normal weight has been maintained for a number of months.

With loss of weight, anorexics develop sleep disturbances marked by early morning waking although, unlike depressed patients, they rarely complain of it. It has been found that initial weight gain with treatment is associated with an increase in slow wave sleep whch tends to decrease as weight is restored to normal.

Half the anorexic patients exhibit bulimia which is the rapid consumption of large amounts of food in a short period of time, referred to as 'bingeing'. This is associated with induced vomiting, laxative abuse, diuretic abuse and intensive physical activity to help to reduce weight. The self-induced vomiting can cause hypokalaemia which can lead to cardiac arrhythmias and sometimes to sudden death. Chronic hypokalaemia can result in kidney damage and polyuria.

A proportion of patients with anorexia nervosa have a late onset and have been designated 'anorexia tardive'. Usually, the disorder develops as a maladaptive solution to a growing marital crisis. Many of the husbands involved were immature men who readily accepted a sick dependent wife.

A sub-group developed anorexia after the menopause and were often depressed with the loss of weight and expressed a desire to die.

It has been suggested that the anorexia nervosa of early onset is a principal symptom of phobia of normal adolescent weight following the growth changes of puberty.

Dieting in response to a dislike of being fat becomes a dominant pursuit for the security and comfort of childhood, with freedom from the demands, particularly sexual, of adolescence.

Bulimia

Some patients suffering from anorexia nervosa actively participate in bingeing and vomiting even when they have regained weight and no longer express a normal weight phobia. The term 'bulimia nervosa' has been suggested for such patients with a previous history of anorexia nervosa.

For patients suffering from bulimia with no previous history of anorexia nervosa, the term 'bulimic syndrome' is proposed.

Bulimia can be distinguished from anorexia nervosa by the fact that bulimia patients maintain their weight within a normal range despite marked fluctuations in weight (as much as 20 kg).

The following criteria are useful in the diagnosis of bulimia:

1 Recurrent episodes of rapid consumption of large amounts of food within a limited time, usually less than two hours.
2 At least three of the following features:
   (a) consumption of high calorie easily ingested food during a binge;
   (b) inconspicuous eating during a binge;
   (c) termination of such eating episodes by self-induced vomiting, sleep or abdominal pain;
   (d) repeated attempts to lose weight by low calorie diets, vomiting or the use of purgatives or diuretics.
3 Feelings of depression and self-depreciation after binge eating.

The bulimic patient is heavier than the anorexic patient and gives a history of being unable to maintain weight loss by carbohydrate avoidance. She tends to have sexual feelings but is terrified of them. She is often more attractive than patients with anorexia nervosa. These patients often have emotional difficulties with a man friend or friends and over a third report being depressed.

If the patient is seen soon after vomiting, she will appear distressed, with marked perspiration and sometimes with a mild pyrexia. Her neck will appear swollen and she may wear a handkerchief or a scarf to mask it. Salivary glands may be swollen but painless, but if the parotid glands are affected she may complain of tinnitus or facial ache. The abdomen would be swollen and painful with stretch marks on the lower abdomen and breasts. If vomiting is frequent, hypokalaemia can occur with cardiac arrhythmias, renal damage, tetany with muscle spasm and paraesthesiae.

Erosion of the dental enamel can occur as well as chronic hoarseness, particularly with persistent vomiting.

Further Reading

Christie, M. and Mellett, P. G. (1986) Psychosomatic Approach: Contemporary Practice of Whole-person Care Wiley, Chichester.

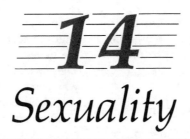

Sexuality

Psychophysiology

Our knowledge of sexual functions has increased tremendously in recent years due to the pioneering work of Kinsey, and Masters and Johnson. This new knowledge has enabled new methods of treatment to be applied to common sexual disorders.

Masters and Johnson have described four successive stages in the male and female sexual response—excitement, plateau, orgasm and resolution.

1   *Excitement* The first stage is associated with erotic feelings, the attainment of erection in men and vaginal lubrication in women. There is also a general bodily reaction consisting of vasocongestion and increased tone of the voluntary muscles. Breathing and heart rate increase and there is an increase in blood pressure. In addition to penile erection, there is thickening of the scrotal sac and the testes begin to elevate due to shortening of the spermatic cords.

In the female, as in the male, there is a local genital and general vasoconstriction of the skin and general increased muscle tone. The skin response in women is more marked and shows a mottling of the skin, and the breasts tend to begin to swell and the nipples become erect. The genital reaction in females consists of engorgement of the tissues deep in the vagina which causes a transudate which enhances vaginal lubrication and this develops within ten to thirty seconds after the beginning of sexual stimulation.

Other changes are some vasocongestion of the clitoris and enlargement of the uterus, which begins to rise from its dormant position on the pelvic floor. Concurrently the vagina begins to enlarge and balloon to accommodate the penis.

2   *The plateau* This stage is a more advanced state

of arousal occurring immediately prior to orgasm. Now local vasocongestion is at its peak in both men and women, the penis is filled and distended with blood to its full capacity, the testicles increase in size due to vascular enlargement and reflex contraction of the cremasteric muscles elevate the testicles in close apposition to the perineum. Two or three drops of clear mucus fluid appear, probably from Cowper's gland.

The labia minora swell and change in colour from bright red to burgundy and form a plateau of congested tissue, which has been called the orgasmic platform, surrounding the entrance of the lower part of the vagina. Just prior to orgasm the clitoris retracts into a flat position behind the symphysis pubis.

3   *Orgasm* In the male, the orgasm consists of ejaculation of semen from the erect penis in three to seven spurts at .8 second intervals. The first component of the male orgasm consists of contractions of the internal reproductive organs (vas deferens, prostate and seminal vesicles) and a feeling of ejaculatory inevitability. Rhythmical contractions of the muscles around the penile base and the perineal muscles follow immediately and constitute the second component and the experience of the orgasm proper.

The female orgasm consists of .8 second reflex rhythmic contractions of the circumvaginal and perineal muscles and the tissues of the orgasmic platform.

After orgasm, the male is refractory to sexual stimulation for a time which becomes longer with age. The female, in contrast, is never physically refractory to orgasm and while she is in the swollen plateau stage, she can be stimulated to repeated orgasms until she is physically exhausted or no longer wishes further stimulation.

4   *Resolution* In this phase the body returns to its

basal state. In the female, the clitoris returns to its normal position five to ten seconds after orgasm, but the vagina may take as long as ten to fifteen minutes to return to its relaxed resting state.

Biphasic Nature of the Sexual Response

There are two distinct and relatively independent components of sexual responses in males and females. The first is a genital vasocongestive reaction producing penile erection in the male and vaginal lubrication and swelling in the female and the second is the reflex clonic muscular contractions which constitute orgasm in both sexes.

The two components involve different anatomical structures and physiological neural mediators. Erection is mediated by the parasympathetic part of the autonomic nervous system, whereas ejaculation is a sympathetic function. The recognition of this distinction is important clinically because the impairment of erection and ejaculation in the male, and lubrication and orgasm in the female, results in clinical disorders of differing causation and responding to different methods of treatment.

Penile erection requires an intact autonomic and sensory nerve supply to the penis. Psychogenic impotence occurs when emotional or other psychological factors interfere with the function of the processes involved in penile engorgement. Anxiety, if severe, may prevent erection during the excitement stage, or may cause failure to maintain erection.

The clinical importance of these mechanisms is shown in disorders of premature ejaculation and retarded ejaculation. Usually men can learn to achieve considerable voluntary control to delay ejaculation but, in some men, anxiety prevents this control and premature ejaculation occurs. Retarded ejaculation occurs despite the development of a satisfactory erection, arousal and achievement of the plateau stage. The occurrence of premature and delayed ejaculation can cause secondary anxiety which increases sexual difficulties and increases the risk of failure to perform satisfactorily.

Sexual Disorders in the Female

The vasocongestive responses are believed to be mediated by the parasympathetic as in the male and, similarly, are subject to functional interference by emotional factors.

Severely inhibited women do not develop genital engorgement, do not lubricate and do not develop the general bodily responses to sexual stimulation. These women are truly frigid, as opposed to women who complain that they get no pleasurable response despite adequate lubrication and other physiological changes, and who describe being 'cut-off' from their erotic sensations. This is a psychogenic mechanism with different possible causes, including hysterical reactions. Many women reach the plateau phase without difficulty and experience high degrees of sexual arousal, but have difficulty in reaching a climax despite continued stimulation. This is not appropriately designated as frigidity, but is more analogous to the retarded ejaculation in the male. Both syndromes can be described as a specific inhibition of orgasm in which the sexual response is arrested at the plateau phase.

Freud's teaching was that, in normal females, orgasm is always triggered by vaginal stimulation and that clitoral orgasm represented an immature form of sexual satisfaction. Recent researches have convincingly revealed the fallacy of this concept and the present consensus of evidence suggests that stimulation of the clitoris may be crucial in producing a female orgasm.

Even though stimulation of the clitoris seems to be crucial for the production of orgasm, it plays no role in its execution which is reflex and consists of rhythmical contractions of the striated circumvaginal muscles.

There are important differences in the sexual response between males and females. Sexual arousal occurs more rapidly in men. The vasocongestive phase is more vulnerable in men than women, hence impotence is a common complaint in men, whereas inhibition of lubrication and swelling is much rarer in women. The female orgasm is far more vulnerable to inhibition than in men and failure to reach orgasm, which is the analogue of retarded ejaculation, is more somatic. Further differences are that the male experiences a refractory period which increases with age, whereas this does not occur in women. Both male and female libido and sexual responses are ultimately dependent on androgens as well as psychic factors. Androgens are responsible for maintaining normal levels of sexual interest, potency and ability to ejaculate. Penile erection is produced by blood flowing into the corpora cavernosa. Blood flow can be impaired by arteriosclerotic changes and stimulation of sympathetic anti-erectile fibres. The parasympathetic is essential for reflex erection but psychogenic and sleep erection may be mediated by parasympathetic or sympathetic erectile fibres.

Androgens enhance sex drives in both males and females. Sex drive and potency decrease when anti-androgen medication is prescribed. This occurs when oestrogen is prescribed for prostatic carcinoma or when the anti-androgenic cyproterone is prescribed for sexual offenders. Libido and potency disappear within three weeks but rapidly return when the medication is discontinued.

The importance of androgens in female sex drives has only been fully recognized in recent years. Women deprived of all sources of androgens by ovariectomy and adrenalectomy lose sex desire and cannot be sexually aroused by what was previously effective erotic stimulation.

Testosterone when prescribed for women causes high sexual arousal and increased assertiveness but its use in women for the management of low sex drives is limited by its masculinizing side effects.

Sexual stimulation and even anticipation of sexual encounters tend to increase the levels of circulating testosterone, whereas depression of mood tends to lower the level of blood testosterone.

Further Reading

Kinsey, A. C. and Martin, C. E. (1948) *Sexual Behaviour in the Human Male*. W. B. Saunders, Philadelphia.

Masters, W. H. and Johnson, V. E. (1966) *The Human Sexual Response*. Little Brown, Boston.

Masters, W. H. and Johnson, V. E. (1970) *Human Sexual Inadequacy*. Little Brown, Boston.

Kaplan, H. S. (1974) *The New Sex Therapy*. Brunner/Mazel, New York.

Trimmer, E. J. (1978) *Basic Sexual Medicine: A Textbook of Sexual Medicine and Introduction to Sexual Counselling Techniques*. Heinemann, London.

Bancroft, J. (1985) *Human Sexuality and Its Problems*. Churchill Livingstone, Edinburgh.

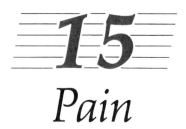

Pain

Pain constitutes one of the greatest challenges in medicine and is the most universal form of distress encountered by humans. There are millions of sufferers with pain associated with arthritis, migraine, other forms of headache and low back pain. It has been estimated that 80% of all visits to a family doctor are for pain-related problems.

Pain has been defined as an unpleasant sensory and emotional experience associated with actual or potential tissue damage. Clinically, pain may be categorized into four different types:

1 Acute pain which is usually self-limiting and of less than six months duration; for example, pain after surgical operations, dental pain and pain accompanying childbirth.
2 Chronic periodic pain—this is an acute or chronic pain with intermittent manifestation; for example migraine headaches, tension headaches and trigeminal neuralgia.
3 Chronic intractable benign pain is present for most of the time, varying in intensity, e.g. low back pain and tension headaches. By definition this is pain which has been present for more than six months.
4 Chronic progressive pain which is often associated with malignancies.

Pain arises as a result of stimulation of nociceptors (which are specialized receptors) or their afferent fibres. These occur throughout the tissues and in the perivascular network and respond to physical and chemical changes. Stimulation of the nociceptors is a physiological phenomenon perceived at a subjective level, either as a sensation (burning or pricking) or as an unpleasant effect (distress or discomfort) which

in turn stimulates pain behaviour such as wincing, grimacing or taking pills.

It has been shown that social, cultural and personality variables may have as much to do with pain behaviour as does the activity in the nociceptor fibres.

The moderation of pain on input from pain receptors can be influenced by both peripheral and central processes. The gate theory of pain proposes that a neuronal mechanism in the dorsal horn of the spinal cord acts like a gate which can increase or decrease the flow of impulses from peripheral nociceptors to the central nervous system. Inhibition of the dorsal horn cell activity can be brought about by concurrent action of low threshold mechanoreceptors synapsing with dorsal horn cells. This provides an explanation for pain relief produced by counter-irritation and massage. Modulaton of the dorsal horn neurons by descending inhibitory pathways from higher centres inhibits the spinal cord and produces analgesia. It is believed that opiate endorphins are probably involved in this system.

Serotonin 5-hydroxytryptamine (5HT) also acts as an inhibitory transmitter in some descending neurons which influence the dorsal horn cells.

Two pain thresholds can be described. The low threshold is when the stimulus changes in nature and is first perceived as pain and the higher threshold marks the point when pain can no longer be tolerated.

The lower threshold remains fairly stable in an individual over a period of time, but the upper threshold can be influenced by personality characteristics, by cultural and environmental factors, the experience of stress and by anxiety, fear and depression.

The Treatment of Chronic Pain

The psychological treatment methods used in the management of chronic pain include biofeedback, relaxation, cognitive therapy and operant contingency management methods. Acupuncture and transcutaneous neural stimulation are also effective in some causes of pain.

There is evidence that different frequencies of electro-acupuncture release two kinds of opiate neuropeptides within the central nervous system. Low frequency stimulation releases metendorphin in the brain where it modulates pain. With high frequency stimulation, a precursor of endorphin, called dynorphin, is set free in the spinal cord, where it also has a gating effect on the transmission of pain stimuli.

Clinical Settings for the Complaint of Pain

Pain is not necessarily due to physical injury. It may sometimes have an organic basis but the degree, intensity and duration of the pain may be influenced by other factors such as anxiety, depression, hysteria and increased muscle tension. If the patient engages in pathological illness behaviour this can greatly determine the complaints of pain.

Anxiety States

Various bodily pains found in anxiety states are often due to increased muscle tension; for example precordial pain, the pain of tension headaches in which the patient complains of pain in the frontal, bitemporal, or occipital regions, or a pain in the neck muscles and this is the basis of the common saying 'a pain in the neck'. Pains may also occur in the shoulders, the back or in the limbs due to increased muscle tension.

This can be investigated by electromyography which shows increased muscular activity, and may be further evaluated by the injection of a small dose of intravenous sodium amytal in insufficient quantity to produce analgesia, but enough to produce relaxation. If it causes immediate relief of pain, this supports the diagnosis that the pain is due to increased muscle tension.

Depressive Illness

Depression often presents with physical symptoms and pain can be one of them. Atypical facial pain and pains in various parts of the body may be the focus of the patient's complaints.

Hysteria

Pain may be based on hysterical mechanisms and usually this does not conform to the pain of organic disease. For example, it does not have the neural distribution of the pain as found in sciatica or the distribution found in trigeminal neuralgia or glossopharyngeal neuralgia. Very often the pain has a distribution which conforms to the patient's idea of where the pain should be and may therefore affect half of the body, a whole limb or some other distribution which does not have a neurological or organic basis. The diagnosis of hysteria should not be made because an organic basis cannot be found for the pain, or because the patient makes a great fuss about the pain. Hysteria should only be diagnosed on positive psychiatric grounds indicating a clear underlying motive of gain.

Psychogenic regional pain is the term applied to pain not due to organic disorder. This is found in many patients, sometimes those with anxiety states, depression and other disorders in which the pain occupies defined regions of the body, such as the forequarter, the hind quarter, half or quarter of the trunk or the whole of the head, and is not necessarily hysterical in origin but has a psychogenic basis.

Many pains, although they may have a physiogenic basis, can be influenced by anxiety, depression or hysterical superadditions. This applies to low back pain and abdominal pains in an irritable colon which are due to spasm of the large intestine. The degree of distress and the degree of complaint will be influenced by the patient's emotional state, attitude and personality.

Learned Pain Behaviour

In many patients psychogenic pain may develop or persist independently of any psychiatric illness; for example, complaints of pain may produce attention and sympathy from a person important to the patient and this may encourage future complaints of pain in the presence of that person. Complaints of pain may also enable the patient to avoid unpleasant activities, thus providing another type of reward for the sick role. Behaviours that are compatible with being well are not rewarded and therefore tend to be extinguished. This leads to the development of the syndrome termed 'operant or learned pain behaviour', as described by Tyrer (1986). It is essential not only to exclude organic disease, but also to interview those closest to the patient and to observe interactions between them and the patient.

It is important to follow clues provided by descriptions of the pain, for example, using emotional words like 'sickening' and 'blinding' to describe pain affecting a region or an extremity; the progression of severity and extent of the pain over time; the patient may produce exaggerated facial expressions of pain and posture, frequent grimacing sighs and rubbing of the affected parts. These patients score highly on questionnaires designed to measure illness behaviour.

Physical examination may elicit evidence of non-organic physical signs, including over-reaction to examination, superficial skin tenderness, distribution of pain which does not correspond to neurological or dermatomal distribution. Excessive bracing movements may also be observed.

Treatment consists of eliminating rewards resulting from pain behaviour and substituting more active and constructive behaviours which are then encouraged appropriately.

Such patients are not easy to help, especially if they have suffered from pain and associated learned behaviour for many years.

Further Reading

Merskey, H. and Spear, F. G. (1967) *Pain: Psychological and Psychiatric Aspects.* Bailliere Tindall/Cassell, London
Sternbach, R. A. (1978) *The Psychology of Pain.* Raven Press, New York.
Tyrer, S. P. (1986) Learning pain behaviour. *British Medical Journal,* **1**, 1.

16
Psychopathology

Psychoanalysis and Related Schools

The historical development of psychological methods of treatment up to the discoveries of Freud was briefly outlined in Chapter 1.

Sigmund Freud, born in 1856, studied physiology after qualifying as a doctor and later devoted his attention to neurology. In 1885 Freud went to Paris to work under Charcot, who had impressed him greatly with the use of hypnosis as a method of treating hysteria.

Freud, however, found hypnotic suggestion by itself to be of limited value. In collaboration with Joseph Breuer who, incidentally, had also started his career as a physiologist, he developed a method of treating patients in which they were allowed to talk out their emotional difficulties under hypnosis.

Under hypnosis the patient was able to remember past experiences more clearly and to release emotions associated with forgotten experiences. Breuer and Freud were impressed by the curative effect of talking out difficulties and referred to the process as mental catharsis. The term abreaction was used to denote the liberation of emotion whilst talking about emotional problems and experiences.

Both Breuer and Freud found that, during treatment by these methods, some female patients appeared to fall in love with them. This alarmed Breuer but Freud soon realized that it was not his own personality that was attractive but merely that he was serving as a substitute for the original person they loved. The love was transferred to the physician and this process was referred to as 'transference' which Freud dealt with by maintaining an impersonal attitude and, in fact, utilized the transference reaction in the resolution of problems and promoting recovery.

Freud discontinued hypnosis and instead instructed patients to relax in a reclining position and to talk freely about their problems. This method was referred to as free association and patients were encouraged to tell everything that came into their minds, even if it appeared embarrassing, ridiculous, irrelevant or unimportant.

In order to facilitate and expedite progress achieved by free association, Freud also used interpretation of the patient's dreams, again using free association. He found that there were many suppressed desires and complexes and that these were often of a sexual nature. Sex desires when in conflict with the requirements of society were repressed.

Freud found that exploring by free association deeper and further back into the patient's history was more effective in treating his patients. Many patients recalled traumatic emotional experiences in childhood, often of a sexual nature, and related sexual assaults by relatives. Freud realized that many of these accounts were fantasy rather than fact.

Ernest Jones describes the major principles of Freudian doctrine as follows:
1 psychic determinism, and goal motivated behaviour;
2 emotional processes have a certain autonomy, and can be detached and displaced.

Topography of the Mind

Freud divided the mind into three regions: the unconscious, the preconscious and the conscious, each of which has unique characteristics.

The unconscious is the repository of instinctive drives together with repressed material from experience. The contents of the unconscious are not accessible to consciousness and can only reach the conscious via the preconscious, which excludes them by censorship or repression. Repressed ideas may, however, reach consciousness when the censor is evaded as in dreams or in psychiatric symptoms or by slips of the tongue and other errors of everyday life.

The **preconscious** develops during childhood in parallel with the development of the ego. The preconscious can be reached by both the conscious and the unconscious. Contents of the unconscious can only gain access to consciousness by being linked with words via the preconscious.

The **conscious** is involved with awareness and attention whereby the individual becomes aware of stimuli from the outside world.

1 *The id* The id is the term applied to basic drives, instinctive drives such as those concerned with survival, sex and aggression. The id demands immediate satisfaction and is ruled by the pleasure-pain principle and is illogical. It is non-verbal and does not enter consciousness.
2 *The ego* is conscious and attempts to be the mediator between the drives derived from the id and the outer world. It is influenced by the super-ego. The ego is concerned with reality testing, discrimination, integration, adaptation, learning, consciousness, reason, intellect, memory, judgment and will power.
3 *The super-ego* arises out of the ego by a process of learning from experience to deal with the needs of society. It is mainly unconscious. The super-ego is composed of the conscience, the ego ideal and is derived from primitive conditioning.

Libido Theory and Psychosexual Development

The term libido is used to describe sexual drives in the widest sense and includes pleasurable sensations relating to bodily functions. The libido can be attached to a variety of objects and undergoes development through different phases. Freud described the following stages of psychosexual development:

1 **The oral phase** which starts at birth and continues for about 18 months. It is divided into a receptive phase followed later by a sadistic phase when the child acquires teeth and becomes more aggressive.

2 **The anal phase** develops during the first year and continues until approximately the age of 3 years. The anal phase has been divided into a destructive expulsive component and a mastering retaining aspect.
3 **The genital erotic phase** begins during the third year of life and continues until the end of the fifth year approximately.

The Oedipus situation evolves during the third to the fifth years in children of both sexes. In the Oedipus situation the child's libido becomes directed towards the parent of the opposite sex. The other parent is seen as a rival and feelings of hostility are engendered. The child anticipates retaliation because of its own aggressive feelings and in boys this takes the form of a castration complex.

Freud regarded the Oedipus situation as being prepotent for the development of later neurosis and symptom formation, and also in the development of character and personality.

In the development of obsessional symptoms, sex drives may be dealt with by displacement into washing activities acting as a purification.

Projection

Projection is the process whereby some attribute of the self or some quality or property of the self is attributed to the environment. It is a common mental mechanism as well as an important pathological process. It is well known that what is perceived is, in part, a function of the motivational structure of the personality. This forms the basis of projective tests.

In experiments it has been found that the frequency with which food is mentioned in speculations about the missing parts of incomplete pictures correlates positively with the degree of hunger.

As a psychopathological mechanism, projection may be a defence mechanism against anxiety and it has been found experimentally that individuals who possess more than an average amount of a particular trait tend to attribute that trait to others, providing that insight is lacking. For instance, people with a strong tendency to dishonesty will suspect others of being dishonest.

Various symptoms of schizophrenia and other mental disorders may be produced by the projection of dissociated complexes; for example, hallucinations, delusions of persecution and grandeur.

Rationalization

This is an attempt to render understandable and logical feelings or actions or attitudes which are emotionally influenced and irrational.

Intellectualization

This is the excessive use of intellectual processes to avoid unpleasant emotional experience or expression.

Denial

Denial is the refusal to admit or acknowledge the presence or existence of something, usually unpleasant reality. This occurs frequently as a normal phenomenon as well as in pathological conditions. Denial may operate in any unpleasant experience including the possibility of illness.

Introjection

Introjection is the process of assimilating or internalizing into the subject's ego qualities of the loved object.

Identification

When a person incorporates within himself a mental picture of another person and then feels, thinks and acts as he conceives that person to think, feel and act, this is **identification** and is largely an unconscious process. Identification with the loved object plays an important part in ego development. It may play an important role as a defence mechanism against anxiety or distress which accompany separation from, or the loss of an object, whether this is real, as in bereavement, or threatened.

Analytical Psychology

Carl Jung of Zurich, born in 1875, was originally a follower of Freud but later developed his own school of psychotherapy and psychopathology.

In treatment, Jung also used the technique of free association and dream analysis but started with the study of the patient's present problem and sought to discover the elements of weakness in his manner of dealing with it. Jungian analysis gives the patient an understanding of his present state as well as of his infantile past.

The concept of libido to Jung is of a general life force. It is the total vital energy seeking the goal of growth as well as of activity and reproduction.

Jung, if anything, makes more of the concept of the unconscious; he distinguishes between the personal unconscious and the collective or racial unconscious. The personal unconscious is formed partly by repression from the conscious and other material that has been acquired unconsciously. The collective unconscious or racial unconscious is inherited and consists of instincts and primordial ideas or archetypes. The instincts are primitive ways of acting and the archetypes are primitive ways of thinking.

Dream interpretation as defined by Freud is carried out in terms of causality and determinism but as defined by Jung, dreams are symbolized accounts of what has happened but also provide symbolic guidance for the present and the future.

Individual Psychology

Alfred Adler, born in Vienna in 1870, also broke away from Freud because of disagreement over the importance of infantile sexuality and the validity of the libido theory of Freud.

Adler placed much greater emphasis on the ego as against the libido and placed more emphasis on the influence of the social environment and, as each person was unique in his psychology, he termed his school that of 'individual psychology'.

The following are some of Adler's concepts:

1 Inferiority feelings are fundamental in the development of neurosis.
2 The study and analysis of the individual patient is designed to discover his pattern of life or Life Style, as Adler calls it, and in particular the goal of superiority which he has set himself and which he still follows in some form or another.

Adler emphasized that individuals tended to cope with inferiority feelings by elaborating compensatory attitudes and patterns of behaviour. He laid great emphasis on the will to power, characterized by strivings for power, dominance and superiority.

Horney's Dynamic Cultural School

Karen Horney developed a theory which differs from the classical Freudian theory in many respects. She did not accept the libido theory and the derivatives therefrom such as the stages of psychosexual development, the Oedipus complex, infantile fixation and regression. While acknowledging the importance of sexual drives, she considered cultural-social influences and disturbances in interpersonal and intra-psychic development to be more important in neurosis in general. She accepted the Freudian concept of psychic determinism and unconscious motivation. However, her concept of the unconscious was broader than that of classical psycho-analytic teaching.

Horney represented one of two main branches within the dynamic cultural school of psycho-analysis, the other being the school of Harry Stack Sullivan.

Sullivan's School

Sullivan emphasized social, cultural and environmental factors rather than biological events as being important in the development of neuroses. He considered present-day interpersonal relationships rather than past experience as being most relevant and important.

Sullivan's therapy was based on his conviction that psychotherapy is the study of interpersonal processes in which the psychiatrist acts as a participant observer.

Rado's System of Adaptational Psychodynamics

Sandor Rado, having worked with Freud, felt the need to reformulate classical psychoanalytic theory on lines of biological science and scientific methodology. He used evolutionary principles in which adaptation to the environment was deemed to be of paramount importance. He interpreted the role of pleasure and pain, emotions and thought, desire and executive action in terms of adaptation to the environment based on concepts of evolution.

He divided his methods of psychotherapy into two groups:

1 Reconstructive, using the adaptational technique of psychoanalytic therapy.

2 Reparative, which is less ambitious and with limited goals, and usually of shorter duration.

Adolf Meyer's School of Psychobiology

Meyer paid particular attention to types of reaction manifested by the total individual in terms of his total life experience. Psychobiology is the genetic, dynamic science which studies personality development in the light of environmental setting and longitudinal growth. His central theme is the mind in action and he stresses the relationship between the conscious drives and the environment. He considered that ideal mental health was the optimum ability to get on with people without the interference of internal conflict or external frictions, this resulting in full mutual satisfaction based on a constant give and take relationship.

The system of treatment, based on Meyer's teaching, is referred to as distributive analysis and synthesis and attempts to adapt the patient to his surroundings both by working with him and, indirectly, via environmental manipulation.

The School of Melanie Klein

The Kleinian or English School of psychoanalyis differs from the classical psychoanalytic school in the following respects.

Klein maintains that the primitive super-ego develops during the first and second years at the stage of infantile anxiety and aggressiveness, in contrast to orthodox theory which postulates the development of the super-ego during the fourth year of life. Klein also believes that aggressive rather than sexual drives are pre-eminent during the earlier stages of development. She considers that the presence of aggressive and sadistic impulses and the fear of retaliation are mainly responsible for the development of the primitive super-ego.

Using special methods such as play, story telling, dreams, etc., Klein maintains that children of two years of age can be treated analytically.

Klein also differs from the orthodox school in that she considers that the answer to the Oedipus situation can be traced to the earliest months of life, and also in her concept of a depressive condition during childhood which she considers of paramount importance in the child's development and its later capacity for love. The child introjects both good and bad objects. The introjection of bad objects is considered to be dangerous to the ego.

She considers that a paranoid condition develops at the age of about two to three months. Projection is employed as a defence and in the earlier stages the aggressive fantasies are turned towards the mother during the later oral phase.

Klein believes that the child develops anxiety lest the loved object be lost due to its own destructiveness. Whenever the mother makes the child angry the good internal object is threatened with destruction. This conflict is the basis of the depressive condition in which guilt forms the precursor of conscience.

Further Reading

Walker, N. (1957) *A Short History of Psychotherapy*. Routledge & Kegan Paul, London.

Hoch, P. H. and Zubin, J. (eds) (1960) *Current Approaches to Psychoanalysis*. Grune and Stratton, London.

Brown, J. A. C. (1961) *Freud and the Post Freudians*. Penguin, Harmondsworth.

Jaspers, K. (trans. Hoenig, J. and Hamilton, M. W.) (1963) *General Psychopathology*. Manchester University Press, Manchester.

Kraupl-Taylor, F. (1979) *Psychopathology: Its Causes and Symptoms*, 2nd end. Quartermaine House, Brookland.

Kline, P. (1981) *Fact and Fantasy in Freudian Theory*. Methuen, London.

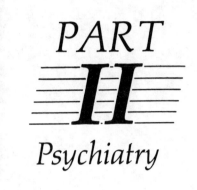

PART

II

Psychiatry

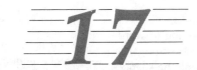

Psychiatric Examination

Psychiatric examination comprises:

1 History-taking
2 Examination of the patient's mental state
3 Examination of physical state and any special investigations that are indicated.

History-taking

The taking of the patient's history is of fundamental importance, both for investigation and for treatment.

The history, when completed, should give a picture of the patient's development and adjustment during his life. It should contain relevant information on possible genetic and family influences on his personality and his illness. It should portray his development from childhood to adult life. It should provide evidence of adjustment to school, work, marriage, society, together with a record of his physical and mental health and previous personality.

Before discussing details of history-taking, we should consider more fully the interview itself.

The Interview

The psychiatric interview is of paramount importance as it is the basis of all treatment and investigation. The psychiatrist, in his conduct of the interview, can demonstrate the art of psychiatry at its best. Interviews can be fact-finding, therapeutic or both. In either type the interview enables rapport to be developed between the patient and the doctor.

The setting of the interview room is important. The patient should not be made to feel inferior or small by the presence of a huge desk by which he is separated from the physician.

The physician must allow adequate time for the interview and have freedom from interruption. Both physician and patient should be comfortable and relaxed. Patients are usually anxious and frightened when coming for a psychiatric interview and they must be put at their ease. If necessary the physician should get up from his chair, go to meet the patient and a handshake is usually very helpful in welcoming and reassuring the patient.

The physician places the chair comfortably for the patient and then himself sits down. He should adopt a listening attitude and should avoid interrupting the patient, at least in the early stages.

The interviewer must not only feel interest but should make it clearly manifest to the patient and be friendly and accepting in manner. Note-taking is generally better left till afterwards as it often puts the patient off and may interfere with the establishment of a good doctor–patient relationship.

The physician must never give the impression that he is in a hurry. He must be flexible in taking the history and in carrying out the interview. It is necessary to have a scheme in mind in order to ensure that important aspects are not overlooked but the course the interview takes will largely depend on what emerges initially, and subsequently the physician should let things come gently and naturally.

Questions which can be answered 'yes' or 'no' should be avoided. Questions containing a lead must not, of course, be given. The wider the question the better, as this will give the patient a chance to reply as he wishes, will not restrict or impede him in so doing and will give the best opportunity of obtaining relevant and important data.

The interview is a two-way process and the physician must convey his interest by nodding the head and by making remarks such as 'surely', 'naturally', 'of course', 'I see', etc. A friendly attitude and demeanour are much more important than the particular words chosen. If there are silences, the physician should show greater interest; leaning forward, repeating the last word or phrase and urging the patient to carry on will often overcome the silence. Emotional expression should be encouraged. The interview should be channelled towards topics of relevance and importance; such topics can be encouraged by increasing one's interest and uttering suitable remarks. Unimportant or irrelevant topics can be discouraged by showing less interest.

Careful note should be made of the patient's facial expression, change of colour, halting evasion of a topic, sudden silences, increased rapidity of speech, pleading or laughing. Points made by the patient should be emphasized to let him know that you understand his feeling. Repeat the patient's statement or reformulate what he has said in order to reinforce the understanding and rapport.

General Rules for Interviews

1 Make no promises. Questions can be countered with other questions for further information.
2 Reassurance must only be given after careful enquiry and investigation. Interpretation is very dangerous unless done appropriately at the right time.
3 Don't take sides with the patient.
4 Don't egg the patient on to action.
4 Don't give advice.

Historical Anamnesis

Ascertain the patient's complaints or difficulties or, if he has no complaints, enquire the reason for his referral. Following this it is usually convenient to start with the history of the present illness.

In recording this, facts should be included rather than technical terms. It is important that the present mental state and the history should not be mixed up.

Whilst the history is being taken, the patient's behaviour and reactions should be observed and should later be recorded under 'general behaviour'.

It is also important that objective and subjective data should not be mixed up. It is undesirable to make the greater part of the record a mere transcript of what the patient has said. The examiner's observations, summaries and conclusions should be recorded as well.

Family History

One usually starts with questions about the patient's parents, enquiring if they are alive and, if so, are they in good health; if not, what is wrong or, if dead, what they died from.

It is important to assess the social position and general efficiency of the family, as well as the occurrence of familial diseases and also a note made of the home atmosphere, particularly any significant happenings among parents and siblings during the patient's early years and the patient's relationship to parents, siblings and others.

It is always wise to obtain a history from a second person as well as the patient, as important additional information may be acquired and, in any event, any discrepancies may be valuable in the assessment and understanding of the patient.

Personal History

Ascertain the date and place of birth, whether the birth was normal or prolonged, instrumental or premature, the mother's health during pregnancy and after birth, whether the patient was breast or bottle fed, brought up by the mother or, if someone else, the reasons for this.

Infancy and Childhood

The age at which the patient passed the milestones of development such as teething, talking, walking, achievement of bowel and bladder control. Note general health.

The occurrence of neurotic traits in childhood such as night terrors, somnambulism, tantrums, enuresis, nail-biting, stammering, fear states, school phobia, model child, chorea, convulsions, etc, should also be noted.

School

Age of starting and finishing, standard reached, attitude to teachers, attitude to school work and success achieved, attitude to school mates, whether he played games, mixed well, was bullied, able to stand up for himself or not.

Work

Age when started work and jobs held, listed in chronological order with dates, reasons for change; (poor work record with unduly frequent changes of employment is often an indicator of personality instability).

Menstrual Functions

Age of menarche, reactions to menarche. Regularity and duration of menses, length of cycle, amount of loss, dysmenorrhoea, premenstrual tension, date of last period, climacteric symptoms.

Sexual Inclinations and Practice

How sexual information was gained and received, prudery, worries about masturbation, homosexuality, heterosexual experiences apart from marriage.

Marital History

Time marriage partner known before marriage and engagement, compatibility. Sex relations—whether satisfactory or not, contraceptive measures used. Any financial, domestic or temperamental difficulties.

Children

Give chronological list of children, miscarriages, with ages, names, etc.

Personal Habits

Amount of alcohol, tobacco, drugs taken recently and previously.

Medical History

Details of illnesses, operations and accidents in chronological order.

Previous Mental Health

History of any previous psychiatric illnesses, whether medical attention sought and treatment given by GP, as an outpatient or inpatient, duration and description of such illnesses.

Personality

Describe the personality before the onset of the present illness and aim to present a picture of an individual and not a type, give illustrative anecdotes and detailed statements rather than relying on a series of adjectives.

Examination of Mental State

General Appearance and Behaviour

When taking the history, a great deal of information about the patient's appearance and behaviour will already have been obtained.

The first thing to observe is whether the patient looks ill, whether he looks his age or looks much older or younger. Note his general posture and facial expression. The tense, anxious patient sits on the edge of the chair, jumps at sudden noises. The depressed patient lacks muscular tone, has a dejected posture.

Is he in touch with the situation? Does he behave appropriately to it? Does he respond to the requirements of the examination? Does he show any oddities or eccentricities in speech, dress or manner?

Motor activity may be diminished, the patient being slow in his movements and in his replies. Marked reduction of activity, with the patient showing no spontaneous activity and little response to stimuli, is termed **stupor**.

Over-activity may be the manifestation of general pressure of activity found in the hypomanic patient, in which there is general psychomotor activity, restlessness, circumstantiality in speech, or it may be in the form of the agitated movements found in agitated melancholia, the patient continually fidgeting, picking his clothes, wringing his hands and walking to and fro.

Are there tics, mannerisms or stereotyped movements? Is the activity abrupt, fitful, erratic or constant?

In catatonic schizophrenics the following phenomena may be found: **automatic obedience, echolalia** (repetition by the patient of what is said to him), **echopraxia** (imitation of actions), **waxy flexibility** with maintenance of posture even in uncomfortable positions, **negativism** in which the patient does the opposite of what is required or resists attempts to help him (e.g. if when you offer to shake hands with him he moves his hand away, when you withdraw your hand his hand will come forward).

Finally, a note should be made of his eating and sleeping habits, whether he is clean and how he spends his time.

Form of Talk

Observe whether he says a great deal or is uncommunicative or retarded in speech, whether he talks spontaneously or only in answer to questions, whether he is hesitant, slow, fast, discursive, disconnected; sudden silences, change of topic, going off at a tangent; whether he uses rhymes, puns or strange words.

Perseveration in speech and in action is found in organic mental states; the patient, when asked to do a certain thing, will continue doing this action even though he is asked to do other things. This is a case of momentum and inertia carrying on and interfering with following events.

Mood

The patient's mood will already have been reflected in his general behaviour, in speech and manner. He should be asked 'How do you feel in yourself? What are your spirits like? What is your mood?' Note the constancy of mood, whether it changes rapidly or whether it is constant, the factors which change the mood and also whether the patient's behaviour and facial expression agree with what he says about his mood.

Mental Content

Enquire about the patient's attitude to himself, to the people around him and to the various things in his environment; does he feel a special reference is made to him, does he feel that people shun him or admire him, does he tend to depreciate himself regarding his past behaviour, morals, possessions and health or, conversely, is he expansive and grandiose about his possessions and personal abilities? Enquire about the predominant thoughts or preoccupations that the patient has; in depressive states these are characteristically painful and unhappy, full of regrets, dwelling on the past, the present or the future in a hopeless and gloomy way.

Disorders of Perception

It will be necessary to know whether the patient has auditory, visual, olfactory, gustatory, tactile or other hallucinations. It is usually convenient to broach this by asking the patient if he ever hears noises, later communications and then definitely voices. It is important to note at what time the hallucinations occur, whether by night or by day, their complexity, their vividness and how they are received by the patient. If they occur when falling asleep, it is usually of little significance. Severely depressed patients report that there are unusual sensations, lack of sensations or lack of organs.

Consciousness (Sensorium)

It is important to note whether the patient is alert, dull, self-absorbed, confused or delirious. Try to discover his grasp of the environment and his judgment. Enquire into his orientation in time and with regard to place and to persons.

Orientation

General orientation can be assessed by questions such as 'Where are you now?' 'What is the name of this place?' 'Where is it situated?' 'What day of the week is it today?' 'What month are we in?' 'What day of the month is it?' 'What is the year?'

If he is in hospital one can ascertain his orientation in the ward, such as 'Show me the nearest lavatory', 'Where is the bathroom?' 'Where is the main entrance?' 'Are there any other ways out?' 'Where is the television?' 'Where is the nurses' office?' etc.

Compulsive Phenomena

Does he get any recurrent thoughts which distress him, which are unwanted and which he finds difficult to dismiss? Does he feel them to be a part of his own mind or to come from without? Does he regard them as inappropriate or irrational? Are they related to his emotional state, e.g. a state of depression or anxiety? Does he feel compelled to carry out actions repeatedly, despite trying to resist, e.g. compulsively touching things or washing his hands unduly frequently?

Memory

The patient's memory functions are assessed by comparing his account of his life with that given by others. It is important to test also for recent events—when he first attended hospital or when he was admitted, whether he had seen another doctor and if so, whom and where the doctor saw him and when.

The patient may be given a name and address to remember and then asked to recall it three or five minutes later. He can be given a series of digits to repeat forwards, then others to repeat backwards.

Grasp of General Information

Questions regarding general information should be varied according to the patient's educational level, his experience and interests. He should be asked the name of the monarch and the immediate predecessors, the Prime Minister and the capitals of France, Italy, Spain and the United States. He should be asked to name six large cities in England. He should be asked to carry out the serial-7 test, i.e. subtraction of 7 from 100, and note the answer given and the time taken.

The purpose of these tests is to give a general idea whether there has been any falling off in a person's former presumptive level of knowledge and intellectual capacity.

Insight and Judgment

What is his attitude to his present state? Is his attitude and assessment of it reasonable for his intelligence and experience? Does he regard himself as being ill or as suffering from a nervous or mental illness or needing treatment? How does he regard his present difficulties or deficits? What is his opinion regarding his previous attacks of mental illness, if any?

Examination of Stuporose or Non-Cooperative Patients

The difficulties of getting information from non-cooperative or stuporose patients should not discourage the student from making and recording observations, which can be done without difficulty and which may be of great importance in presenting a record of the clinical state at the time in case the patient's clinical condition should change suddenly.

Observations can be made under the following headings:

1 *Posture and general reactions* Whether his posture is natural or awkward; whether he maintains his limbs when they are placed in awkward positions; whether his behaviour is negativistic, evasive, irritable, apathetic or obedient; whether he exhibits any spontaneous actions; his behaviour with regard to dressing, eating and personal hygiene. Describe his facial expression—whether it is vacant, placid, perplexed, depressed, distressed, any tears, flushing etc.; whether the eyes are open or closed; if the eyes are closed whether they resist attempts to raise the lid; reaction to sudden approach or threat to touch the eye.

2 *Reactions to commands* The patient should be asked to show his tongue, close his eyes, open his eyes, move limbs, shake hands. Notice whether there is negativism, echopraxia, echolalia or automatic obedience.

3 *Muscular functions* Note whether the muscles are tensed, rigid or show waxy flexibility.

Test how the patient reacts to passive movements, of the head and neck and of the limbs, and whether it is possible to influence these reactions by commands or distractions.

Physical Examination and Special Investigations

It may cause surprise to include physical examination as an important part of treatment. Physical examination and any additional investigations that may be necessary must be carried out thoroughly, not only to detect, assess or exclude the presence of organic disease but also to give weight and conviction to the reassurance and explanation given by the physician at the appropriate time to the patient concerning his illness. The patient will be impressed by a thorough physical examination and thus more likely to accept the physician's opinion about his physical state.

It will only antagonize a patient to tell him there is nothing wrong with him. He may be told that there is nothing physically wrong but this must be followed by an explanation of his symptoms, in terms suitable to his intelligence and his personality.

Similarly, when special investigations are necessary, the reasons and nature of the investigations should be explained to the patient beforehand. Wherever possible, he should be told about the outcome of these results, otherwise feelings of anxiety and apprehension will be fostered.

Once a physician is reasonably satisfied with a patient's physical state, he should avoid repeating the physical examination unless this is dictated by the patient's medical condition. Repeated examination usually has a harmful effect on the patient, suggesting to him that the doctor is not sure of his case and reinforcing his fears that there may be something seriously, physically wrong with him. Prolonged and exhaustive clinical and laboratory investigations also may make the patient very apprehensive. Special investigations, when necessary, should be reduced to the minimum and always given with adequate explanation and, when possible, strong reassurance.

Further Reading

McKinnon, R. A. (1971) *The Psychiatric Interview in Clinical Practice*. W. B. Saunders, Philadelphia.

Institute of Psychiatry, Department of Psychiatry Teaching Committee (1973) *Notes on Eliciting and Recording Clinical Information*. Oxford University Press/Institute of Psychiatry, London.

Kendell, R. E. (1975) *The Role of Diagnosis in Psychiatry*. Blackwell, Oxford.

Leff, J. P. and Isaacs, A. D. (1978) *Psychiatric Examination in Clinical Practice*. Blackwell, Oxford.

American Psychiatric Association (1980) *Diagnostic and Statistical Manual of Mental Disorders*, 3rd edn. American Psychiatric Association, New York.

Neill, J. R. and Sandifer, M. G. (1980) *Manual of Psychiatric Consultation*. Williams and Wilkins, Baltimore.

18

Advanced Technology in the Investigation of Psychiatric Disorders

Biochemical Techniques

Gas chromatography, using electron capture for detection, has greatly increased the sensitivity of measurements of biochemical and biological compounds. Radio-immuno-assay techniques and related radio-receptor techniques utilize highly specific biologically derived immunoglobulin molecules or receptors. This method has been used successfully in the study of endorphins in body fluids. Gas chromatography, combined with mass spectroscopy, has been used in the measurement of neural transmitter metabolites. High performance liquid chromatography, gas chromatography, mass spectroscopy, radio-immuno-assay and radio-receptor assays have greatly increased sensitivity and precision in the measurement of chemical and biological actions of drugs and chemical compounds important in neural transmission.

Electroencephalogram (EEG)

The electroencephalogram records electrical potential differences between a variety of points on the surface of the scalp. The EEG is valuable in the diagnosis of epilepsy, organic psycho-syndromes, including presenile dementia, such as Alzheimer's disease, Huntington's chorea and the Jacob Creutzfeld syndrome, and also drug and metabolic encephalopathy. In Alzheimer's disease there is a slowing of the alpha rhythm and appearance of diffuse theta activity which eventually becomes dominant as cerebral degeneration progresses. Huntington's chorea is characterized by a marked absence of all rhythmic activity. The EEG is also useful in the diagnosis of states of stupor and can distinguish those due to organic causes from those due to depression or hysteria. Evoked potentials to auditory stimuli can be summated by computer and have a diagnostic value in studying deafness in children who are unable to speak or who are too young to communicate.

Computerized Tomography

The introduction of computerized tomography (CT) a decade ago provided the first opportunity for brain function to be studied *in vivo*. In psychiatry this enabled the association between neuroanatomy and psychopathology to be investigated.

The CT image can detect lesions larger than 0.5 cm in diameter. It can measure the thickness of the cerebral cortex, basal ganglia, the size of a subarachnoid space and the size and shape of the ventricles. CT scans can detect lesions such as tumours, abscesses, demyelination, cerebral atrophy, infarcts, subdural haematoma and hydrocephalus.

In alcoholism, ventricular enlargement, sulcal widening, atrophy of the cerebellar vermis and reduced cerebral density have been reported. There has been some evidence that the changes associated with alcoholism can eventually be reversed with abstention from alcohol. In schizophrenia enlarged ventricles, dilated sulcal widening and cerebellar atrophy have been reported. Such changes tend to correlate with schizophrenia characterized by negative symptoms and which tend to show a poor response to the majority of neuroleptics.

Brain Electro-activity Mapping (BEAM)

This is a method of presenting EEG and evoked potential data derived from twenty or more electrodes topographically in the form of colour maps. Recent evidence has shown that in schizophrenia both medicated and drug-free patients showed an increased delta activity compared with normal controls. This is particularly notable in the increased frontal delta. This finding is in keeping with evidence of frontal dysfunction in schizophrenia derived from blood flow measurements and positron emission tomography.

Positron Emission Tomography (PET)

In contrast to CT which measures structure, PET can provide information on physiological and biochemical changes within the central nervous system.

The procedure involves intravenous administration of a bolus of radioactive substance. Scanning starts thirty minutes after the administration, and the measurements obtained permit calculation of local cerebral metabolism for a given region. PET provides a unique opportunity for studying regional brain activity in normal psychiatric patients during rest and functional activity. Studies using PET scans in schizophrenia have shown a hypofunctioning of the frontal lobes and basal ganglia.

Magnetic Resonance Imaging (MRI)

This is a non-invasive technique for the study of structure and pathophysiology of the brain, and provides useful information in suspected metabolic and neurotransmitter defects. The technique uses powerful magnets to align or polarize the random spinning nuclei in their natural environment so that they tend to be parallel with the magnetic field. This new method is being utilized in the studies of epilepsy, organic psychosyndromes, presenile dementia, senile dementia and schizophrenia and promises to be a rewarding method of investigation which is much cheaper than positron emission tomography.

Dexamethasone Suppression Test

Dexamethasone, which suppresses cortisol levels in the blood, has been found to be abnormal in this respect in depressive patients. The test consists of giving 1 mg of dexamethasone at 2000 hours, and blood samples are taken between 1500 and 1600 hours the following day for the estimation of cortisol. About 70% of depressed patients show an abnormal DST, compared with 11% controls.

However, the test is not specific for depression and abnormal responses occur in a proportion of schizophrenics, abstinent alcoholics, neurotics and patients undergoing prophylactic lithium therapy.

The Tyramine Challenge Test

The tyramine challenge test consists of giving 125 mg of tyramine hydrochloride (equivalent to 100 mg of tyramine) orally at 0900 hours immediately after voiding the bladder and collecting a complete urine sample during the three-hour period following the ingestion of tyramine.

Depressed patients excrete significantly lower amounts of urinary tyramine as sulphate following oral administration of tyramine hydrochloride, compared with normal subjects.

The test appears to be a reliable trait marker for depression.

19
Principles of Aetiology

Aetiology is the science or the philosophy of causation of disease.

Throughout the ages attempts have been made to determine the causation of mental illnesses and psychiatrists, like other physicians, have been tempted to look for a single cause for each disease. This approach, however, was found to be inappropriate and unhelpful and nowadays it is necessary to consider a complex interaction of forces within the individual and between the individual and the environment.

The search for causality in medicine always involves a concept of factors, each of which has as good a claim to the title of cause as any other. For example, if we stated that the tubercle bacillus is the cause of tuberculosis, this implies that the presence of the tubercle bacilli in the body is a sufficient condition for the occurrence of the disease tuberculosis but, as is well known, this is not so. A person can experience the invasion of tubercle bacilli into the body without developing tuberculosis. On the other hand, we could not say that the person was suffering from tuberculosis if he did not have, or never had, any tubercle bacilli in his body. It may be said, therefore, that the presence of tubercle bacilli in a person's body is a necessary condition but we cannot say it is a sufficient condition for the development of tuberculosis. It may be termed *a* factor or *a* cause but not *the* cause. It is known that a variety of factors may determine whether invasion of the tubercle bacillus into the body will develop into tuberculosis. Nutritional state, overcrowding, stressful experiences and many other conditions may determine the actual development of tuberculosis at a particular time. These factors are the *sufficient* causes; the tubercle bacillus itself is the *essential* cause.

Thus, the aetiology of diseases may be discussed in terms of essential causes, without which a disease could not develop, and sufficient causes which enable the essential cause to be clinically manifested as the disease.

One may also regard causes as predisposing and precipitating.

In studying the causes of illness, there are three fields of observation:

1 The field of the person, which includes observations on the characteristics of the person before he becomes ill.
2 The field of the environment, including observations on the features of the environment which the person met at, or just before, the time he became ill.
3 The field of mechanism. This includes observation on the structural, physical, chemical and psychological mechanisms brought into action by the encounter of the individual with his environment which, ultimately, bring about the particular mode of behaviour which we refer to as illness.

Aetiology is therefore concerned with ascertaining which features of the individual and the environment are relevant and causal and which mechanisms in the body are involved in the illness.

We need to know the factors which determine the onset of the illness, the course of the illness and the factors which determine its outcome.

One can therefore discuss an aetiology of onset, an aetiology of the course of the illness and an aetiology of the outcome of the illness.

We can ask a number of questions about anybody who becomes ill:

1 Why has he become ill?

2 Why has he become ill in the way in which he has become ill?

3 Why has he become ill at this time of his life?

Thus, we can consider intrinsic causes residing in the individual and extrinsic causes arising from his environment.

Intrinsic causes may be classified as follows:

1 genogenic
2 constitutional
3 personality
4 critical stages of development

Extrinsic causes include psychosocial stresses, infections, trauma etc.

A psychiatric illness is the result of the interaction of a number of factors residing within the individual (intrinsic factors) and in the environment (extrinsic factors).

Multiple causation is the rule. The relative importance of intrinsic and extrinsic factors varies according to the type of illness as well as the individual.

There is a continuous interaction between intrinsic and extrinsic factors.

Genetic Factors

As discussed in Chapter 20, a number of psychiatric illnesses are genetically determined, some with a specific predisposition determined by a single gene.

Certain minor disorders and personality disorders appear to be determined by a large number of genes of small effect, i.e. they are multifactorially determined.

It should be remembered that more than one type of predisposition to mental illness may occur in the same person, e.g. a person may carry the gene for schizophrenia as well as that for endogenous depression.

Genes are influenced by the genotypic milieu as well as by the internal environment of the body, in addition to the effect of environmental influences.

Genes produce their effects by controlling enzyme systems and, therefore, the chemical status of the body. It is believed that many of the severe psychiatric illnesses like schizophrenia and depressive illness will probably be demonstrated to have an underlying biochemical disturbance, and possibly many different types of disturbance for the subtypes of schizophrenia and depressive illness.

Certain changes in the internal environment occurring at puberty, premenstrually, at childbirth and the menopause are well known to pre-dispose to the manifestation of psychiatric disorders.

Physical Constitution

Physical constitution shows some correlation with schizophrenia, manic-depressive psychosis and certain psychosomatic disorders as discussed in Chapter 10.

The assumption here is that the genes determining body build influence the genes determining schizophrenia and manic-depressive illness.

Personality

Personality types show some but not complete correlation with particular disorders, such as schizothymic and schizoid personality, cyclothymic obsessional, hysterical, etc.

The correlation is not a close one as there are many people with these types of personality who never fall mentally ill or, if they do, do not necessarily develop the type of illness to which they are allegedly predisposed.

Extrinsic Causes

Infections, physical injury, intoxication, malnutrition and avitaminosis may all affect the person's mental state by altering the internal environment of the body.

Certain infections, traumatic conditions and anoxic states may result in permanent damage to the brain and cause dementia.

Psychosocial Stresses

The experience of various psychosocial stresses such as bereavement, loss of a loved person, financial catastrophe, loss of status and prestige may all act as non-specific stresses for making manifest the predisposition to psychiatric disorders.

It is important in assessing the role of psychosocial stresses to take into account the effect of stresses immediately preceding the appearance of the precipitating stress, and also the fact that patients show specific susceptibilities to certain stresses.

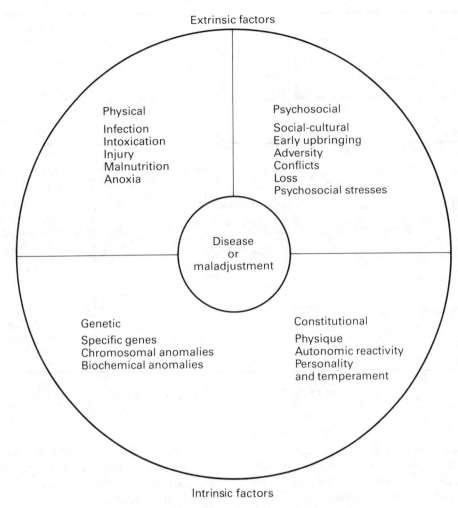

Extrinsic factors

Physical

Infection
Intoxication
Injury
Malnutrition
Anoxia

Psychosocial

Social-cultural
Early upbringing
Adversity
Conflicts
Loss
Psychosocial stresses

Disease
or
maladjustment

Genetic

Specific genes
Chromosomal anomalies
Biochemical anomalies

Constitutional

Physique
Autonomic reactivity
Personality
and temperament

Intrinsic factors

Figure 19.1 *Multifactorial aetiology of psychiatric illness.*

Classification

It is not possible in the present state of knowledge to achieve an accurate aetiological classification of psychiatric disorders, but it is possible to separate the organic mental states from those in which no demonstrable organic pathology is at present known.

The acute organic mental states (toxic infective mental states) comprise the syndromes, delirium, subdelirious state, Korsakov's syndrome and neuraesthenia.

The next group are the organic dementias in which there is damage to the brain due to a variety of causes.

In the acute organic mental states (toxic con-fusional states), the predominant clinical features are clouding of consciousness and disorientation. In the dementias the predominant feature is loss of mental capacity mainly affecting memory functions.

The remaining disorders are often subdivided into psychoses and neuroses. The term psychosis refers to the more severe mental illnesses such schizophrenia, manic-depressive psychosis, whereas the neuroses refer to conditions such as hysteria, obsessional state, etc.

The distinction between whether an illness is psychotic or neurotic is not very sensible and serves no useful purpose, and very often the term psychotic is loosely used synonymously with schizophrenia. What the users of these terms usually have in mind is that the psychotic may lack insight into his illness

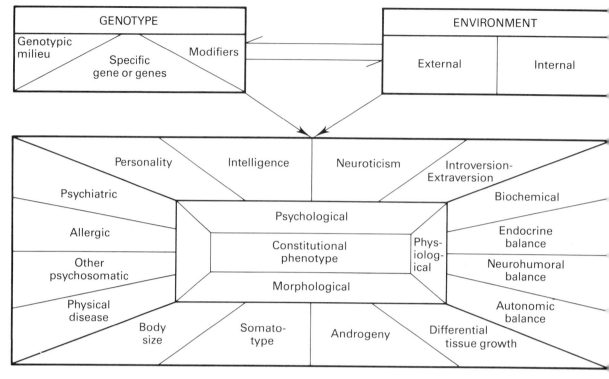

Figure 19.2   *Relationships of genotype to phenotype.*

and may need care in a psychiatric hospital, whereas the neurotic is alleged to have reasonable insight into his illness and can be cared for in the community; but these criteria are by no means satisfactory because some schizophrenics have good insight and can be cared for in the community, whereas some hysterics lack insight and may need institutional care. There would be no loss to psychiatry if these terms were discarded.

With regard to personality disorders, these may occur as problems by themselves or may occur in any psychiatric illness. Similarly, intelligence of all ranges may accompany all varieties of psychiatric illness.

Classification of Psychiatric Disorders

1 **Psychosomatic and somatopsychic interactions**
2 **Organic states**
   Acute—Delirium, Korsakov's syndrome, subdelirious state, toxic confusional state.
   Chronic—Including dementia due to degener-

ative, infective, cardiovascular, neoplastic, traumatic, demyelinating, epileptic or metabolic disorders; drugs and other intoxicants.
3 **Affective disorders**
   Depressive illness
   Hypomanic and manic states
   Anxiety states
   Phobic states
4 **Schizophrenia**
5 **Hysteria**
6 **Obsessional states**
7 **Personality abnormalities**
8 **Psychopathy**
9 **Psychosexual anomalies**
10 **Mental subnormality**

Further Reading

Wing, J. K. (1974) *Measurement and Classification of Psychiatric Syndromes.* Cambridge University Press, Cambridge.

20

Genetical Aspects

The fruitless discussions of the past as to whether a particular disease or attribute was either genetically determined or due to environmental influences have been superseded by the modern concept of a continuous interaction between genes and the environment.

Genes may be influenced by three distinct environments:

1 external environment
2 internal environment of the body (milieu interieur)
3 the environment of other genes, collectively called the genotypic milieu

The observable manifestation of an inherited attribute is referred to as the phenotype. The phenotype is the resultant of interaction of the genetic make-up of the individual (genotype) and environmental influences.

Genes

The gene is the basic unit of heredity and consists of large and elaborately constructed molecules of deoxyribonucleic acid (DNA). Genes are transmitted from one generation to the next unchanged unless altered by mutation.

Mutation is a rare and rather haphazard event and may occur spontaneously or be brought about by chemicals, radiation or physical agents. Genes have two functions, being able (1) to replicate themselves, and (2) to determine the architecture of protein molecules. Genes exert their effects through their control of biochemical reactions, accelerating some and retarding others, or inhibiting some reactions until the chemical environment is such as to set it into action.

Although genes are transmitted as independent units, it is necessary to think of the genetic constitution (genotype) as acting as a whole, with the cumulative effects of minor influences of many genes sometimes being just as important as the major effects of single genes.

Genes can only act in the framework of their environment and their effects will be influenced to a greater or lesser degree by environmental factors.

Genetical research aims at discovering how much of the total variance occurring in a given population can be attributed to genetical and how much to environmental factors.

Chromosomes

Genes are found in chromosomes which are contained in the nucleus of the cell. In the human being there are 46 chromosomes in each cell excluding the gametes. The set of 46 chromosomes consists of 22 matched pairs (autosomes or non-sex chromosomes), and one pair of sex chromosomes. In the male the sex chromosome pair consists of an X-chromosome and a smaller Y-chromosome. In the female the sex chromosome pair consists of two X-chromosomes.

Chromosomes exist in pairs, each member of which is homologous to the other. The genes of which they consist are also homologous and paired and are known as alleles. Each member of a pair is either chemically identical with its partner or differing slightly.

Chromosomes are, in appearance, thread-like structures with the genes ranged along their length. In experimental animals, it is possible to identify the individual gene by its position in a particular chromosome.

Chromosome Abnormalities

During recent years, there has been a great expansion of research on human chromosome abnormalities. In 1949 Barr and Bertram discovered the sex chromatin body in the nucleus of cells of females. Later sexual dimorphism was also found to be expressed in the configuration of the polymorphonuclear leucocytes, a club-like attachment on the nucleus seen in cells of females but rarely, if ever, in males.

The discovery of nuclear sex led to enquiries regarding the possibility that the anatomical expression of sex, i.e. the sexual phenotype could, in some clinical states, be at variance with the sex of the individual person as determined at conception.

This line of enquiry, coupled with the discovery of techniques of chromosome analysis, led to the discovery of a number of sex chromosome abnormalities in the human.

Many of the chromosome abnormalities are the results of errors of cell division and chromosome partitioning, either during gametogenesis, during cleavage of zygote or, occasionally, later.

Mitosis is the regular repeated cell division which leads to the formation of tissues in organisms and animals from a single original cell.

Meiosis, on the other hand, is the process involved in preparing the gametes, each of which will contain half the chromosome number of the original mother cell, and takes place only in the gonads. Its objective is achieved through two cell divisions, the first of which halves the chromosome number by separating the homologous chromosomes from each other into two daughter cells.

The abnormal phenomena whereby two chromosomes migrate together to the same part of the dividing cell and are both included in one daughter cell and excluded from the other is called non-dysjunction.

Sex chromosomes may be abnormal in number or in structure.

The first anomalies to be discovered were Klinefelter's syndrome (i.e. chromatin positive males), and ovarian dysgenesis (i.e. chromatin negative females).

Autosomal Chromosomal Anomalies

Any of the 22 matching pairs comprising 44 autosomes may be abnormal in size and morphology or in number. They may be over-represented (trisomy) or under-represented (monosomy).

The following are the most important syndromes due to autosomal chromosome anomalies:

1 Down's syndrome (mongolism) due to trisomy G.
2 Edward's syndrome, trisomy E.
3 Patau's syndrome, trisomy D.
4 Cri-du-chat syndrome due to deletion of part of a short arm of B group chromosomes.

In the first three there is an extra chromosome, 47 instead of 46 (2 sex and 44 autosomes). The extra chromosome may be fused on to another chromosomal fusion and is abnormal in size and shape.

Single Gene Inheritance

A number of disorders, particularly certain forms of mental deficiency with specific clinical features or biochemical characteristics, are transmitted by single genes. The mode of transmission may be dominant, recessive or intermediate.

Dominant transmission needs only one specific gene, the other being normal, i.e. a heterozygote, and is characterized by a 50% incidence in relatives of index case parents, 50% in siblings and 50% in children.

Recessive transmission depends on two matching genes, one from each parent, i.e. a homozygote, has a 25% incidence in siblings and a higher frequency of consanguinity than expected by chance. Recessively transmitted disorders usually have an early age of onset, are usually severe and present as a clear-cut syndrome. Dominantly transmitted disorders often have a late age of onset, and often have a variable clinical presentation.

Sex-linked Inheritance

One of the 23 pairs of chromosomes is anomalous in that the two members of the pair are not the same size and hence not strictly homologous. These are the sex chromosomes of which the X-chromosome is full-sized, whilst the Y-chromsome is hardly more than a fragment containing very little genetic material in proportion. The female can only produce ova of one kind with one X-chromosome, whereas the male can produce two kinds of spermatozoa—one with an X and one with a Y-chromosome. As the X-chromosome is so much bigger than the Y-chromosome, the greater part of it in the male has no matching partner. Any gene, dominant or recessive, in this part of the X-chromosome will have its full effect in the male but, if recessive, will be liable to be repressed in the female.

Conditions determined in this way have a very characteristic pedigree, with transmission occurring through the female but manifestation being confined to males. An example is red-green colour blindness.

Multifactorial (Polygenic) Inheritance

Some characteristics show quantitative variation and usually are distributed along the normal frequency curve, as in the case of intelligence, height, weight, body build, etc.

These are usually due to a large number of genes and, in fact, it may be said that when we find distribution of a normal frequency type we should think of multifactorial inheritance.

Methods of Human Genetic Research

In the past the principal method of studying heredity was the investigation of isolated family pedigrees. This was of value only for marked abnormalitytransmitted by dominant genes having a high penetrance and the method is quite unsatisfactory for studying the inheritance of common disorders.

The main methods used nowadays for investigating the inheritance of psychiatric illnesses and other common disorders are:

1 *The Statistical, Genealogical Proband Method* This method involves taking a random sample of patients suffering from the disease to be studied, who are referred to as probands, and the incidence of the disorder is ascertained in the relatives of the probands. This is compared with the incidence in the relatives of a normal control group of probands of similar age and sex distribution which will give the incidence of the disorder in the general population.

If the results show a statistically significantly higher incidence of the disease among the relatives of the disease probands than among the relatives of the normal probands, it is highly probable that the disease is due to inherited factors in the absence of exogenous differences between the disease probands and the control probands series.

2 *Twin Studies* Genetic twin studies are based on the fact that the genetic equipment in uniovular twins is the same and that any differences found between the pairs are considered to be due to environmental influences. In binovular twins, as the genetic equipment is different, any intrapair differences could be due to heredity and/or the environment. Stated in another way, the high degree of similarity among pairs of uniovular twins for a specific trait indicates a heredity factor. Binovular twins, on the other hand, are no more alike than ordinary siblings as regards genetical endowment.

Intelligence

Intelligence, in the normal population, is distributed along the normal frequency curve and is considered to be of multifactorial (polygenic) inheritance.

Mentally handicapped people with IQs above 50 represent the lowest part of the normal variation in intelligence and here the mental handicap is also multifactorially determined.

Below an intelligence quotient of 50, mentally subnormal patients cannot be accommodated into this scheme and, in these instances, the mode of inheritance is by means of single major genes.

This is borne out by the fact that the correlation of intelligence between siblings and the mental defective whose IQ was above 50 has been found to be $+0.5$ which corresponds to the correlation for the general population, whereas in the low grade mentally subnormal patients, i.e. with an IQ below 50, the correlation was zero.

Personality, Character and Neurosis

Animal breeding experiments provide strong evidence of a genetic basis for behavioural characteristics in mice, rats, dogs and rabbits, particularly differences in aggressiveness, emotional stability and temperament.

Identical twins have been studied by means of tests of intelligence, personality and autonomic nervous system functioning. The results showed that intelligence, autonomic lability and extraversion–introversion were genetically determined; extraversion is determined by heredity to as large an extent as intelligence.

Uniovular twins brought up apart still show a significant similarity, even when they are brought

similar personality traits in the near relatives of ulcer patients. The evidence suggests that the predisposition to duodenal ulcer is associated with certain personality characteristics and a narrow physique.

There is also evidence that the predisposition to peptic ulceration is correlated with a high level of pepsinogen in the blood; pepsinogen level is considered to be genetically determined.

Single Dominant	Single Recessive	Multifactorial
Endogenous depression	?Schizophrenia	Intelligence
?Bipolar affective disorder		Personality
?Schizophrenia		Neurosis
Huntington's chorea		Physique
Pick's presenile dementia		Senile dementia
Congenital dyslexia		Alzheimer's presenile dementia
?Asthma		
Migraine		Some forms of nocturnal enuresis
Some forms of nocturnal enuresis		?Schizophrenia
		?Manic depressive
		?Asthma

up by dissimilar types of parents—dissimilar in mode of upbringing, attitude and personality.

Family studies of the relatives of patients suffering from anxiety states, hysteria and obsessional states had a significantly higher incidence of neurosis than corresponding normal control groups.

Studies on identical and binovular twins revealed that about 80% of individual differences in neuroticism was due to heredity and 20% to environment.

It has also been found that uniovular twins were twice as likely as binovular twins to have a similar degree of difficulty in adjustment.

Psychosomatic Disorders

It has been found that peptic ulcer patients had a higher incidence of narrow physique and autonomic imbalance than control groups and there was good reason to believe that these had existed before the onset of illness.

Genetic studies revealed a preponderance of

Careful genetic studies carried out in Sweden have revealed that specific dyslexia, or **congenital word blindness,** is transmitted by a single dominant gene with a manifestation of practically 100%.

Nocturnal enuresis has also been studied genetically in Sweden and was found to be aetiologically heterogeneous, but that there was probably a group of patients in which it was genetically determined, although subject to environmental influences. The mode of inheritance is not clear; it may be a simple dominant with reduced penetrance or polygenic.

Mental Subnormality

The genetical aspects of mental subnormality are dealt with in Chapter 32.

Various forms are determined by autosomal recessive or dominant genes, a variety of cytogenic aberrations and associated biochemical disorders, as well as the important high grade group which is mainly multifactorially determined.

Mental Illness

The role of genetic factors is discussed in the text on each disorder. The table opposite gives a summary of the mode of inheritance of some mental disorders.

Further Reading

Slater, E. T. and Cowie, V. (1971) *Genetics of Mental Disorders*. Oxford University Press, Oxford.

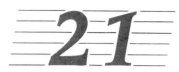

Epidemiology, Social and Transcultural Psychiatry

Social psychiatry deals with the social causes and consequences of mental illness, and the various social methods which can be utilized in treating such illness.

Psychiatric illnesses are multifactorial in origin and arise from an interaction between genetic, constitutional, biological, psychological and environmental factors.

Epidemiology is the study of health and disease in the community.

The ways in which epidemiology can be applied are as follows:

1 To delineate the historical trend of diseases.
2 To estimate the incidence of diseases in the population.
3 To assess the working of health services.
4 To estimate the risk of the individual developing a particular disease.
5 To complement the clinical picture of disease of which only a part is visible to the clinician.
6 To describe and distinguish syndromes and search for causes of disease.

The principles of epidemiology as a science were established over a century ago by Snow who demonstrated that cholera was conveyed by sewage-contaminated water.

The application of epidemiological methods to infectious diseases was also applied to non-infectious disease, e.g. the discovery that pellagra was due to dietary deficiency and, more recently, the discovery of a causal relationship between cigarette smoking and lung cancer.

The following terms are relevant in considering epidemiological and social aspects of psychiatric illness.

Prevalence is the number of cases present during a given time in a unit of population ('point prevalence'), or during a given period of time ('period prevalence').

Expectancy is the probability that an individual will develop the illness during a given period.

Incidence is the number of new cases in a unit population during a given period of time, which is usually one year. Sometimes, lifetime incidence is calculated and this relates to the lifetime expectancy for development of the disease.

Incidence relates to new patients and is more likely to provide relevant data regarding causal factors than the data of prevalence or expectancy.

Two major practical problems in epidemiology are the definition of what constitutes a case, and the identification of patients suffering from the illness.

Hospital statistics only provide evidence of the more severe forms of psychiatric illness requiring hospital admission, and they are an underestimate. Case registers established in various parts of the country contain more information on patients who have been in contact with various psychiatric agencies, but these do not provide a full and comprehensive picture of the prevalence of psychiatric illness in the community.

Surveys of general practice have revealed that during one year 14% of the population have consulted their doctor because of psychiatric illness, and only one-fifth of these are referred to a psychiatrist. Even this figure is an underestimate of the true prevalence of psychiatric morbidity, since only about one-third of psychiatric disorders in general practice are detected by the doctor.

Using questionnaires, such as general health questionnaires or a modified Cornell medical index, surveys of random samples of the general population for all psychiatric illness indicate that the rates per 1000 population range from 184 to 203 with females having twice the prevalence of males. These figures refer to 'point prevalence'.

Surveys in Sweden revealed a history of mental disorder (so-called 'life prevalence') of 1.7% for psychoses (including schizophrenia and manic-depressive illness), 13.1% for neuroses and 1.2% for mental deficiency. The risk of developing mental illnesses during a ten-year period was 11.3% for men and 20.4% for women.

Suicide

Statistics from the World Health Organization have shown that suicide rates tend to remain relatively constant for each country, although differing considerably between different countries.

The rate per 100 000 population in England and Wales is roughly 11.5, Sweden 17, the United States 10.5, Northern Ireland 5, Republic of Ireland 3.2, Israel 6.4, Australia 11.9, France 15.9, West Berlin 37, Hungary 24, Japan 20.

It has been shown that the incidence of suicide in various London boroughs was correlated with indices of social isolation, mobility, divorce and illegitimacy but not with unemployment or overcrowding.

Suicide rates are higher in the upper social classes except in the older age groups when the rate is greatest in the lowest social classes. This suggests that different factors operate in the older groups where social isolation has been shown to be an important factor.

Psychosomatic Disorders

It has been estimated that a man aged 35 will run the risk of 1 in 8 chances of coronary heart disease, 1 in 10 of peptic ulcer; 33% of men reaching 35 will die before they reach 65 compared with just over 20% of women.

Epidemiology can sometimes help in the identification of syndromes. This was shown clearly in the

case of peptic ulcer; mortality rates in different social classes showed that there were two conditions to be studied, namely gastric ulcer and duodenal ulcer.

Coronary disease has a particularly high mortality in Class 1. Although diet was considered to be the important factor, recent investigations have suggested that the differences are the product of a connection between coronary heart disease and physical activity of work. The higher the status the less active the job.

The class distribution seems to be mainly dependent on the proportion of light and heavy workers in each class.

Social Class

It has been known for many years that schizophrenia is relatively more common in unskilled workers than in professional or business men. It has been found in USA that the rate of schizophrenia was ten times as great in the lowest as in the highest social class. The figures for England and Wales for first hospital admissions indicate that schizophrenia is four times greater than in the highest social class.

The two possible reasons for this association are that the stresses associated with the conditions in Social Class 5 are conducive to the development of schizophrenia or that schizophrenic patients, as they deteriorate, drift downward into these areas.

The main evidence of an individual downward drift is the ability of schizophrenic patients to win high places in schools, although they end up in semi-skilled or unskilled jobs.

The discrepancies in social performance between father and son could be mainly attributable to the effects of the disease process.

The social drift appears to affect the highest and lowest social classes most severely.

The findings suggest that gross socio-economic deprivation is unlikely to be a major aetiological factor in schizophrenia.

Marital Status

It has been shown that there is a higher proportion of single people amongst those admitted to mental hospitals as compared with the general population, with a considerable proportion of this excess due to those admitted with a diagnosis of schizophrenia.

There are two possible explanations for this; firstly

that the pre-admission states of the disease militate against marriage or that marriage protects the individual against the psychosis.

Transcultural Psychiatry

An aspect of social psychiatry which has gained increasing attention and research enquiry in recent years is transcultural psychiatry, which is concerned with the influence of different cultures on the aetiology, manifestation and course of psychiatric illnesses.

The term 'culture' used in this context refers to the values, customs, institutions and social organization of a particular community.

Reports of differences in incidence and prevalence of psychiatric illnesses in different cultures are difficult to interpret because, in addition to the environmental components of culture, other factors such as genetic influence, malnutrition and infections also have to be taken into account when differences in rates of incidence and prevalence of psychiatric illness are reported.

It should be borne in mind that culture also defines normality and abnormality in a particular community and influences the ways in which mental illness is recognized and labelled. Socio-cultural and traditional influences may also affect the content and the symptomatology of psychiatric illnesses. People from more primitive cultures who suffer from anxiety and depression may report that they are possessed by devils or influenced by supernatural forces, or that they can hear the voices of ancestral spirits. These may simply be benign culture specific and standardized modes of explaining distress or misfortune, and the pitfall of assuming that these are symptoms of schizophrenia has to be avoided.

The belief that psychiatric disorders are non-existent or extremely rare in primitive cultures is no longer tenable. Psychiatric illnesses occur in all communities throughout the world and investigators have been more impressed by the similarities than the differences.

Schizophrenia

The World Health Organization carried out an outstanding study entitled *The International Pilot Study of Schizophrenia* in which standardized methods of diagnosis were used, and it was found that patients with an identical pattern of symptoms could be recognized in all parts of the world, including Colombia, Czechoslovakia, Denmark, India, Nigeria, Taiwan, USSR, Britain and the United States. These findings support the view that schizophrenia is a disease or group of diseases and not merely a label applied to social deviants, as some writers have suggested.

In a follow-up study covering a two-year period, wide differences were found in course and outcome. About one-third of patients re-examined were totally free from symptoms, whereas one third were still severely affected by schizophrenia, and one third showed some improvement, but not amounting to total recovery.

In three developing countries, Nigeria, India and Colombia, schizophrenia had a better outcome than the other six countries. These differences could be due to social factors, but might also be due to the possibility that schizophrenia is not a single disease, but a group of disorders with differing biological and, perhaps, genetic bases, whose distribution varies in different ethnic groups.

Depressive Disorders

Earlier reports about the rarity of depression in developing countries are not correct. Depression in the past was under-diagnosed because of the application of European criteria.

Depression in Nigeria, for example, is not usually associated with feelings of guilt, unworthiness and self-depreciation and, as a consequence, suicide is relatively rare.

Paranoid delusions, somatic complaints and hypochondriacal preoccupation with bodily symptoms are more common. Neuroses and various neurotic manifestations are found in all cultures, but it appears that somatic symptoms, hysterical conversion or dissociative symptoms are more common in developing countries.

Studies of immigrants in the United Kingdom and other parts of the world have shown that they often exhibit a higher incidence of mental illness than their country of origin and the country to which they have immigrated. This may be due in part to factors of selection in which the urge to migrate may be due to an actual or developing psychiatric disorder. This is not likely to be the entire explanation because when migration is associated with difficulties, the healthier and more able members of the community are more likely to migrate and therefore are expected to have a lower rate of psychiatric morbidity. A more likely factor is that stresses of moving to a different culture, including difficulties of language, overcrowding, shared dwellings, unemployment and other problems, may tax the adaptive capacity of the immigrant to the maximum and lead to a psychiatric disorder.

Culture-bound Psychiatric Disorders

We have noted that similarity in major psychiatric illnesses is more striking than differences in various parts of the world. Nevertheless, culture can influence the early diagnosis, determine the content of the illness, the form of symptoms and the behaviour pattern. Thus culture may be more pathoplastic than pathogenic.

The pathoplastic influence of culture is most marked in specific culture-bound disorders such as koro, amok, latah and windigo. **Koro** is a panic state occurring among males from the southern provinces of China and from Malaysia, in which the patient becomes convinced that the penis is shrinking and retracting into the abdomen with fatal results. The patient will try to prevent retraction by placing a clamp on the penis or by tying string around it.

Amok occurs in South East Asia and in other parts of the world. It occurs almost exclusively in men, following a period of depression and outburst of murderous rage in which the patient violently attacks people, animals or inanimate objects, usually ending in suicide or being killed or, sometimes, ending in exhaustion with amnesia.

Latah is found in Malaysia and North Africa and characteristically affects middle-aged or elderly females, and develops as a state of dissociation following severe stress. During this state the sufferer exhibits echolalia, echopraxia or automatic obedience, but schizophrenic symptoms do not develop.

Piblokto is also a dissociative state, occurring in Eskimo women. It follows depression and is associated with self-destructive or homicidal behaviour, with amnesia for the episode.

Windigo occurs in certain Indian tribes in North America and Canada. The windigo, which is a cannibalistic monster with a heart of ice, is a part of the mythology in these cultures and the patient, during depression, believes he has been transformed into a windigo and attacks of cannibalism on the other members of the tribe may follow.

Further Reading

Barker, D. J. P. and Rose, D. (1979) *Epidemiology in Medical Practice*, 2nd edn. Churchill Livingstone, Edinburgh.

Knox, E. (1979) *Epidemiology in Health Care Planning*. Oxford University Press, Oxford.

Lipsedge, M. (1979) *Aliens and Alienists* (out of print). Penguin, Harmondsworth.

Rose, G. and Barker D. J. P. (1980) *Epidemiology for the Uninitiated*. British Medical Association, London.

Rack, P. (1982) *Race Culture and Mental Disorder*. Tavistock, London.

22

Psychosomatic Relationships

Definitions

The term psychosomatic has two main usages:

1 It is applied to an approach to illness in general, in which the physician pays due attention to psychological and social as well as physical factors. Used in this sense the term is applicable to all illnesses.
2 It is also applied to denote a group of disorders in which emotional factors have a demonstrable role in aetiology. These are disorders manifesting a physical lesion in which emotional and physical factors may have a causative role.

Characteristics

A list of these disorders is given in Table 22.1. They have certain features in common.

1 Emotions precipitate attacks of the illness; this may be demonstrable by clinical observation or reproduced under experimental conditions. Emotional changes may increase the severity of an attack, if already present, or prolong its duration.
2 A correlation is observable between the occurrence of stressful life experiences and the onset of these disorders, or with recurrence of attacks during the course of the illness.
3 They exhibit a differential sex incidence. For example asthma before puberty is twice as common in boys as in girls, whereas after puberty it is more common in women than in men. Chronic urticaria and thyrotoxicosis are more common in women; peptic ulcer, coronary thrombosis and arterial hypertension more common in men.

Table 22.1   Some common psychosomatic disorders

1 *Respiratory Disorders*
  (a) Asthma
  (b) Vasomotor rhinitis
  (c) Hay fever
2 *Gastro-intestinal Disorders*
  (a) Peptic ulcer
  (b) Colonic disorders
3 *Skin Disorders*
4 *Disorders of Muscles and Joints*
  (a) Rheumatoid arthritis
  (b) 'Fibrositis'
5 *Endocrine Disorders*
  (a) Hyperthyroidism
  (b) Diabetes mellitus
6 *Cardiovascular System*
  (a) Essential hypertension
  (b) Coronary disease
  (c) Cerebrovascular disease
  (d) Migraine
7 *Disorders associated with Menstrual and Reproductive Functions*
  (a) Amenorrhoea and oligomenorrhoea
  (b) Dysmenorrhoea
  (c) Menorrhagia
  (d) Premenstrual tension
  (e) Menopausal disturbances

4 Psychosomatic disorders often run a phasic course.
5 Most of the disorders fulfilling the above criteria show evidence of a genetic and constitutional predisposition. Not infrequently other members of the family suffer from the same or allied conditions.

Respiratory Disorders

Asthma

Asthma is characterized by recurrent attacks of dyspnoea, with difficulty and prolongation of the expiratory phase and accompanied by wheezing and, usually, with intervening periods of freedom.

The mechanism underlying an attack is a narrowing of the lumen of the smaller bronchi, arising either from constriction of the circular muscle of the bronchus and/or swelling of the bronchial mucosa. An additional factor in some patients is increased muscular tension of the muscles of the larynx and chest wall, which can also influence the degree of dyspnoea.

Studies of a random sample of asthmatic patients of all ages reveal a multiplicity of causal factors, the three most important being:

1 Infections, particularly of the upper and lower respiratory tract.
2 Allergic factors. In asthma the allergens commonly found are house dust, pollen and sometimes ingestants and injectants.
   A convenient method of investigating the role of suspected allergens is to measure the patient's respiratory movements with a spirometer and to introduce the allergen by means of an aerosol. If ventilation is reduced by more than 10%, it is diagnostic of an attack of asthma.
3 Psychological factors. Emotional tension is the most important of the various psychological factors. It may be of any form—anxiety, indignation, resentment, humiliation, grief, joy, laughter and even pleasurable anticipation of going out on a desired social occasion.

Vasomotor Rhinitis

Vasomotor rhinitis is characterized by paroxysmal attacks of rhinorrhoea with sneezing and nasal blockage. During the attack there is profuse secretion of the glands of the nasal mucosa and an increase in the thickness and vascularity of the mucous membrane.

As with asthma, the three most important factors are allergens, infections and emotional factors and multiplicity is the rule.

Hay Fever

Hay fever is an allergic disorder par excellence. It is, by definition, an allergic reaction to pollen by the nasal mucous membrane, conjunctivae and mucous membranes of the pharynx and upper respiratory tract. It is seasonal and the attacks are closely correlated with the amount of circulating pollen.

Allergy and Emotions

Under experimental conditions, subjects have been investigated in a specially prepared room in which a constant amount of pollen was circulated by means of a fan and the nasal mucosal reactions were recorded by objective methods including vascularity, thickness and amount of secretion. It was found that the reaction to a given amount of pollen was greater if the patients were in an emotionally tense state or if they had a preceding infection.

Similar observations have been demonstrated in asthma, when a known allergen was introduced by an aerosol and the reactions measured by a spirograph.

The reaction to a given amount of allergen is much greater when the patient is tense than when he is relaxed.

This summation of effects between emotions and allergy was noted a long time ago by the famous French physician Trousseau, who was an asthmatic sufferer. One day he caught his coachman stealing oats from his stable; Trousseau was very angry and wanted to tell him off but was unable to do so because he was seized with the most severe attack of asthma that he had experienced and, when describing it later, he realized that it must have been a combination of his anger plus the dust in the stable which had caused such a severe attack because, previously, he had been exposed to similar quantities of dust in the stable and in the streets of Paris without getting such a severe attack.

Interrelationships also exist between emotions and the development of infections and it has been demonstrated experimentally that emotional tension can produce swelling, hypersecretion and hyperaemia of the nasal mucosa.

Prolonged action of emotional factors results in a boggy, swollen state of the nasal mucosa, with impairment of ciliary activity and lymphatic

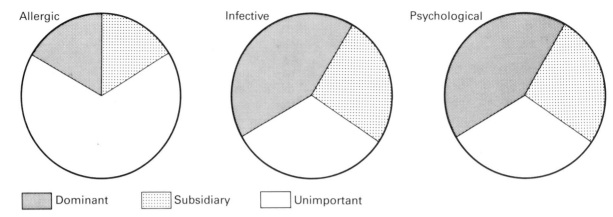

Figure 22.1   *Aetiological factors in asthma.*

stasis. These changes are conducive to the development of a super-imposed infection.

Sometimes patients will develop attacks of asthma due to the combined effect of infections with emotional stress. One patient, a girl aged 10, who had suffered repeated attacks of bronchitis for many years without any wheezing or asthmatic attacks, developed her first attacks of asthma when she was suffering from bronchitis and a burglar broke into the house, causing her alarm and fright.

Thus allergy, infections and emotions can interact in various ways, creating vicious circle effects which can result in a continuous disease process.

The Role of Suggestion and Conditioning

Many published accounts of asthma tend to describe the role of suggestion as being one of the most important of the psychological factors operating in asthma.

Suggestion very often can have potent effects; it can both relieve attacks and precipitate attacks. Similarly, various stimuli associated with allergic precipitation of asthmatic attacks may subsequently produce asthmatic attacks themselves, even without the allergen.

For example, people who were sensitive to pollen have been known to visit an art gallery and when they saw a painting of a cornfield they had an immediate attack of hay fever or hay asthma.

Other patients, sensitive to dust, have been known to develop an attack of asthma when watching a cowboy picture in which a stampede of buffaloes produced a dust storm. Others sensitive to

flowers have gone into a room and had an attack of asthma, only to discover later that what they had seen were artificial flowers.

Suggestion may sometimes relieve attacks. There is the well known example of a physician who suffered from asthma and who went to stay in a remote hotel in the countryside one weekend. He woke up in the middle of the night with a severe attack of asthma; he groped for the electric light switch but was unable to find it and, in desperation, caught hold of his shoe, felt for the window and, on feeling glass, smashed it. He breathed in deeply, the attack passed off and he had a peaceful night, but he was horrified to find in the morning when he woke that he had broken the mirror instead of the window.

There are now many authenticated cases of asthma developing as a conditioned response to stimuli originally associated with direct precipitants of asthmatic attacks, such as allergens.

Pathogenetic Mechanisms

The neural mechanisms mediating the effect of emotional tension in precipitating attacks of asthma, vasomotor rhinitis or aggravating hay fever are parasympathetic pathways.

Parasympathetic over-activity produces all the local changes which form the pathophysiological basis of the attacks. For example, a stellate ganglion block on one side will produce swelling, hyperaemia and increased nasal secretion on the same side. Interruptions of the parasympathetic nerve supply on one side will stop the manifestations.

Gastro-intestinal Disorders

Peptic Ulcer

Clinical observations for many years have shown that peptic ulcer symptoms may be precipitated or exacerbated by emotional changes in the patient or by the experience of various stressful conditions.

The first reports of direct correlations between the reactions of the stomach and emotional changes were made by Beaumont on his celebrated patient Alexis St. Martin, who had a gastric fistula resulting from an old gunshot wound. Beaumont described the course of digestion of various articles of diet under different conditions and various emotional states.

More recently, work of outstanding importance was carried out by Wolf and Wolff, who carried out a study of gastric functioning on a gentleman called Tom, who is now famous throughout the world. He had a gastric fistula which enabled Drs Wolf and Wolff to carry out observations and investigations on the functioning of the gastric mucosa of the stomach under various conditions. On one occasion, as part of a planned experiment, Tom was in a roundabout way accused of overcharging for some work he had carried out for his employers; he resented this accusation greatly but, being an employee, was unable to express his resentment outwardly to those responsible and went around in a state of bottled up indignation and resentment. During this emotional state it was observed that the gastric mucosa became redder due to greater engorgement with blood and that gastric juice was produced in higher volume and of greater acidity. The gastric mucosa in this state when touched with a glass rod was found to be very friable and bled easily.

These changes are precisely those which are conducive to the development of chronic peptic ulceration. Thus, emotion can produce changes in the function of the stomach which are conducive to the formation of peptic ulcers. The increased friability of the mucosa is conducive to the development of acute ulcers or abrasions from mechanical stimuli. Gastric juice produced in greater volume and acidity prevents such ulcers from healing, tending to make them chronic.

Emotional factors are not the only ones concerned in the genesis of peptic ulceration. For example,

recent work by Mirski showed that the level of pepsinogen excretion was much higher in patients with peptic ulcer. It was found that the level of blood pepsinogen tended to remain relatively constant and was determined early in life and may be predominantly genetically determined.

In a study of many thousands of individuals called up for the United States Army, it was found that ulcers tended to develop in persons with a sustained high rate of gastric secretion, as indicated by the level of serum pepsinogen together with the presence of certain conflicts, personality difficulties or environmental circumstances which evoke emotional reactions which, in turn, affect autonomic, neuro-endocrine mechanisms.

The Large Intestine

Certain disorders of the large intestine, such as irritable and spastic colon, have been shown to be largely determined by psychogenic factors. Direct observations on the functioning of the large intestine in patients with colostomy or caecostomy have demonstrated the marked changes which occur in vascularity and lysozyme secretion during certain emotional states.

One series of experiments showed that certain emotional states increased motility in the bowel, increased vascularity and increased the production of the enzyme lysozyme, which has been suggested by some workers as a possible factor for causing ulcerative colitis. Lysozyme, by depriving the colonic mucosa of its protective layer of mucus, makes it more vulnerable to other noxic agents, including infective and mechanical factors. Others have suggested that prolonged spasms of the muscles of the colon, resulting from emotional tension, produces an ischaemia of the colonic mucosa and that on relaxation of the muscular tension, a necrosis of the epithelium results in bleeding.

Other theories are that the liquid contents of the small intestine are carried into the colon as a consequence of emotionally induced hypermotility of the small bowel, that the enzymes of this liquid have a greater digestive action than normally and that anything which lowers the natural protective powers of the colonic mucosa could lead to digestion of its surface, permitting bacterial invasion and ulceration.

Although the evidence is very clear that

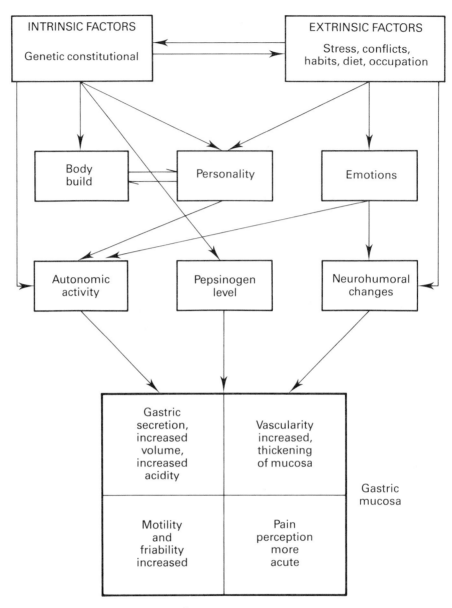

Figure 22.2   *Factors involved in the development of a peptic ulcer.*

emotional factors can aggravate ulcerative colitis, the relationship between emotional and other aetiological factors has not been fully elucidated. The aetiology of the condition remains obscure and infective, allergic, nutritional and psychological factors have all been implicated.

It is, however, clear that anything which can relieve the patient's emotional distress would be of potential therapeutic value in the management of ulcerative colitis. Some physicians have reported in the early stages that group psychotherapy has apparently been beneficial but in many instances, particularly when the disease has been present for a long time, tissue changes may occur to such an extent that they become irreversible and psychotherapeutic measures then can have little effect.

Anorexia Nervosa (see also p. 65)

Anorexia nervosa is a disorder which is almost confined to young women; it occasionally occurs in older women and, exceptionally, in men.

The term anorexia is a misnomer. At first there is usually a deliberate restriction of eating; the patient takes minimal quantities usually of the most slimming foods and will secretly dispose of food or vomit it afterwards or hide it in various places.

Anorexia nervosa often does not come to medical attention until the patient has lost 12 kg or more in weight.

With the decrease in food intake anorexia will occur but at times the patients often have ravenous appetites and occasionally will gorge large amounts of food, then feel very guilty and either vomit what they have eaten or take a great deal of exercise to work it off.

Progressive loss of weight makes the patients emaciated and some look like victims of Belsen. They however remain characteristically active and energetic. Sometimes a growth of fine, downy hair appears over the body which is similar to that found in other types of intense starvation. Amenorrhoea is characteristic and the basal metabolic rate is low.

The onset of the disorder is usually associated with some emotional conflict, the most common being conflicts about accepting the female role or, during the engagement period, if the patient has conflicts about accepting the responsibilities of marriage. Other conflicts relate to the parents, particularly the mother. Often the restriction in diet starts because the girl regards herself as too fat and may have been teased about her weight. More rarely the condition starts in a setting of depressive illness.

Differential diagnosis

The condition superficially resembles Sheehan's syndrome but, in practice, the differential diagnosis between the two conditions is not difficult. The loss of weight in Sheehan's syndrome is not marked. Sheehan's syndrome usually comes on after childbirth. In anorexia nervosa, the 17-ketosteroid excretion will not be decreased to a level 2–3 mg per 24 hours. Similarly, the marked insulin sensitivity found in Sheehan's syndrome is not found in anorexia nervosa.

Treatment

Admission to hospital is essential, with one nurse assuming responsibility for the patient's supervision who should personally assist at every meal and, by persuasion, encourage the patient to eat.

With skilled nursing, weight can be gained with ordinary food but sometimes highly concentrated foods in small bulk are helpful in recovering lost weight.

Chlorpromazine is a useful drug for relieving tension and facilitating regain in weight. Recently, amitriptyline has been even more helpful.

When weight has been regained, psychological investigation and treatment may be necessary and may be indispensable in order to achieve lasting recovery. In some patients, whose motives for losing weight were mainly for appearance's sake and who have no deeper conflicts, psychotherapy may not be necessary.

The first essential step in treatment is the regain of lost weight and then the need for psychotherapy will have to be assessed in each individual on the merits of each case.

In practice, one cannot be satisfied that recovery has occurred until the menstrual periods return.

Without treatment, or after unsuccessful treatment, the patient's condition may become extremely serious and death can occur due to inanition or intercurrent infection, such as pneumonia or tuberculosis.

Skin Disorders

It is everyday knowledge and observation that emotional factors affect the skin, as shown by the blushing of embarrassment, the pallor of fear and the pallor or redness of rage, depending on the subject and his emotional state. Experiments have demonstrated that emotional states can affect the following, which are of direct relevance in the aetiology of certain skin disorders:

1 Control of vascularity of the skin
2 Control of sebaceous gland secretion
3 Control of sweat
4 Influencing of the degree of exudation
5 Influencing of the tendency to pruritus

In urticaria, for example, it has been demonstrated that acetyl choline and histamine are involved in the production of the characteristic wheals and constitute the final common pathway for a large number of causative agents such as physical stimuli, infections, allergic reactions, emotional factors and certain changes in the internal environment. Emotional tension, by increasing vascularity, exudation and itching, can exacerbate the majority of skin disorders. The itching mechanism is of particular importance, as pruritus tends to lead to scratching which in turn stimulates the itching mechanism in the skin further, thus creating a vicious circle.

In skin disorders emotional factors are only one of many causative factors. Constitutional predisposition, allergy, mechanical factors, dietetic, hormonal and many others can all play a part in determining the onset and course of these illnesses.

Disorders of Muscles and Joints

Fibrositis and muscular rheumatism are rather vague diagnostic labels which probably cover a variety of conditions. They are characterized by a dull aching and stiffness which is worse in the mornings and tends to wear off during the day. Sharp twinges of pain are brought on by sudden movements or by pressure on particular spots.

Undoubtedly a proportion of these symptoms are mainly psychogenically determined. They are often local manifestations of tension in a strained, tense, anxious individual. They may also occur in depressive states, whereas some pains are hysterical. In pains due to localized increased muscular tension, it is possible to demonstrate this objectively by measuring action potentials in these muscles.

Rheumatoid Arthritis

Whether rheumatoid arthritis should be regarded as a psychosomatic disorder is still controversial. Selye has shown that arthritis can occur as a result of an imbalance between the mineralocorticoids and the glucocorticoids. It is possible that rheumatoid arthritis may develop as a result of prolonged stress leading to the changes of the general adaptation syndrome with an imbalance of the various fractions of adrenal corticoids as described by Selye.

The role of emotional factors, is, however, obscure and further research is necessary in order that they may be elucidated.

Endocrine Disorders

Hyperthyroidism

In patients suffering from hyperthyroidism, psychosomatic and somatopsychic effects are often intermingled. Although some patients have been emotionally disturbed before developing hyperthyroidism, once the thyroid becomes over-active the patient's emotional instability is increased and anxiety symptoms, tension and various bodily manifestations similar to those of anxiety are very frequent. These effects of hyperthyroidism often lead to increased interpersonal tensions and problems, thereby increasing the patient's emotional difficulties and again worsening the condition.

For very many years physicians have reported the development of thyrotoxicosis following emotional upsets, stresses and shocks of various kinds. A variety of psychosocial stresses may be associated with the onset of thyrotoxicosis, e.g. bereavement, financial, domestic, marital problems and crises, traumatic experiences etc.

Although there is strong evidence that psychosocial stresses and emotional disturbances can exert a precipitating action at the onset of thyrotoxicosis, this does not necessarily mean that the concatenation of processes occurring in thyrotoxicosis can be reversed by psychotherapeutic measures. The immediate need in treatment is to diminish thyroid over-activity by medical or surgical means. It has often been found that patients who have been so treated and now have their thyroids functioning normally, still suffer from a large variety of emotional, autonomic symptoms and still have considerable disability. Psychotherapy at this stage can, of course, be valuable.

Diabetes Mellitus

Physicians supervising the treatment of diabetics by insulin, drugs, diet, etc. have observed that the metabolic balance in the patient can be readily upset by emotional disturbances. Possible mechanisms involved are:

1 The autonomic nervous system, through the sympathetic, which is mediated by adrenalin which increases the level of blood sugar, or the parasympathetic through the vagus nerve, stimulating

the production of insulin which lowers blood sugar.

2 Neuro-endocrine mechanisms, particularly the adrenal cortex. Many of the hormones of the adrenal cortex are concerned with carbohydrate metabolism.

3 The effects of diuresis provoked by stressful anxiety, which can occur in normal as well as diabetic subjects. In diabetic subjects the diuresis can lead to marked loss of sugar, ketones and chlorides, accompanied by a marked decrease in fixed base and in glycogen storage. These effects can lead to acidosis, particularly when the anxious patient neglects his dietetic regime or other treatment, as he often does.

Cardiovascular System

Essential Hypertension

High blood pressure when not due to arterial disease or kidney disease or to other physical causes is known as essential hypertension.

In some cases it can be demonstrated that emotional factors can play an important role. Clinical and experimental observations demonstrate the effect of emotions on blood pressure. Every physician knows that the first blood pressure reading is usually much higher than subsequent ones because of the patient's state of apprehension initially. States of bottled up anxiety, tension, aggression, hostility, resentment and many others can result in a sustained rise of blood pressure.

The mechanisms responsible include:

1 Stimulation of the sympathetic division of the autonomic nervous system.

2 Prolonged emotional tension evoking manifestations of the General Adaptation Syndrome (GAS) which, in certain circumstances, results in disorders such as arteriosclerosis, hypertension and thrombosis of the coronary and cerebral vessels.

3 Noradrenaline release from the adrenal medulla by emotions and stress.

4 All the above mechanisms can produce constriction of the arterioles of the kidney giving rise to ischaemia and release of a chemical substance which is now believed to play an important role in the development of hypertension.

Cerebrovascular Accidents

Cerebral haemorrhage and cerebral thrombosis are determined by multiple factors, one of which can be emotional tension arising in response to difficulties, conflicts or stresses.

The interrelationships between psychosomatic and somatopsychic processes can be seen clearly in the development of stroke and associated disabilities (see Fig. 22.3).

Coronary Disease

Coronary thrombosis and angina pectoris are disorders of great medical and social importance because of the frequency with which they cause suffering, disability and death. The role of emotional factors in the development of coronary disease is still rather controversial. Other factors such as the amount and type of fat in the diet, the level of blood cholesterol, the amount of exercise engaged in by the individual and the degree of atheroma of the arteries have been implicated.

Many authors have reported that the onset of coronary heart disease is not infrequently preceded by severe strain associated with occupational, domestic or financial anxiety, by depression or fatigue. Studies in which a group of persons were observed working under great intellectual pressure revealed a rise in serum cholesterol with decrease in the clotting time of whole blood. During times of rest and relaxation the clotting time was normal and serum cholesterol was lower. These changes were independent of individual variations in weight, diet and physical activity.

An increase in serum cholesterol has also been found to accompany the mental and emotional stress of examinations.

Disorders Associated with Menstrual and Reproductive Functions

Amenorrhoea and Oligomenorrhoea

Emotional disturbance may cause scanty menstruation (oligomenorrhoea) or may cause complete amenorrhoea for months or years.

The emotional factors are varied and arise from a variety of psychological stresses such as illness, injury or the death of a loved person; a frightening

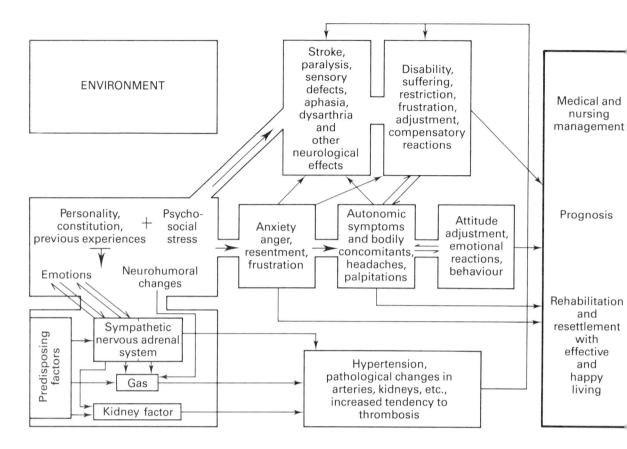

Figure 22.3   *The interaction of psychogenic factors in stroke.*

experience, accidents, radical change of environment or occupation, fears of pregnancy after intercourse in unmarried persons, as a manifestation of depressive states or as a result of addiction to morphine or heroin.

Amenorrhoea can occur in an interesting disorder known as **pseudocyesis** or false pregnancy which is not uncommon in animals and which can occur in young women and at all ages, including women approaching the menopause. The disorder provides a striking illustration of the powerful action of psychological factors on female behaviour and endocrine function.

Pseudocyesis in women is characterized by a cessation of menstruation accompanied by nausea, vomiting, enlargement and sometimes pigmentation of the breasts. The patient reports quickening and has swelling of the abdomen and may have simulated labour pains.

Underlying the disorder there is often a wish for pregnancy, sometimes linked with a desire to please the husband or to retain his attention and affection. Sometimes the wish for pregnancy is motivated to prove youthfulness or health and, more rarely, it occurs in unmarried women as an attempt to force marriage.

The diagnosis is made by repeated negative pregnancy tests, absence of an abdominal tumour on examination of the abdomen, disappearance of the abdominal swelling under anaesthesia and a normal size uterus on bimanual examination.

Functional Dysmenorrhoea

Primary functional dysmenorrhoea starts with menarche and secondary functional dysmenorrhoea develops after the establishment of normal menstruation.

A number of factors are usually involved, e.g. a lowered pain threshold, emotional tension, intolerance of discomfort or pain. Other possible factors are the greater intensity of muscular uterine contractions due to hormonal or other causes during menstruation.

Menorrhagia, in some cases, may be determined by stress and emotional tension.

Pregnancy and Childbirth

During early pregnancy, if there is conflict or doubt about having a baby or if it is definitely unwanted, a reactive depression or an anxiety state may precipitate attempts at suicide or self-induced abortion.

There is little evidence that the incidence of psychiatric disorders, apart from those reactive to the pregnancy, is significantly greater than what would be expected by chance.

Post-partum reactions, however, are not uncommon and some are very severe. Post-partum psychiatric illnesses must not be confused with the 'maternity blues' which is very common and occurs usually within the first week after delivery. It consists of transitory depression and tearfulness lasting a few days only. This occurs in about a third of normal women and does not cause any significant disability.

There is a group of women who get depression following childbirth which continues for weeks or months but is of mild degree and does not necessarily come to medical attention or necessitate treatment.

Surveys carried out on all deliveries in the general population show that the incidence of severe post-partum psychiatric illness is about 1 per 1000 deliveries. In Bristol, a survey revealed an incidence of 1.7 per 1000 deliveries. 1 per 1000 were sufficiently ill to require admission to a mental hospital.

Most post-partum illnesses start within 6 weeks of birth and the large majority appear before the end of the third week after birth, the peak incidence being between 7–20 days after birth. There is usually a latent period during which the patient may appear normal. A smaller number of patients develop their symptoms within the first few days after birth.

The most common types of post-partum psychiatric illness are depressive states, schizo-affective states, schizophrenia and, only rarely nowadays, a toxic confusional state.

Even patients who eventually turn out to be suffering from schizophrenia may initially show symptoms and signs of depression and it is only after two or three weeks' observation that the underlying schizophrenia becomes more clearly manifest.

The Registrar General has shown that post-partum patients constitute about 1% of all female admissions of all ages to mental hospitals, and that post-partum patients tend to stay in hospital 4–6 months as against an average length of stay of 2.2 months for all admissions.

In general, post-partum psychiatric illnesses do well, recovering either spontaneously or with treatment with electroconvulsive therapy in the case of depressions and schizo-affective disorders. In the schizophrenic illnesses, combined therapy by phenothiazines and ECT gives good results. Some regrettably remain ill for years and prove resistant to all forms of treatment.

The author has observed a subgroup of patients suffering from post-partum psychiatric illnesses who, having recovered completely from their post-partum psychiatric illness, subsequently, when the periods become re-established, develop a premenstrual recurrence of their post-partum psychiatric symptoms similar qualitatively but quantitatively less marked. In post-partum schizophrenic patients, for example, the same delusions may reappear but are less marked and less disturbing. They appear about 7–10 days before the menses and usually clear up at the onset of the period, the patient remaining free from psychiatric manifestations until the next period. This premenstrual recurrence following a post-partum psychiatric illness in many cases spontaneously clears up during the course of a year or so or responds to progestogen therapy.

Follow up studies have shown that the chances of a further post-partum illness with subsequent births are of the order 1 in 5 to 1 in 7.

Treatment of post-partum psychiatric disorders

The treatment of these disorders will depend on the the type of illness and its degree of severity.

Depressive illnesses will respond to antidepressant drugs but, if severe, electroconvulsive therapy will be needed.

Schizophrenic illnesses will require phenothiazine drugs, with or without electroconvulsive therapy.

Large doses of progestogens have been tried but the results have been, on the whole, disappointing.

For premenstrual recurrence of post-partum illnesses, the treatment is that for premenstrual tension syndromes.

Premenstrual Tension

Premenstrual tension is a syndrome occurring during the second half of a menstrual cycle and consisting of a number of mental and physical symptoms. The syndrome is composed of feelings of anxiety, tension and irritability, with one or more of the following symptoms: depression, bloated abdominal feelings, swelling of the subcutaneous tissues, nausea, fatigue, painful swelling of the breasts, headaches, dizziness and palpitations. Less frequently there may be increased sex desire, excessive thirst, increased appetite and hypersomnia.

The symptoms usually start about seven to fourteen days before menstruation and pass off soon after the onset of the period, although some patients continue to have symptoms throughout the period.

The aetiology of the condition is still obscure. The most generally accepted view is that it is due to the unantagonized action of oestrogens resulting from faulty luteinization. Oestrogens produce many of the manifestations of the premenstrual syndrome and oestrogens given to ovariectomized women or after the menopause will produce similar symptoms.

The syndrome is somatopsychic rather than psychosomatic but there is a complex interplay between psychological factors and physical factors. It is interesting to note that, in many women, their conflict and problems become manifest during the premenstrual phase and at other times of the cycle may not significantly affect them.

The syndrome can occur in normal, stable women but when it coexists with neurosis, it is more severe the more neurotic the woman.

Treatment

Dehydration therapy consisting of restricting salt and water and giving diuretics produces some relief particularly in physical comfort, but does not help emotional symptoms significantly. Treatment by progesterone injections or orally active progestogens gives the best results.

Menopausal Disturbances

It is well known that in many women the menopause is associated with a variety of nervous symptoms and manifestations of emotional instability. Increased nervousness, irritability, depression, hyperaesthesias, paraesthesia, vertigo and many other symptoms associated with a lowered threshold to nervous stimuli results in an increase in emotional tension and organ response. The autonomic nervous system is more labile, particularly the vascular apparatus, giving rise to hot flushes, night sweats, chills, fainting, palpitations and cardiac arrhythmias.

The most striking feature is the hot flush. The woman suddenly experiences a sensation of heat, more or less violent, which sweeps like a wave over her body to her head. This may come on spontaneously or may be provoked by emotional upsets. Along with the subjective sensation of heat there is an intense flushing of the face. Following this there is a feeling of depression accompanied by pallor and profuse sweating, especially on the head, sometimes so copious that sweat drops from the skin. Finally, there may be cold or shivering sensations.

The syndrome, therefore, is a rushing of warm blood to the skin, particularly face and neck and the upper part of the body i.e. the areas which are particularly concerned with controlling heat loss by the body.

A number of factors will precipitate the attacks. Flushes will be aggravated by physical effort, by eating or drinking warm foods or beverages, by intense emotions, by excitement, by a warm environment, too many bedclothes at night or heavy clothes in the day. All of these factors are ones which give rise to excessive heat production or retention. It is believed that the hot flush is hypothalamic in origin and represents a disturbance of the heat regulating mechanism.

Somatopsychic Sequences

We have considered the role of emotional changes and stress in the production of lesions and dysfunctions in psychosomatic disorders where the sequence is a psychosomatic sequence.

We now need to consider the effect of an illness, disorder or disability on the person's reactions, i.e. somatopsychic sequence.

Even in those psychosomatic disorders which have important psychogenic factors, with emotions or stress having a demonstrably contributory role in their aetiology, somatopsychic sequences may also be important. This is well exemplified in the case of stroke due to a cerebrovascular accident (see Fig. 22.3).

A patient's reactions and the consequent psychological burden he has to carry with regard to a stroke derives from three main sources:

1 The symptoms, i.e. the sudden onset of paralysis, sometimes aphasia, dysarthria and sensory defects is naturally a frightening, perplexing and frustrating experience.
2 The threat inherent in the diagnosis of the underlying cause of the stroke, e.g. high blood pressure and/or arteriosclerosis.
3 The strain imposed by the limitations due to his physical disability resulting from the stroke and which evoke increased anxiety, depression, anger or frustration.

Such reactions are important as they evoke emotional changes which by different mechanisms can, by a psychosomatic sequence, worsen the disorder. For example:

1 Stimulation of the sympathetic nervous system, by increasing heart rate and causing arterial vasoconstriction, causes an increase in blood pressure.
2 Prolonged states of emotional tension evoke the General Adaptation Syndrome and, under certain conditions, the adaptive mechanisms of the syndrome fail which may result in arteriosclerosis, hypertension and thrombosis.
3 The mechanisms described under (1) may result in a decrease in the blood supply to the kidney, releasing a chemical factor now known to play an important role in the development of arterial hypertension.
4 Emotional tension and stresses are known to increase coagulability of the blood and, therefore, increase the tendency to cerebral thrombosis.

The psychosomatic and somatopsychic mechanisms involved in a stroke are shown in Figure 22.3.

Reactions to Onset of Symptoms and Diagnosis

The patient's reactions will depend partly on his personality make-up and partly on the suddenness or unexpectedness of the development of symptoms and, also, the threat to security which may be caused by the onset of an illness and by knowledge of the diagnosis.

Anxiety is the most frequent reaction. Anxiety arises because the illness threatens the patient's bodily safety and security. The illness incapacitates him temporarily or for a long period from his usual work; this may lead to financial worries.

Some patients react to illness by becoming apathetic with loss of interest; this may sometimes cover an underlying anxiety.

Some patients will resent the enforced dependency due to an illness and they particularly resent being in a position of being looked after by other people and may react to this by becoming tense, anxious, irritable or even aggressive, truculent and generally awkward.

To other people, illness and bed rest satisfy their dependency needs and they almost welcome the opportunity of being dependent.

Thus, the reaction to a diagnosis, to disability and to enforced dependency may evoke in some people anxiety, in others hostility and in others an increase in dependency needs, in some a non-acceptance and non-recognition of the diagnosis or the illness.

Undesirable forms of reaction to a disability may take the form of:

1 Rebellious, aggressive attitudes and unwillingness to conform to medical regimes and treatment. This attitude impairs the chances of successful rehabilitation and its emotional effects may aggravate the disorder or, at least, the degree of disability associated with it.
2 The patient may react by becoming vindictive, spiteful and tending to belittle other people in order to elevate himself or he may succumb to the disability, using it as an excuse for avoiding responsibility or possible failure.

In general, patients when they come into hospital are anxious and frightened about three things. First of all what is wrong with them, secondly, what is going to be the outcome of the illness and thirdly, what residual effects are likely to occur after the illness or following the operation.

Patients sometimes give the impression that they do not want to know anything about the illness and that they are happy to remain ignorant; but this is only applicable to a small number of patients and the majority, and sometimes even those who pretend they do not want to, in fact wish to know something about the illness. They want to know how long they are going to be in hospital, because they have to make necessary arrangements, and they want to know what implication the illness has for the present and for the future.

Communication with doctors and nurses is an important need to alleviate patients of these anxieties. It is important for a patient to be treated as an individual, as a person; one should remember his name and one should take him into one's confidence with regard to the various procedures, diagnostic or therapeutic, which are going to be carried out to help him.

If the patient can express his various fears this in itself is often a great relief. So the nurse or doctor should listen and give whatever comfort possible to the patient.

Principles in Treatment and Management of Psychosomatic Disorders

The first step is the thorough investigation of each patient to assess the relative importance of various physical as well as emotional factors.

In asthma, for example, infections and allergy and other factors may play a dominant or subsidiary role to psychogenic factors. Teamwork is important and every method of treatment to deal with as many factors as possible is the correct approach.

In some patients emotional factors may be playing a very important part and special consideration has to be given to how these can be helped.

It is necessary to study each patient to assess which personality attributes are conducive to the development of states of tension which may precipitate attacks of the psychosomatic disorder under consideration. The next step is to ascertain the setting in which the attacks occur and the third step is to help the patient to understand how the relationship between his personality disposition, his

life situation, his conflicts and emotional problems makes him react in the way he does and predisposes to the arousal of an emotional state which leads to an attack of his disorder.

Patients suffering from psychosomatic disorders are not necessarily unstable or neurotic in the usual sense and frequently are well adjusted, successful persons. However, certain personality characteristics which are common in psychosomatic disorders tend to lead to emotional states which, in turn, can produce the various manifestations.

Psychosomatic patients are often tense, anxious, self-driving persons who are rigid, ambitious, perfectionistic, always highly competitive in their outlook, always trying to do better than their fellows. They are usually reliable, conscientious persons so responsibilities and duties are thrust on them and characteristically they may have great difficulty in delegating responsibility.

Such patients readily become resentful when they cannot keep up to their own expectations or what others expect of them. The inevitable outcome is the development of tension, fatigue and exhaustion.

Psychotherapeutic Management

The interview is the medium whereby the patient, with the help of the physician, gains an understanding of the factors and situations which provoke attacks of the psychosomatic disorder the patient suffers from.

Attacks may be precipitated by sudden traumatic experiences or may be the result of a gradual build-up of tension due to everyday problems and difficulties, determined largely by the patient's attitudes and personality make-up.

The direct relationship between attacks and stressful experiences is important but it is also necessary to realize that some disorders such as migraine, urticaria and asthma may occur during the 24–48 hours immediately following a stressful period.

The patient needs to be advised to modify his attitudes; he must avoid becoming extremely perfectionistic and avoid imposing on himself expectations to get greater amounts of work done in a given time. He should aim at getting three-quarters of the work that he usually attempts done in a given period of time. He has to learn to delegate responsibilities and to have adequate periods of rest and recreation. He should be encouraged to deal with each day as it comes, rather than to anticipate problems and meet them half-way. He will need frequent and strong reassurance and it will probably be some time before he realizes that greater spontaneity, productivity and effectiveness will come with less anxiety and tension.

In the case of children with asthma or other psychosomatic disorders, the best way of helping the child is usually to devote one's main attention to the parents, particularly if they exhibit over-anxious, over-protective, perfectionistic or rejecting attitudes.

The best way to get the parents' co-operation is not to condemn them or pass judgment but to try to get them to discuss their problems freely, with the interviewer adopting an accepting, listening attitude. This often results in their spontaneous realization of the effect of their attitudes on the child's well-being and attacks of asthma.

The over-anxious parent can be turned to the advantage of the child because often the mother is quite willing to learn how to manage the child more satisfactorily. By letting the parents speak, express their feelings regarding the child—sometimes aggressive feelings, sometimes anxiety or fear—they increasingly come to realize the effect that their attitudes have and therefore to realize their importance, and this may help to achieve a modification in attitude and upbringing.

Improvements in the child, when such attitudes can be improved, are sometimes quite dramatic.

Consultation and Liaison Psychiatry

During recent years considerable advances have occurred in the utilization of psychiatric knowledge and expertise in the management of medical and surgical patients.

Consultation psychiatry is the provision of expert advice for the diagnostic assessment and management of a patient's mental state and behaviour at the request of a non-psychiatric physician or surgeon. Liaison psychiatry refers to the association and cooperation of groups for the effective delivery of relevant aspects of psychiatric care to the medically or surgically ill.

Consultation and liaison psychiatry serve the comprehensive diagnostic assessment of the medically or surgically ill patient, contribute to man-

agement treatment and after-care, and also serve the purpose of instruction and research.

In the field of operative surgery, the patient is usually assessed to discover whether there are any psychiatric contraindications to the proposed surgical intervention, e.g. in plastic surgery and other non-urgent surgical conditions. Services are also required for the care of those who develop emotional or psychiatric disorders post-operatively.

The best results are achieved with a good therapeutic relationship, established pre-operatively and continued into the post-operative phase. A psychiatrist will then be able to deal not only with minor emotional difficulties, but also more effectively help in the more severe post-operative disorder, whether it is schizophrenia, depression or delirium.

The possible psychological impact of the dialysis situation and of the psychiatric syndromes which may develop as a consequence are well recognized. The patient's reactions will be influenced not only by emotional and stress factors, but also physical factors and medication as well. The psychological reactions of the caring team must not be overlooked because they undergo a great deal of stress which is inherent in the total situation of haemodialysis.

Patients receiving renal transplants have been found to run a risk of developing post-operative psychiatric problems, mainly depression and anxiety, but some develop organic brain syndromes in which the use of steroids play an important part, which is further aggravated by emotional and stressful factors.

In cardiac surgery, post-operative delirium is usually multifactorial, but supportive therapy from a psychiatrist and his team before and after the operation have been valuable. Similarly, the psychiatrist working as a member of a multidisciplinary team is becoming more common in various departments of medicine, surgery and paediatrics, e.g. pain clinics, orthopaedic departments, gastroenterology, respiratory medicine, rheumatology and endocrinology. In fact it could be said that consultation and liaison psychiatry would be appropriate in any medical or surgical department when requested by the physician or surgeon, and where a good working collaboration exists.

Further Reading

Hamilton, M. (1955) *Psychosomatics.* Chapman and Hall, London.

Engel, G. L. (1963) *Psychological Development of Health and Disease.* W. B. Saunders, Philadelphia.

Rachman, S. and Philips, C. (1975) *Psychology and Medicine.* Temple Smith/Penguin, London.

Hill, O. W. (1976) *Modern Trends in Psychosomatic Medicine 3.* Butterworths, Sevenoaks.

Lipowski, Z. J., Lipstitt, D. R. and Whybrow, P. D. (eds) (1977) *Psychosomatic Medicine: Current Trends and Clinical Applications.* Oxford University Press, New York.

Sandler, M. (ed) (1978) *Mental Illness in Pregnancy and the Puerperium.* Oxford University Press, Oxford.

Carenza, L. and Zichella, L. (1986) *Emotion and Reproduction.* Academic Press, London.

Christie, M. and Mellett, P. G. (1986) *Psychosomatic Approach. Contemporary Practice of Wholeperson Care.* John Wiley, Chichester.

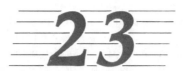

Organic Psychosyndromes

Organic psychosyndromes are a result of anatomical and physiological disturbance in the central nervous system caused by physical disease, trauma, intoxication or degeneration.

Organic psychosyndromes may be conveniently subdivided into:

Acute and Subacute Organic Psychosyndromes

(1) Acute delirium.
(2) Subacute.
   (a) Dysmnesic syndrome (Korsakov's)
   (b) Subacute delirious state

Chronic Organic Psychosyndromes

These are classified according to the underlying pathogenic processes, e.g. inflammatory, degenerative, traumatic etc.

Delirium

The following are the characteristic features of delirium:

1 Varying degrees of clouding of consciousness. This is associated with (a) disorientation for time, place or person, (b) difficulty in grasping what goes on in the environment.
2 Attention is disturbed and it is difficult to secure the patient's attention for more than a short time. The patient is easily distracted by stimuli, moving objects, shadows and noises which he often misinterprets.
3 Disorders of perception, such as illusions and hallucinations, particularly visual hallucinations.

4 Mood varies from mild unease to frank terror and perplexity. Fear and suspicion are the predominant aspects.
5 Mental content. Sometimes thinking is disconnected and speech is incoherent. Occasionally talk and actions are concerned with daily tasks; this is referred to as occupational delirium—the bus conductor calling for fares and handing out imaginary tickets.
6 Misidentification of people.
7 There is a tendency for the symptomatology to become more marked as darkness falls.
8 Sleep is disturbed. There is a tendency for the patient to be drowsy during the day and to be awake as night comes on. Occasionally there is marked restlessness by day and night.
9 On recovery from delirium, the patient's memory for the period is vague or sometimes absent. This is because attention and registration have been significantly impaired during the acute phase.

Diagnosis

The diagnosis of acute delirium usually presents no difficulties. Occasionally acute mania and acute schizophrenia may appear to be like delirium but in these there is no clouding of consciousness and the patient's awareness of his surroundings is usually intact. The main problem of diagnosis is to ascertain the underlying toxic, metabolic, infective or other factors responsible for the delirium.

A large number of disorders may be complicated by delirium, e.g.

1 Systemic infections.
2 Inflammatory conditions of the central nervous system, such as tubercular cerebrospinal menin-

gitis, cerebral abscess, meningo-vascular syphilis, etc.

3 Non-inflammatory lesion of the brain, such as concussion, contusion, neoplastic deposits, raised intracranial pressure, haemorrhage, embolism, hypertensive encephalography, senile and pre-senile dementia, epilepsy.

4 Barbiturates, bromides, amphetamines, hysocine, atropine, cocaine, hashish, alcohol. Imipramine, amitriptyline and nortriptyline in elderly patients.

5 Sudden withdrawal of drugs such as barbiturates, and alcohol.

6 Cerebral anaemia due to any cause.

7 Metabolic and endocrine conditions. Uraemia, liver failure, ketosis, alkalosis, vitamin deficiency, acute porphyria, hyperinsulinism, hypoglycaemia, thyrotoxicosis and hypopituitarism.

The severity of delirium is determined by the patient's constitutional make-up and by the severity of the toxic, infective or other noxic agent. Some patients will become delirious with an infection of the finger. Children and elderly patients more readily become delirious, probably due to difficulty in maintaining homeostatic mechanisms.

Two approaches have been made to analyse and interpret the manifestations in terms of cerebral function:

1 Certain elements of the delirium may be viewed as reflecting dysfunction of particular parts of the brain, such as agnosia, dysphasia, amnesia, auditory and visual hallucinations.

2 In Korsakov's syndrome, the confusional state is notable for the breakdown in memory mechanisms and the orientation of memory in correct temporal sequence; the hypothalamic region and its interconnections with the frontal lobes are usually involved. Thus, a lesion in this situation should be considered when temporal disorientation is a distinct feature of delirium.

Treatment

The first step in treatment is to ascertain, treat or alleviate the underlying physical condition. Nursing care is of paramount importance and if possible a nurse should be specifically designated to the patient and change avoided. If the patient is very disturbed, markedly distressed or agitated, medication may be necessary. Barbiturates are contraindicated; pheno-thiazines such as chlorpromazine and thioridazine have a useful place or butyrophenones such as haloperidol. In alcoholic and elderly patients the benzodiazepines or carbamazepine may be given. In delirium tremens large doses of vitamin B complex are also desirable.

Subacute Delirium

The causes which can result in delirium may also produce states of lesser severity in which the degree of clouding of consciousness is less marked and less constant. The patient shows incoherence of thinking and is more interested and eager to get in contact with his environment than in delirium. The EEG is theta dominant with delta components, but little or no alpha activity. The treatment is as for delirium.

Dysmnesic Syndrome (Korsakov's Syndrome)

Korsakov's syndrome is characterized by failure of recent memory with preservation of immediate recall, remote memory and other cognitive functions. The commonest cause is chronic alcoholism. It is also found in lead and carbon monoxide intoxication, uraemia, vitamin B deficiency, arteriosclerosis, cerebral syphilis, thiamine (B1) deficiency or it may follow a delirious state or head injury. Bilateral damage to the mammillary bodies is the neurological basis for the disorder. Treatment is of the underlying condition in the case of alcohol-induced Korsakov's syndrome. High doses of vitamin B1 (thiamine) can be given, although there is only a limited penetration to the brain. A fluoryl derivative of thiamine has much greater degrees of penetration of the blood brain barrier and achieves somewhat better results.

Transient Global Amnesia

This is characterized by episodes of loss of recent memory and is due to transient ischaemia of the medial aspects of both temporal lobes caused by vertebrobasilar insufficiency.

Frontal Lobe Syndrome

This is characterized by a tendency to live for the moment without due regard for the future. The patient is thoughtless, unreliable and untrustworthy

The mood is usually shallow, euphoric and inappropriate. It occurs in many disorders in which there is diffuse cerebral damage.

Post-infective Depression

This may follow any severe infection, especially virus infections. The patient complains of weakness, headaches, irritability, hypersensitivity to light and noise, tends to be anxious, unduly reactive to noise and to lack concentration. Emotional lability, depression and retardation are common.

The duration of post-infective depression shows little correlation with the course of the underlying infective illness and depression and hypochondriasis may continue for months after all signs of bodily illness have cleared up.

Dementia

Definition

The term dementia denotes a loss of mental capacity due to organic damage to the brain. It is characterized by:

1 A failure of memory mainly for recent events at first, and subsequently for remote events as well.
2 Difficulty in grasp and comprehension.
3 Emotional instability with emotional outbursts on minor provocation.
4 Difficulty in forming judgments.

Classification

The dementias may be classified on an aetiological basis into:

1 Primary degenerative conditions, e.g. senile dementia, Huntington's chorea, Pick's disease and Alzheimer's disease.
2 Cardiovascular disorders e.g. multi-infarct or arteriosclerotic dementia, cerebral embolism, sub-arachnoid haemorrhage, subdural haematoma.
3 Inflammatory conditions, e.g. cerebral syphilis, other forms of encephalitis, encephalomyelitis etc.
4 Demyelinating disorders.
5 Neoplastic disorders.
6 Metabolic, endocrine and nutritional disorders.
7 Intoxications, poisoning and anoxia, e.g. carbon

monoxide poisoning or arrest or decrease of blood supply to the brain.
8 Trauma.

Clinical Features of Dementia in General

The loss of mental capacity and deterioration may be diffuse as in senile dementia or focal as in arteriosclerotic dementia. It may be gradually progressive or it may be arrested, with a limited degree of improvement; or may be rapidly progressive.

Dementia denotes deterioration of a person's mental capacity affecting mainly memory, comprehension and judgment, and secondarily, affecting feeling and conduct, due to damage to the cerebrum.

We have noted that different pathological agencies can produce dementia and the clinical picture will vary, according to (1) the nature of the underlying pathological condition, (2) the age of onset, (3) the previous personality, (4) the localization of lesions, (5) the rate of progress.

The following are the principal manifestations of dementia:

1 *Memory impairment* Recollection of recent events is first affected and usually the condition becomes progressively worse and more remote events are affected as well. The memory failure is mainly due to difficulty in retention.
2 *Judgment and reasoning* Impaired judgment and the failure to grasp the situation as a whole, and hence the failure to react to it appropriately, may be an early sign of dementia.
3 *Emotional reactions* Emotional instability manifested by irritability, impulsive conduct, occasional acts of violence, alcoholic excess or sexual aberration can occur.

   A variety of mood changes can occur in dementia, e.g. euphoria, depression, anxiety and perplexity. In some patients apathy predominates.
4 *Disorientation* This occurs mainly at night but also depends on the underlying condition; for example, it is more common in arteriosclerotic and hypertensive disorders because of interference to the blood supply of the brain.
5 *Delusions* are the outcome of the impairment of judgment, the defective appreciation of reality and the person's emotional state. The form of the delusion is often influenced by the person's previous personality.

6 *Personal care* Carelessness in dress, cleanliness and finally complete disregard for personal cleanliness and hygiene with incontinence occur.

7 *The physical concomitants* will depend on the underlying causal disorder, but there is usually a general physical deterioration with loss of weight and depression of endocrine functions.

8 *Catastrophic reaction* is the term applied to the sudden change in behaviour, with anger and hostility, when a patient with dementia fails to cope with a task beyond his intellectual capacity.

Primary Degenerative Conditions

Old Age

During the past 60 years the proportion of elderly people in the general population has steadily increased, and the incidence of psychiatric disorders has shown a disproportionately greater increase.

Senescence

The term senescence is applied to the normal process of growing old and is characterized by a gradual falling off in mental and physical capacity, a decrease in ability to cope with new situations, a tendency to become rigid and fixed in outlook, movement becoming slower, more tremulous, less accurate and a decreased tolerance of physical effort. Gradually there develops some impairment of memory for recent events and an increasing tendency to dwell in the past; a narrowing of interests, a decrease in adaptability and a tendency to become possessive and rigid.

It should be noted that there is considerable variation among people in the rate at which normal processes of senescence take place. Although many people lose speed and ability to adapt to new situations this is often offset by gains in persistence and quality as well as accuracy of performance. This is particularly relevant to the question of employment of elderly people.

Senile Dementia

In senile dementia the changes of senescence develop to such a degree that it interferes with a person's well-being and adjustment. Senile dementia is characterized by a progressive deterioration of memory, thinking and stability, by blunting and lack of responsiveness in emotional reactions and reduction in interest and initiative.

Senile dementia is a disease with a fairly well defined course and, when the diagnosis has been made, it carries a prognosis of death within a few years from clinical onset.

The onset is gradual and later becomes more rapidly progressive. The keystone of the understanding of senile dementia is that memory for recent experience is impaired, whilst the person retains the ability to remember remote experiences. This failure of memory for recent events tends to recede progressively backwards until ultimately it involves early life.

There is a decrease of interest and the person becomes increasingly egocentric, irritable and difficult, intolerant of any change and suspicious of things which are modern. Judgment is defective, emotions tend to be generally blunted and the patient tends to be irritable and quarrelsome. At night there is a tendency for confusion to develop and the patient will wander about the house, often causing domestic difficulties by turning the water taps on and possibly flooding the house, turning the gas on and sometimes lighting a fire and forgetting about it. The patient has difficulty in grasp and comprehension, he tires easily and finds it difficult to follow conversation, particularly when it deals with new or unfamiliar topics. Patients may become deluded because of difficulty in comprehending and grasping what goes on around them. Delusions that people are stealing their property or possessions are a common form. Any sudden change in the environment, such as moving house, may precipitate severe ideas of persecution.

Huntington's Chorea

Huntington's chorea was first described in 1872 by George Huntington in America and is characterized by progressive dementia associated with choreoathetoid movements.

There is evidence that at least some of the American families with Huntington's chorea came from Suffolk and it has been reported in many parts of the world in different races.

Huntington's chorea is transmitted by a single dominant gene with a manifestation rate of practically 100%. Therefore 50% of the children of one parent with Huntington's chorea will develop it if they live sufficiently long.

The onset usually occurs between the ages of 30 and 50 years but sometimes it starts earlier. Psychiatric anomalies often precede the development of neurological manifestations. The patient becomes irritable, moody, ill-tempered, quarrelsome and very sensitive and may develop delusions of persecution. Occasionally the illness may first present itself as dullness, apathy, lack of initiative and occasionally as depression. The onset of the physical symptoms is gradual and subtle; the patient appears fidgety but he soon develops the characteristic jerking, abrupt movements which usually start in the face, hands and shoulders. Sometimes the movements are choreic but more often are a combination of slow, writhing movements combined with a jerking movement, i.e. choreoathetoid movements.

Speech becomes abrupt and staccato. Involvement of the diaphragm causes irregularity of breathing. Involvement of muscles concerned with swallowing may sometimes cause choking.

The most common psychiatric syndromes associated with it are (1) depression, which may be associated with impulsive suicidal attempts, (2) paranoid tendencies and (3) sometimes a definite paranoid psychosis. It has been stated that some patients who develop the disease earlier show evidence of Parkinsonism as well as the choreoathetotic movements. The average duration is 10 to 15 years.

The pressing problem with Huntington's chorea is to find some means of ascertaining the carrier of the dominant gene. Investigations have been directed towards studies of premorbid personality, electroencephalogram and other abnormalities which might be associated with the carrier of Huntington's chorea.

Management

The recent finding that GABA and its biosynthetic enzyme glutamic acid decarboxylase are markedly reduced in the globus pallidus substantia nigra, the caudate nucleus and the plutamen, and the finding that GABA receptors are intact, suggested the possibility that GABA-mimetic drugs might be useful in the management of the involuntary movements. However, treatment with sodium valproate which increases brain GABA in animals has not been suc-

cessful. In order to reduce the increased dopaminergic activity caused by the loss of the inhibiting action of GABA, thioridazine and tetrabenazine are found to be the most useful drugs in the management of Huntington's chorea.

Alzheimer's Disease

Alzheimer's disease usually develops in the fifties or sixties but sometimes earlier. The average duration of the disease is about seven years.

Alzheimer's disease usually starts with memory failure for recent events. Marked lack of spontaneous activity and lack of initiative is common in the early stages.

Quite frequently extrapyramidal manifestations or akinetic hypotonic symptoms occur. Reading difficulties occur and there is marked disorientation in space, whereas orientation in time is not so much affected. The loss of spatial orientation causes patients to wander and lose themselves, even to get lost in the house in which they live.

There is a tendency for patients to stare with a forward gaze which is associated with a marked inability to change the position of their eyes.

After two or three years dementia becomes well established and focal symptoms appear in the form of aphasia, apraxia and agnosia. Gait disturbances become noticeable, gait being slow, unsteady and clumsy.

The terminal stages of the illness are characterized by a very severe dementia and a vegetable existence, with progressive deterioration in speech and a rapid physical deterioration with flexion contractures, bed sores and cachexia. Forced grasping and groping sometimes occur and also the sucking reflex. The genetic basis of Alzheimer's disease is considered to be multifactorial.

Neuropathology

Diffuse atrophy occurs mainly in the frontal and temporal lobes and sometimes in the parietal lobes. There is a marked loss of ganglial cells, particularly in the outer parts of the cortex, and degenerative changes which are characteristic of the disease and referred to as Alzheimer's fibrillary change, together with argentophile plaques.

There are at least two types of Alzheimer's disease which share certain features but which differ in significant pathological and biochemical characteristics.

Type I

Alzheimer's disease usually begins in the late seventies. Cell loss in the brain is not increased in comparison with aged matched controls but other features of Alzheimer's disease are found, including senile plaques and neurofibrillary tangles, the latter being found in the neocortex, a distribution which is not seen in the normal aged brain.

Type II

Type II Alzheimer's disease usually begins earlier than Type I and substantial cell loss is evident in many areas, including the main noradrenergic and cholinergic subcortical nuclei. Senile plaques and neurofibrillary tangles are widespread and much more numerous than in Type I.

Very recent work has identified an aberrant natural protein which is stable and accumulates causing the neurofibrillary tangle to develop. Research is in progress to discover ways of preventing the formation of this protein.

The limbic system controls behaviour including memory while the association cortex deals with the higher functions of thought and perception. Both are affected in Alzheimer's disease. Recent research has shown decreased cholinergic, serotoninergic and noradrenergic activity.

The finding that there is a decrease in CAT (choline acetyl transferase) has stimulated the use of cholinergic drugs like physostigmine, and cholinergic agonists like arecoline. Attempts have also been made to give precursor loading by administering choline and lecithin. The results on the whole have not been consistent and are rather disappointing. The use of stimulants such as amphetamines and methylphenidate improve learning, particularly when the learning involves active participation by the patient. Nomifensine has been found to be helpful in the treatment of memory difficulties in a depression associated with dementia. Neuropeptides have also been used because ACTH has been found to help learning in experimental animals. DDAVP (argenin vasopressin) has also been used and the results have not all been in agreement but somewhat encouraging.

Nootropic drugs refer to compounds which act on cognitive functions and are aimed at facilitating learning and memory and preventing impairment of cognitive functions induced by disease and brain insults.

Research into the biochemical basis of senile and presenile dementias is just beginning and holds exciting prospects for the future.

A rare form of presenile dementia, with a rapidly deteriorating course and variable neurological features (Creutzfeldt-Jacob disease), has recently been shown to be associated with a transmissible agent, possibly a slow virus.

Pick's Disease

Pick's disease is a form of presenile dementia which is transmitted by a single dominant gene.

It has an average age of onset between 52 and 57 years and an average duration of six to seven years. In the early stages there is lack of initiative and drive and memory failure for recent events, with a tendency to be fatuous and to have diminished control over impulses and behaviour.

Later there is severe progressive dementia with aphasia. Patients do not show the typical disturbance of gait found in Alzheimer's disease.

The final stage is one of marked dementia, the patient being bedridden with contractures of the limbs and cachexia similar to Alzheimer's disease. Spatial disorientation occurs much earlier than in Alzheimer's disease.

Pathologically there is a marked atrophy of the frontal and/or temporal lobes with narrow sulci. There are no Alzheimer's fibrillary changes or senile plaques and the parietal lobe is very rarely affected.

Cardiovascular Disorders

Hypertension does not necessarily cause any psychiatric symptoms. In those patients who ultimately develop signs of dementia there is usually a history of episodes of disturbance of consciousness, which may vary from transient interruptions of consciousness to periods of confusion or twilight states.

Eventually symptoms of dementia with memory failure and difficulty in comprehension supervene. Bouts of hypertensive encephalopathy with vomiting, loss of vision, epilepsy and monoplegia may occur.

Multi-infarct and arteriosclerotic dementia usually start in the sixth decade but may occasionally begin in the forties or fifties.

The presence of arteriosclerosis in itself, even in the fundal arteries, does not mean that the patient is suffering from arteriosclerotic dementia. The diagnosis of arteriosclerotic dementia must first be made on the evidence of dementia and secondly on the characteristic features of arteriosclerotic dementia itself.

It should be remembered that the underlying pathology is an ischaemia of parts of the brain causing anoxia and necrosis. As the disorder is vascular, the characteristic features are its fluctuating course, with periods of exacerbation and intervening periods of improvement. At first the personality is well preserved with good insight into the condition. The memory loss for recent events tends to be transient, variable, patchy and lacunar.

There may be periods of impairment of consciousness, which may be transient or may last for days.

The presence of focal neurological signs clinches the diagnosis, e.g. paralysis, aphasia and apraxia.

Epileptiform seizures occur in about 20% of cases. The fluctuating course of the disease is maintained until a late stage.

Eventually there is a disintegration of personality with marked dementia.

The treatment of arteriosclerotic (multi-infarct) dementia by cerebral vasodilators has so far been disappointing.

In carefully selected patients, surgery involving the redirection of extracranial arteries to areas of the brain with diminished blood flow due to arterial disease is promising.

Inflammatory Conditions

Cerebral Syphilis

Neurosyphilis occurs in some 10% of people infected with *Spirochaeta pallida*.

Psychiatric symptoms may occur with other manifestations of neurosyphilis, e.g. severe meningovascular syphilis may give rise to clouding of consciousness or delirium. Mental disturbances sometimes accompany tabes and are due to the syphilitic changes in the brain.

The most important inflammatory condition in clinical practice is general paralysis.

General Paralysis

GP is three times as common in men as in women and the incubation period ranges from 10 to 24 years after initial infection.

The most common type of disorder is a simple dementing form; other types are the manic-expansive-grandiose type and the depressive variety. Negative blood WRs are found in 8% but the WR is always positive in the CSF.

Early diagnosis and prompt penicillin treatment produces clinical improvement and ability to return to work in more than 80% of cases and has nearly eliminated deaths from neurosyphilis. Even in severely affected patients needing treatment in a mental hospital, there is a 1 in 3 chance of improvement and re-ablement for work.

However, in very few cases is recovery complete; impairment of judgment, insight and speech usually persist.

A total of 6 000 000 units of penicillin is usually adequate. Further courses of penicillin are indicated if clinical improvement is followed by deterioration or if the CSF cell count was greater than 5 per cubic millimetre in the first post-treatment years.

The pre-treatment CSF findings are of some value in forecasting the response to treatment. A marked increase in the cell count, indicating an active inflammatory process, will tend to improve with treatment, although there might be residual symptoms due to damage of the brain before treatment was started. Absence of pleocytosis in the CSF indicates a relatively static process and is less likely to be improved by treatment but also less likely to deteriorate.

Encephalitis Lethargica

During the acute phase of the illness the patient may exhibit involuntary movements of the choreiform and athetoid type, and show insomnia and mild delirium.

Usually some years after the initial attack various extrapyramidal phenomena occur, including Parkinsonism and dystonic reactions and oculogyric crises. Patients with these extrapyramidal conditions are often slow and may develop a reactive depression on account of their disability and its long duration.

Encephalitis lethargica affecting children and

young adults often results in marked personality difficulties. The patients may become social problems, be cruel and may also show lack of restraint in sexual and social behaviour. If it occurs very early in childhood it may cause an arrest of development of the mind and cause mental subnormality.

Sydenham's Chorea

The early symptoms of Sydenham's chorea are irritability, disobedience and misbehaviour or sometimes unusual placidity, apathy and lack of attention; emotional lability varying from depression to hilarity, distractability and absent-mindedness also occurs.

Following the illness, tics, twitches and compulsive utterances may persist into adult life.

Demyelinating Disorders

Multiple sclerosis may be associated with emotional instability, hysterical tendencies and, extremely rarely, may lead to dementia.

Schilder's disease causes marked dementia along with blindness, deafness, aphasia and agnosia.

Neoplastic Disorders

Cerebral Tumour

Cerebral tumours may produce effects as a result of increased intracranial pressure when the common symptoms are headaches and vomiting, both being worse in the morning and associated with papilloedema.

The effects of infiltration of the tumour into the brain will vary according to the area affected but certain symptoms are common. A change of personality, a lack of control and suppressed earlier tendencies, such as homosexuality, may now become manifest; sometimes hysterical mechanisms are released. The development of hysteria for the first time in middle age or later should make one suspect an underlying organic lesion.

If the tumour is rapidly growing, disturbances of consciousness, clouding of consciousness or the dysmnesic syndrome may occur; dementia, loss of mental capacity with memory failure and difficulty in comprehension also occur.

Tumours in the frontal lobe tend to be associated with fatuousness and cheerfulness, but this can occur with other cerebral tumours as well. The patient tends to be inattentive, distractable, dull and apathetic.

Temporal lobe tumours may give rise to temporal lobe epilepsy and behavioural and emotional changes which are referred to in Chapter 24.

Parietal lobe lesions produce defects at the highest levels of sensory and perceptual integration.

Metabolic, Endocrine and Nutritional Disorders

Vitamin Deficiency

Thiamine (vitamin B₁, aneurin)

Thiamine plays an important part in the oxidation of carbohydrates and has a fundamental role in the process of oxidation in the living cell.

Thiamine deficiency may result in the following syndromes:

1 *A neurasthenic syndrome* This is the earliest and most frequent manifestation of thiamine deficiency. Anorexia, fatigue and insomnia are common; irritability, mild depression etc. may also occur.
2 *Wernicke's encephalopathy* This syndrome often has an abrupt onset and may occur with alcoholism or as a terminal complication of disease, particularly chronic gastro-intestinal disorders such as gastric carcinoma.

   The features include clouding of consciousness, varying ophthalmoplegias and ataxia. The clouding of consciousness may vary from drowsiness or apathy to delirium or coma. There is paralysis of conjugate eye movements, nystagmus is often present, polyneuritis of the lower limbs is common.
3 *Korsakov's syndrome.*
4 *Delirium tremens.*

Treatment is the provision of a balanced highly nutritious diet of natural unrefined foods and the administration of vitamin B complex.

For mild cases the dose should be 10 mg–30 mg a day, for severe cases with polyneuropathy the dose may vary from 10 mg–100 mg twice daily for Wernicke's encephalopathy 50 mg–100 mg three times daily for seven days.

Nicotinic acid

The following syndromes occur with nicotinic acid deficiency:

A neurasthenic syndrome.

Pellagra The diagnostic triad of dermatitis, diarrhoea and dementia is out of date. The features of pellagra are mental abnormality, loss of weight, stomatitis, glossitis, porphyrinuria, diarrhoea, tachycardia, peripheral neuropathy and vomiting, in relative order of frequency.

Encephalopathy, characterized by clouding of consciousness, cogwheel rigidity in the extremities and uncontrollable grasping and sucking reflexes.

Treatment includes an abundant high-calorie diet together with the specific vitamin.

In the early stages, owing to painful mouth lesions and gastric disturbances, milk and meat juices may have to be the mainstay.

Nicotinamide is given in a dose of 15 mg–30 mg every hour for 10 hours a day. The addition of brewer's yeast 15 g–30 g daily is advisable, owing to the danger of precipitation of latent deficiencies in other B factors such as thiamine or riboflavine. A maintenance dose of 25 mg–50 mg three times a day should be given for a prolonged period, in addition to the continued enriched diet.

Anaemia

Sometimes a disturbed mental state may precede evidence of megaloblastic anaemia. An abnormal EEG is one of the positive findings.

Much larger doses of Vitamin B_{12} are needed in treating this type of case and care must be taken to ensure that an associated encephalopathy is not missed in a patient who presents with severe anaemia.

Severe iron deficiency anaemias may result in fatigue, irritability and mild depression.

Thyroid Disorder

Hypothyroidism

The features of hypothyroidism are mental torpor, lack of spontaneity, retardation in thinking and motor activity, intense fatigue associated with emotional lability.

In some patients marked memory difficulties may occur and in others delusions, hallucinations and disturbances of behaviour may be present. The most frequent accompaniment is depression and retardation.

Hyperthyroidism

Hyperthyroidism is associated with excessive activity, emotional instability, difficulty in interpersonal relationships due to irritability, excitability, impatience and liability to explosive rage.

In predisposed subjects a schizophreniform picture may occur, which is usually of short duration. Depressive and manic states also occur

Miscellaneous Intoxications

Bromide

Bromide intoxication is an iatrogenic disorder which is often unrecognized.

Delirium, confusional states with delusions of persecution, amnesic states with emotional lability are the usual forms. Acne and physical signs of intoxication are not always evident.

Diagnosis is made by a history of administration of medicine containing bromide and a level of blood bromide greater than 50 mg per 100 cm^3.

Treatment consists of withdrawal of the drug and giving large quantities of sodium chloride to promote its excretion.

Lead Poisoning

The mental symptoms associated with lead poisoning may be acute or chronic.

Acute poisoning may cause delirium, tremors, visual hallucinations and delusions.

In the chronic progressive form apathy, depression, memory impairment, speech difficulties and Korsakov's syndrome may occur.

Mild intoxication may give rise to a clinical picture of irritability, weakness and dizziness.

Mercury Poisoning

This includes irritability, loss of confidence, anxiety symptoms and depression. There is a coarse tremor of the lips, tongue and hands.

Manganese Poisoning

Prolonged exposure to manganese gives rise to Parkinsonism and uncontrollable laughing and crying.

Carbon Monoxide Poisoning

This may occur accidentally as a result of improperly burning combustion stoves, inhalation of exhaust gases from petrol engines and working in coal mines.

Acute poisoning occurs with suicidal attempts with coal gas. A gradual onset of carbon monoxide poisoning leads to lowering of efficiency and self control without insight, leading eventually to loss of consciousness.

Acute poisoning results in disorientation, confusion, amnesia, headache, giddiness.

Only about 50% of cases recover completely. In some, chronic symptoms may follow directly on the acute intoxication, whereas other develop symptoms after an interval of 1–3 weeks; they then become disorientated, confused, amnesic with headaches, giddiness, pains in the extremities and sometimes a Parkinsonian syndrome develops.

Normal Pressure Hydrocephalus

This form of hydrocephalus is obstructive yet communicating. The block is in the subarachnoid space, allowing free passage from the ventricles but preventing its upward flow over the hemisphere for absorption to the superior saggital sinus. Pressure in the ventricles is usually normal, and headache is usually absent

The clinical picture is the occurrence over several weeks or months of memory failure, physical or mental slowness, unsteadiness of gait and urinary incontinence.

Lumbar CSF pressure is normal. Air encephalography shows symmetrically enlarged ventricles with little or no air in the cerebral subarachnoid space above the basal cistern.

Surgical treatment by shunt operation to lower the CSF pressure in the ventricles is often very successful.

Trauma (Head Injury)

A patient who suffers from immediate unconsciousness as a result of head injury goes through stages of stupor and confusion before regaining clear

consciousness. Though this recovery can be complete in a matter of minutes it can take hours or days

The term concussion should not be confined to instances in which there is immediate loss of consciousness with rapid and complete recovery; it should also include the very many cases in which the initial symptoms are the same but which subsequently have a long continued disturbance of consciousness which is often followed by residual symptoms.

Concussion in this wider sense depends on the diffuse injury to nerve cells and fibres sustained at the moment of the accident. The effects of such an injury may or may not be reversible.

Acute Stage following Brain Injury

It is customary to divide the symptoms in the acute stage into those seen in mild cases, moderate cases and severe cases.

In the mild case the patient loses consciousness for a few seconds to an hour or so, or he may be dazed and walking around in a confused manner with amnesia for the accident and just before it. Within a few hours the mental symptoms will have disappeared in most cases.

In the moderate case unconsciousness lasts for several hours and, before awakening, the patient shows clouding of consciousness followed by a dysmnesic state. Sometimes acute delirious states occur before recovery.

In severe head injury unconsciousness lasts for several hours to several days. The delirious and dysmnesic stages may last for days or weeks. Mortality in severe injury is high.

The severity of the injury can be gauged from the duration of post-traumatic amnesia, which is best measured from the time of the injury to the time of the occurrence of continuous awareness. The longer the post-traumatic amnesia, the longer the period of convalescence before return to work. If the post-traumatic amnesia is greater than seven days it usually takes four to eight months for the person to get back to work.

Chronic State

The following disabilities can occur: post-concussional syndrome, dementia, epilepsy, chronic subdural haematoma, focal neurological lesions and precipitated endogenous illnesses or organic mental disorders.

The post-concussional syndrome starts within a few days or a week or more after the accident. The syndrome consists of headache, giddiness and nervous instability with undue fatigue of body and mind, intolerance of noise and light, insomnia, anxiety and depression.

The manifestations of the post-concussional state are similar to those of anxiety states. Psychological factors and predisposition to psychiatric breakdown, as well as litigation factors, may influence the symptomatology.

Nevertheless, the syndrome would appear to have some organic basis which is often reversible and variable in severity. The severity of the disability is largely influenced by the patient's predisposition together with the influence of psychological and environmental stresses.

Post-traumatic Dementia

The degree of the loss of mental capacity or dementia shows infinite variation from mild forgetfulness, impaired concentration and lack of spontaneity to severe dementia with personality change, sometimes showing evidence of the frontal lobe syndrome when the patient becomes disinhibited, tactless, expansive, jocular and euphoric.

Post-traumatic Epilepsy

This is more common with penetrating wounds, particularly where there is penetration of the dura.

Patients who develop epileptic fits soon after the injury do not usually have recurrent attacks, whereas epilepsy starting months or years afterwards tends to persist. Grand mal attacks are the most common but other forms can also take place.

Chronic Subdural Haematoma

This is a late sequel of head injury and occurs after some weeks or months. The injury is often slight; the patient is sleepy and his condition fluctuates in severity.

Focal neurological lesions may also occur as sequelae to head injury.

Further Reading

Mayer-Gross, W., Slater, E. and Roth, M. (1960) *Clinical Psychiatry*. Cassell, London.

Post, F. (1965) *The Clinical Psychiatry of Later Life*. Pergamon Press, Oxford.

Pitt, B. M. M. (1974) *Psychogeriatrics: Introduction to the Psychiatry of Old Age*. Churchill Livingstone, Edinburgh.

Whitehead, J. A. (1974) *Psychiatric Disorders in Old Age; A Handbook for the Clinic Team*. Springer, New York.

Brocklehurst, J. C. (ed) (1978) *Textbook of Medicine and Gerontology*, 2nd edn. Churchill Livingstone, Edinburgh.

Isaacs, D. and Post, F. (1978) *Studies in Geriatric Psychiatry*. Wiley, Chichester.

Lishman, W. A. (1978) *Organic Psychiatry. The Psychological Consequences of Cerebral Disorders*. Blackwell, Oxford.

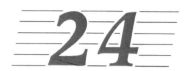

Psychiatric Aspects of Epilepsy

Epilepsy may be defined as a disorder of the brain, expressed as a paroxysmal cerebral dysrhythmia. This dysrhythmia is symptomatic and is associated with seizures composed of one or more of the following recurrent and involuntary phenomena:

1 Loss or derangement of consciousness or memory
2 Excess or loss of muscle tone or movement
3 Alteration of sensation, including hallucinations
4 Disturbance of the autonomic nervous system
5 Other psychic manifestations, including abnormal thought processes and moods

It should be noted, however, that a person with clear cut seizure discharges in the EEG but without these symptoms is a potential epileptic but not, in fact, an epileptic. Genuine epileptics may have normal brain-waves on some occasions when recording of the electroencephalogram is taken and repeated EEG examination may be necessary to reveal the epileptic dysrhythmia. Special techniques such as hyperventilation, photic stimulation or recording during sleep may be required.

Classification of Epilepsy

Classification of epilepsy on clinical grounds is traditionally into petit mal, grand mal and psychomotor seizures. Lennox gives a more detailed classification.

1 *The petit mal triad*
  (a) True petit mal
  (b) Jerk
  (c) Atonic
2 *Convulsive triad*
  (a) Generalized (grand mal)
  (b) Focal (localized, partial)
  (c) Jacksonian (Rolandic)

3 *Temporal lobe triad*
  (a) Automatic
  (b) Subjective
  (c) Tonic focal
4 Autonomic
5 Unclassified

The Petit Mal Triad

The three varieties classified under petit mal include an absence or true petit mal, a jerk and a fall (atonic form).

They frequently co-exist in a given patient. They all show a spike and wave in the electroencephalogram and improve with forms of medication which are not effective for convulsions. They also are characterized by marked frequency, brevity, an abrupt onset and ending; and occur predominantly in childhood. In the pure petit mal (absence) the period of unconsciousness varies between five and thirty seconds. Muscular movements take the form of small, rhythmic clonic movements. Facial movements are usually twitching and in the extremities are usually in the form of jerks. The twitch and the jerk coincide with the spike of the electroencephalogram and occur at the rate of three per second.

The Convulsive Triad

1 *Grand mal epilepsy* The tonic phase of the convulsion lasts 20 seconds, the clinic phase 40 seconds, the period of relaxation 1 minute and recuperation 3 minutes.

2 *Focal or partial convulsions* Represented by convulsive movements confined to one side of the body. Movements may be limited perhaps to the facial

muscles of one side or to an arm or leg. Muscles with bilateral innervation, as those of the chest, are not involved unilaterally. Consciousness is usually retained if movements remain unilateral.

3 *Jacksonian or Rolandic epilepsy* This is a focal seizure characterized by a march of spasm or sensation with preservation of consciousness; however, some authorities use the term Jacksonian to cover all forms of focal seizures. The march of the spasm or sensation usually appears in distal portions of the extremity and travels upwards.

Temporal Lobe Epilepsy

Temporal lobe seizures vary in severity and complexity. They vary according to the situation of the epileptic focus within the temporal lobe, according to the violence of the local epileptic discharge and the extent to which it spreads, not only within the temporal lobe but to other regions of the brain.

Auras in temporal lobe epilepsy may be of various kinds:

1 Crude perceptual disturbances including epigastric sensation like the 'stomach turning over', sudden crude sensations of smell or taste of an unpleasant character, experience of roaring, rushing or ringing noises or sudden disturbance of balance.
2 Emotional phenomena, sudden change in mood such as fear, anger, excitement or pleasure.
3 Perceptual disturbances based on memory mechanisms. Here the patient may experience a sudden feeling of familiarity with surroundings, or conversely, a sudden unreality or strangeness. He may be in a dreamy state in which surrounding objects seem small and receding or appear unduly large and near. He may suddenly feel that he is witnessing a scene which has already taken place before, viz. the 'déjà vu' phenomenon.
4 Auras arising from adjacent regions of the brain.

Sometimes, before losing consciousness, the patient with a lesion of the temporal lobe exhibits symptoms which indicate that the epileptic discharging process has already spread into adjacent regions of the brain, e.g. the occurrence of twitching movements, numbness of one side of the face or body, aphasic difficulties.

Varieties of temporal lobe seizure

1 Minor seizures without loss of consciousness
2 Amnesic attacks without convulsions
3 Major convulsive seizures.

1 *Minor seizures* These are usually sudden and transient sensory auras lasting for one or two seconds.

2 *Amnesic attacks without convulsions* The patient is dazed and exhibits confused or semi-purposive behaviour but not generalized convulsions. The EEG at the onset of these amnesic seizures usually shows a suppression of electrical activity over both hemispheres for a few seconds, followed by more or less symmetrical and rhythmical bilateral 6–8 cycles per second waves. The motor phenomena are usually masticatory, grimacing or semipurposive movements of the limbs.

3 *Major convulsive seizures* Unless the initial aura has been witnessed, these major convulsions may be indistinguishable from grand mal attacks resulting from lesions in other parts of the brain. These have a particular tendency to occur during sleep.

Investigation of suspected temporal lobe epilepsy

It should be noted that the recent appearance of temporal lobe seizures may signal the presence of a cerebral tumour. The diagnosis becomes clear if neurological signs or evidence of increased intracranial pressure are present. In cases in which the fits are of long standing and there is nothing obvious in the clinical picture that would suggest tumour, an attempt should be made to control the seizures by drugs such as phenobarbitone, phenytoin sodium, primidone or carbamazepine. In cases in which the fits cannot be properly controlled and are disabling, or in which there is severe personality disorder, recourse should be made to full neurological, radiological and EEG investigations. The electroencephalographic examination which is most likely to give the decisive answer, and may have to be repeated over a long period, is that recorded during induced sleep using sphenoidal electrodes.

A history of intractable epilepsy and an EEG demonstration of an epileptic focus which is confined to one temporal lobe or, if bilateral, predominantly on one side, constitute the usual indications for temporal lobectomy.

Emotions and Epileptic Attacks

Both petit mal and grand mal attacks may be precipitated by emotional changes.

Petit mal may be precipitated as an immediate response to sudden unpleasurable emotions such as surprise, embarrassment or the arousal of competitive feelings.

Temporal lobe epileptic attacks may also be precipitated by stress but usually the stress is more prolonged than in petit mal.

Emotions may also be aroused by the epileptic process and there is a clear relationship between these and focal abnormalities in the temporal lobe. The commonest emotions are depression, anxiety, pleasure and displeasure.

The emotions are vivid and seem to arise automatically and are, as it were, foreign to the patients; they do not feel them to be a part of their normal emotional reactions; they are simple rather than complex. Pleasant emotions are uncommon but unpleasurable emotional states are very common. The emotions appear to be experiences which are unrelated to the external world of reality or the person's internal world.

It must also be realized that the epileptic's various difficulties, caused by fits or other unrelated factors and involving his relationships and social interactions, may, by arousing emotions which can precipitate attacks, influence this frequency.

Aetiology of Epilepsy

Epilepsy is of varied and multiple aetiology with genetic influences, brain damage, biochemical and psychogenic factors all having a potential role.

Precipitants of Attacks

It is well known that hydration increases cerebral dysrhythmia and increases the tendency to produce epilepsy. This is the basis of the water vasopressin test for epilepsy.

Over-breathing may also precipitate attacks in the epileptic person. Various photic stimuli and, in some, music may precipitate attacks. Alcohol also increases the tendency and the frequency for epileptic attacks to occur.

Epilepsy and Schizophrenia

Recent work has shown that there is often a close link between schizophrenic-like disorders and epilepsy. This occurred more often with temporal lobe epilepsy and the psychotic onset occurred more often with a decrease in fit frequency rather than with a rising fit frequency.

The onset of schizophrenic symptoms was often insidious. Delusional beliefs in clear consciousness occurred in the majority. Compared with the ordinary run of schizophrenic patients, the epileptic schizophrenics showed less catatonia and more normal affective responses, and usually had a negative family history for schizophrenia.

Abnormal Behaviour in Relationships to Fits

Abnormal behaviour occurring during the actual fit (ictal) is usually spontaneous and the result of the epileptic disturbance of the brain, tends to be stereotyped, short-lived and without relation to circumstance.

Post-ictal activity, whether restlessness, aggression or a fugue, is due to the state of confusion so it is simple in form. It may be evoked by stimulation, or when purposeful, is often determined by past experience.

It appears automatic. The confused person walks and fumbles with clothes, undresses routinely or blindly, resists help or interference.

It can be said that there is no real purpose in the ictal activity and that any purpose in the post-ictal activity is immediate and very crude.

No prolonged, elaborate and intelligently purposeful fugue state is epileptic.

It may be noted that in status epilepticus (focal or general) abnormal states of movement, sensation or consciousness may last for many hours. It is usually possible to recognize the individual attacks during the status and so establish responsibility of epilepsy for a prolonged behavioural disorder. Prolonged amnesic states, fugues, stupor, coma or aggressive or antisocial behaviour are unlikely to be epileptic in the absence of status, for even post-ictal confusion lasts for minutes only rather than hours.

It must be emphasized that activity which is motivated and which uses past learning cannot be epileptic.

The soldier absent without leave who finds his way home by road and rail with no memory of the process could not have done so in an epileptic attack. Neither can a criminal who has amnesia for an act of violence directed against a selected subject with an appropriate weapon, however obscure the motive or violent the act.

Employment of Epileptics

Surveys of epilepsy in general practice have revealed that three quarters of all chronic epileptics are fully employed; 12% are in sheltered employment and 6% unemployed for reasons other than epilepsy and 8% unemployed because of the fits or social difficulties arising from epilepsy. Sixteen per cent of all cases presented a social problem.

The importance of suitable employment for the epileptic cannot be over-emphasized. If unemployed the epileptic tends to become depressed, morose, apathetic, aggressive and demoralized. Work helps to bring financial security, provides interests and fosters a suitable sense of independence and responsibility which facilitates proper social adjustment.

Certain occupations are unduly hazardous for the epileptic; for example, those associated with fire, water, vats, ladders, e.g. painting and window-cleaning, machinery, motor driving. The question should be asked, are serious hazards likely to be met if there is sudden loss of consciousness?

It is usually advantageous for the epileptic to register under the Disabled Persons Act 1944. He will then benefit from the services provided by the Department of Employment.

Further Reading

Lennox, W. G. and Lennox, M. A. (1960) *Epilepsy and Related Disorders*. Churchill Livingstone, London.
Reynolds, E. H. and Trimble, M. R. (1981) *Epilepsy and Psychiatry*. Churchill Livingstone, Edinburgh.

25

Schizophrenia

Under the term schizophrenia are included those illnesses, in all age groups, which are characterized from the outset by fundamental disturbances in personality, thinking, emotional life, behaviour, interests and relationships with other people.

Schizophrenia involves a tendency for the person to withdraw from the environment and to show an internal disintegration of thinking, feeling and behaviour, resulting in an incongruity between his emotional state and his thoughts and actions, a tendency to form characteristic associations in thinking and a tendency to morbid projection.

The disintegration of mental functions in schizophrenia is 'molecular' and quite different from the 'molar' dissociation found in hysteria and multiple personality.

It is convenient to describe the clinical features of schizophrenia under the following headings:

1 Withdrawal
2 Splitting
  (a) thought disorder
  (b) emotional disconnection
  (c) conduct disconnection
3 Paranoid disposition
4 Abnormalities of perception.

Withdrawal

The withdrawal in schizophrenia includes a generalized loss of interest in the environment and a diminution in response to external influences, particularly in affective responses.

There tends to be loss of natural affection for relatives and friends and the patient may react to happenings of great importance as if they were of no concern.

Answers to questions are brief and uninformative. Inertia towards external activities and general failure of will with lack of drive and initiative are other manifestations of withdrawal.

The most marked form of withdrawal is stupor, in which the patient shows marked decrease in responses to stimuli. There is lack of spontaneous thought and action but with awareness of passing events. Consciousness is clear and registration and retention of memories are unimpaired.

Thought Disorder

Disorder of thinking is a characteristic feature of schizophrenia. The patient in the early stages of the illness may exhibit a general vagueness and woolliness in his speech which tends to lack coherence and to be uninformative. After talking to a patient for some considerable time, it becomes apparent that very little information has been given by him. There is a feeling of a glass wall between oneself and the patient or, in other words, a difficulty in establishing rapport.

Thoughts and ideas tend to be disconnected and the patient seems unable to continue a normal sequence of his thoughts and speech. Replies to questions may be irrelevant.

Thought blockage, which makes the patient stop in the middle of a sentence or sometimes in the middle of a word may also occur. This may be described by the patient as thought deprivation, i.e. as if his thoughts are suddenly taken away.

There is a general paucity of ideas and repetitive and stereotyped themes may continue throughout the conversation. Thought interpolation may occur whereby the patient feels as if thoughts are inserted into his mind as if from outside. He may also experience a 'crowding in' of many simultaneous thoughts which interfere with his conversation and with the course of his thinking.

Associations may be determined by sounds, assonance ('clanging'), alliteration or any chance irrelevant connection.

Some patients show relative loss of conceptual (categorical) thinking with a tendency to think in concrete terms. This can be shown by interpretation of proverbs, which tends to be literal with the patient having great difficulty in seeing the deeper meaning or wider application of the proverb. It may also be seen in his difficulty in categorizing objects into a particular class; he tends to see them all separately. It may also show itself in literalness, in that he tends to take everything quite literally and will transform metaphors into their literal meaning.

Concrete thinking and literalness may not be present in all patients or may be only observable in the patient at certain times but when they are present, in combination with other manifestations of schizophrenic thinking, they are of considerable diagnostic importance.

Sometimes condensation occurs; a number of different concepts, ideas or words may be fused together.

Cause and effect may be interchanged; things linked by chance association or by any characteristic are taken to be the same. Associations may appear not to proceed in a straight line but may jump from one course to another, exhibiting what has been referred to as the 'Knight's move' in association.

The patient has a tendency to talk in riddles; he counters a question by asking another question and deals with things in a rather philosophical and mystical manner, e.g. when asked about the health of his mother, he may reply by asking some philosophical question about what is meant by health or the understanding of relationships between people.

The patient may invent new words (neologisms) to describe experiences or the way he views things. In some schizophrenic patients, particularly paranoid schizophrenics, the characteristic thought disorder may only become manifested after a long interview and only when they become emotionally disturbed when talking about their delusions. At other times they may show little evidence of thought disorder in ordinary conversation.

Change in Affect

The patient tends to become emotionally flattened and to show a loss of natural affection and appropriate emotional reactions to people he formerly loved. He may become insensitive, inconsiderate or even callously indifferent to other people's feeling and experiences. He takes offence readily and tends to isolate himself from his environment and increasingly develops a state of apathy.

Emotional incongruity is one of the most important aspects of the disturbed affect in schizophrenia. There is a lack of agreement between what the patient says and thinks and how he behaves, and how he feels. He may describe intense persecution in a state of indifference or even with cheerfulness. He may show in his facial expression and demeanour a picture of dejection and misery and yet he may feel happy, elated or may have no feeling at all.

Schizophrenic patients may also experience an extremely rapid change of emotion within a matter of seconds or minutes; they may be angry, depressed, perplexed, ecstatic and anxious all in rapid sequence. Emotional responses may be quite inappropriate, the patient may smile fatuously in a far-away dreamy state. A knowing smile gives the impression that he understands things that the interviewer knows nothing about.

Emotional reactions may be disproportionate and inappropriate to the stimulus and sometimes severe emotional outbursts may appear spontaneously and without any apparent provocation. These may take the form of anger, violence or marked terror and characteristically come out of the blue without warning.

Ambivalence may also be found; the person may hold contrasting and antithetical feelings to the same person or object, concurrently or within a short space of time, e.g. he may have feelings of love and hate for a person at the same time.

Disturbances in Behaviour and Motor Functions

The general demeanour of a schizophrenic patient is often awkward. The patient may show grimacing, twitchings and stereotyped movements of various parts of the body.

In some patients there may be a marked absence of activity, so-called akinetic states, which may last for a few seconds or longer.

Conduct may be disconnected from other aspects of the patient's mental life and one may get evidence of automatic obedience, in that the patient may show waxy flexibility (flexibilitas cerea) in which he will maintain imposed postures for periods of time. He may repeat actions carried out by the interviewer (echopraxia) or repeat things that are said to him (echolalia). He may impulsively utter things in a meaningless fashion. He may exhibit spontaneous fixed attitudes and expressions or exhibit a stereotopy of speech and conduct. He may show negativism, i.e. doing the opposite of what is requested. Some patients show typical negativism in operation when one goes to shake hands with them; they withdraw their hand and, when one puts one's hand down, they bring their hand forward and so on.

Delusion Formation and the Paranoid Disposition

A delusion is a false belief which is not amenable to persuasion or argument and which is out of keeping with the patient's cultural and educational background.

Delusions are characteristic of schizophrenia; they may be primary or secondary. Primary delusions are almost pathognomonic for schizophrenia and characteristically appear suddenly, fully developed and immediately carrying a strong and overwhelming feeling of conviction. They occur in a setting of clear consciousness and the patient is convinced that a particular happening or stimulus is of great significance. For example, a patient on going into the house and perceiving that the window was left partly opened, considered that this indicated that he was Jesus Christ and that he was destined to save the world.

Secondary delusions may occur on the basis of primary delusions or may arise as delusional interpretations of symptoms, such as feelings of passivity or other manifestations of intellectual, emotional or conduct abnormalities found in schizophrenia.

In its strict sense the term paranoid refers to a disturbance of the individual's relationship to the world, so that it would include both delusions of persecution and delusions of grandeur but there is a tendency, generally, among psychiatrists to use the word paranoid as being equivalent to persecutory.

The paranoid disposition is the tendency to attribute to the outside world things which really arise from within the person.

Morbid projection is the basis of the paranoid disposition, i.e. the attribution of something to the outside which arises from within the person, and is a fundamental tendency in paranoid schizophrenia and in the genesis of paranoid delusions.

Morbid projection may vary in form and degree from ideas of reference to completely systematized delusions. The person may believe that he is the subject of special reference, either in people's conversations or from what is said on the radio or seen on television. Delusions of reference are when these beliefs are held with conviction.

Delusions of persecution may be changeable and fleeting or they may be partly systematized to form a system of delusions around a central theme, e.g. that the person is being persecuted by the Jesuits, the Freemasons, the Communists, the Co-operative Society, the Police, MI5 etc. The systematization may range from being partial and variable, to a fully systematized fixed series of delusions as seen in some forms of paranoid schizophrenia.

It is often stated that delusions of grandeur are compensatory to delusions of persecution but there is no evidence for this. They may arise spontaneously without delusions of persecution and, even when both are present, a compensatory relationship is often assumed rather than demonstrated.

Hypochondriacal delusions are very common in schizophrenia and are characteristically bizarre. Sometimes sensations of bodily change, feelings of passivity or interference and other bodily sensations form the basis of hypochondriacal delusions.

Hypochondriacal delusions based on hallucinatory phenomena are diagnostic of schizophrenia.

The patient's complaints are often bizarre but, in assessing bizarreness, it is important to remember the patient's cultural background and intelligence. For example, a depressed mental defective may express hypochondriacal complaints which are extremely bizarre.

In the management of a patient suffering from delusions, the appropriate manner of dealing with him is to do nothing which would confirm the delusions; on the other hand, it is useless trying to argue with the patient about his delusional beliefs because it only tends to make the patient antagonistic and resentful and make him lose faith in the doctor.

Disorders of Perception

Hallucinations may occur in any sensory modality, but by far the most common form of hallucinations in schizophrenia are hallucinations of hearing. In schizophrenia the patient hears voices in a state of clear consciousness, whereas if the patient suffers from visual hallucinations in a setting of clouding of consciousness, one should think of an acute toxic confusional state. Auditory hallucinations vary in clarity and intensity. Sometimes the patient is unable to give a clear description of them because of their vagueness, and at other times they are so clear and intense that they dominate the patient's attention. The voices may be perceived as coming from any part of the patient's body, e.g. from inside the head, or from the heart, the stomach, the limbs or the patient may perceive them as coming from outside himself. He may attribute them to telepathy, electricity, radio waves, television, etc. Especially characteristic of schizophrenia are voices which talk about the patient in the third person or voices which make a running commentary on the patient's actions and the thought echo when the patient hears his own thoughts spoken aloud. Patients vary with regard to the tendency to be influenced by their hallucinatory voices; some patients feel compelled to carry out the commands of their hallucinatory voices; whereas other patients describe the voices as being vague, incoherent or a lot of rubbish.

The voices very frequently are abusive. In men, voices often refer to them as rakes, thieves or other uncomplimentary things; in women that they are prostitutes or are unclean or have venereal disease.

Sometimes the patients feel compelled to answer their voices back and become angry in response to their hallucinations. They often adopt listening attitudes and sometimes smile, sometimes get puzzled and at other times get angry.

Visual hallucinations are uncommon; they are often fragmented in contrast to the complex visual hallucinations one sees in some hysterical states.

Bodily hallucinations, tactile sensations, passivity feelings, sensations of heat, cold, pain, electricity and sexual interference are not infrequent in schizophrenia.

Olfactory hallucinations sometimes occur, e.g. patients complain of odours of decomposition, chemicals, rotting substances, gas etc. These experiences may be woven into their delusional experiences, patients believing that they are being persecuted or drugged.

Varieties of Schizophrenia

It is customary to classify schizophrenia into the following forms:

1 simple
2 hebephrenic
3 catatonic
4 paranoid

In addition, there are the following clinical varieties:

5 schizo-affective
6 periodic catatonia
7 late paraphrenia

The use of customary subtypes—simple, hebephrenic, catatonic, paranoid—has become well established in clinical practice but clinical experience shows that the boundaries between these types are not clear and that an individual patient may change from one subtype to another during the course of the illness.

Simple Schizophrenia

This is characterized by an insidious onset, with a gradual deterioration socially and very often a difficulty in establishing the exact time of onset because of its insidious development.

Clinically, it mainly takes the form of withdrawal of interest from the environment, apathy, difficulty in making social contacts, poverty of ideation, a decline in total performance with marked sensitivity and ideas of reference.

Simple schizophrenics go downhill socially and many become tramps, beggars, thieves or dupes for criminals; women may become prostitutes.

It is distinguished from schizoid pyschopathy by the fact that it is an illness with an onset and a definite change and deterioration in personality, whereas schizoid psychopathy has been present throughout the patient's life.

Hebephrenia

This also has an insidious onset in early life and is characterized by thought disorder and emotional abnormalities.

Characteristically the affect is inappropriate and fatuous, with meaningless giggles and often a self satisfied smile. Thought disorder and delusions, which are often changeable, are common. Hallucinations occur, particularly auditory hallucinations. Behaviour is often silly, mischievous, eccentric, showing much grimacing and mannerisms, or the patient may be inert and apathetic.

Catatonic Schizophrenia

This often has an acute onset and the clinical picture is dominated by disturbance of behaviour and motor phenomena.

The onset is in adolescence or early adult life, but occasionally in the fourth decade or later. The course of the illness often shows extreme alterations in behaviour, varying from stupor to excitement.

Catatonic schizophrenia provides the best examples of disconnection in conduct, ranging from mannerisms, constrained attitudes, automatic responses to stimuli including automatic obedience, echolalia, echopraxia, spontaneous over-activity, the maintenance of imposed postures, negativism. Hallucinations, delusions, thought disorder and emotional disorder are also present but are less prominent than motor phenomena.

Paranoid Schizophrenia

This is characterized by the development of delusions, particularly delusions of persecution. It usually has a later age of onset and patients have a better preservation of personality than in other forms of schizophrenia. The delusions are most often persecutory but grandiose delusions and hypochondriacal delusions may occur. The delusions may be variable, transient and poorly held in some patients whereas in others delusions are systematized, highly complex and relatively fixed.

It was customary in the past to regard paraphrenia and paranoia, which are really subtypes of paranoid schizophrenia, as distinct diseases.

Paraphrenia is characterized by a late age of onset with the existence of semi-systematized delusions occurring with hallucinations, thought disorder becoming more apparent when the patient talks about his delusions or when he gets emotionally disturbed.

Paranoia was the term given to patients showing a fixed delusional system without evidence of thought disorder and without hallucinations and good preservation of personality.

Follow-up studies of patients so diagnosed usually revealed that they later became transformed into clear cases of schizophrenia, with thought disorder and hallucinations.

Schizo-affective Disorder

This term tends to be over-used and ill-used and is sometimes used for cases of schizophrenia with an affective component to the clinical state.

The term schizo-affective disorder should be confined to those cases in which depression or mania occur concurrently with schizophrenia in the patient.

The Relationship between depression and schizophrenia

In recent years increasing importance has been attached to associations between depression and an unequivocal schizophrenia.

The onset of schizophrenia may be associated with depression or even masked by depression. Depression may occur intermittently during the course of the illness and in some patients depression or hypomania may occur as a major constituent of the illness and these are the schizo-affective disorders, which are forms of schizophrenia in which clear affective illnesses occur concurrently.

It is not infrequent for depression to appear during the recovery from a schizophrenic illness; some authorities believe that this occurs with the restoration of insight into the illness but this is not established. In some patients a reciprocal relationship may be seen between the appearance of schizophrenic manifestations and depression. Finally, the recovery from schizophrenia may be followed by an affective disorder, usually depression, which may continue for some considerable time. This may occur as a part of the natural history of the schizophrenic illness but it may also occur as a complication of the parenteral administration of long acting neuroleptics in the maintenance treatment of schizophrenia, and the possibility that this may be a pharmaceutically induced depression cannot be ruled out.

Treatment for depression arising during the course of prolonged phenothiazine therapy may need urgent application because sometimes the depression can be of suicidal intensity and admission to hospital and convulsive therapy may be needed. In milder depressions one of the tricyclic anti-depressants, such as amitriptyline or trimipramine, which are less stimulating in action, should be used.

Periodic Catatonia

This is an interesting condition in which Gjessing found clear correlations between metabolic disturbances and the onset of psychiatric symptoms.

The illness is characterized by phases of stupor or excitement and the metabolic changes are nitrogen retention followed by excretion.

Late Paraphrenia

This occurs more frequently in women than in men and more often in widows or spinsters living alone. Twenty five per cent have some defect of sight or hearing.

Delusions of persecution, for example of being raped and gassed or being affected by strangers, are frequent. Hallucinations of smell, hearing and visual phenomena are common.

Capgras Syndrome

Also known as the syndrome of 'doubles' or illusions of false recognition. The patient is usually a paranoid schizophrenic and claims that strangers around him are friends or relations (positive double) or that they have changed their appearance so that he will not recognize them (negative double).

Aetiology of Schizophrenia

The Influence of Genetic and Environmental Factors in Schizophrenia

In recent years a number of authors have put forward the view that genetic factors play no significant role in the causation of schizophrenia and that environmental factors are prepotent.

Whereas certain environmental factors may, in fact, be important in the precipitation or exacerbation of schizophrenia, very little research work has been carried out to elucidate this. It must be remembered that genetic factors always interact with environmental ones and it is really a problem, in essence, of determining in what ways the genetic factors interact with the environment and particularly to ascertain what features in the environment are relevant and important in this respect. The evidence of genetic factors in schizophrenia is strong and is derived from studies of the occurrence of schizophrenia in the relatives of schizophrenics and from twin studies. The expectation of a member of the population becoming schizophrenic is approximately 1.1% in the United Kingdom. Data, based on investigations in many countries, give an average expectation of 0.86%.

The figures for relatives are as follows: parents 6%, siblings 10%, children 14%, uncles and aunts 3%, nephews and nieces 3%, first cousins 3%. In dizygotic twins of opposite sex, schizophrenia occurs in both twin members in 5.6% and, if the dizygotic twins are of the same sex, in 12%. In monozygotic twins the concordance rate is 45%. Thus the relatives of schizophrenics carry a much greater risk of developing schizophrenia than normal expectation. It is ten times greater in siblings and in children and also increased in remoter relatives. The relatively low figures in parents may be related to the fact that being sufficiently healthy to produce a family and falling ill with schizophrenia are to some extent antagonistic. It is interesting to note that the husbands and wives of schizophrenics and their unrelated step-brothers and sisters, brought up in the same home, have only a slightly increased risk of developing schizophrenia of the order of 2%. Thus the common environment does not appear to have a very strong effect.

If the same family environment accounted for similarity within pairs of twins, the risk of schizophrenia should be the same for a monozygotic as for a dizygotic twin of the same sex brought up with the patient, but actually the difference between monozygotic and dizygotic twins is very marked. Studies of trends of monozygotic twins who have been reared apart again show a similar degree of concordance as monozygotic twins brought up together. A very interesting study has been carried out by Heston, who compared the fate of two series of children taken from their mothers in early infancy. There were 47 children born to schizophrenic mothers in a mental hospital and taken from them to a foster home. These were compared with 50 control children from the same foster institution and matched for sex, and type of eventual placement, whether with adoptive foster family or institutional care and for the length of time in child care institutions. All the members of both groups were followed through childhood and school life, through adult life to a mean age of 36 years. Five of the experimental group developed schizophrenic illnesses whereas none of the control group did so. This is an excellent study in which the early environment is controlled while observing the effect of genetic differences.

The mode of genetic transmissions is still a matter of controversy. A single recessive gene, a single dominant gene, as well as polygenic theories have been put forward.

In conclusion, one could say that the role of genetic factors now is incontrovertible, but further research remains, to elucidate the nature of the genes predisposing to schizophrenia and the way in which the environmental factors operate in the manifestation or the suppression of a genetic predisposition to schizophrenia.

Physical Constitution

Kretschmer in 1921 propounded his hypothesis that there was a biological affinity between manic-depressive psychosis and the pyknic or relatively broad and rounded physique, whereas schizophrenia had a biological affinity to narrow types of physique—athletic and certain dysplastic physiques.

A great deal of research has been carried out to test Kretschmer's hypothesis and the results indicate that schizophrenics, in general, tend to be narrower in physique than normal controls and manic-depressives, that the pyknic or physique of manic-depressives is in part due to increase in age but that the age factor does not entirely invalidate Kretschmer's theory.

There is also some evidence that the narrower the physique the more marked are the manifestations of disconnected thinking, the earlier the age of onset and the more insidious the type of onset.

An explanation of the effect of the correlations between physique and schizophrenia and its course

and prognosis probably rests in the fact that the genes determining body build exert an influence on the operation of the gene or genes determining schizophrenia.

Endocrine and Metabolic Factors

As is well known, genetically determined conditions are manifested or are brought about by the control of chemical systems in the body by genes.

For many years research workers have been searching for the biochemical abnormality or abnormalities which are presumed to exist in schizophrenia.

The most striking finding is that of Gjessing on the rare type of schizophrenia named periodic catatonia, and these findings have been confirmed by other workers in other forms of recurrent schizophrenia.

Gjessing carried out painstaking studies on patients with periodic catatonia who, because of the development of attacks of stupor or excitement at a definite point in time with intervening periods of normality, were admirable for study as they could serve as their own controls. It was found that the onset of the abnormal phase, whether stupor or excitement, was correlated with changes in nitrogen metabolism. Furthermore, Gjessing found that if these patients were kept on a low protein diet and given adequate doses of thyroid, the nitrogen retention–excretion balance became normal and the patients remained symptom-free.

This provides a possible look into the future when the precise nature of biochemical abnormalities in schizophrenia, etc. may be discovered and when means may be found to control and correct these.

The fact that many of the hallucinogenic drugs, which produce syndromes somewhat similar to schizophrenia, contain an indole nucleus, led to the belief that an abnormal metabolite with an indole nucleus may be a factor in schizophrenia and a number of workers have recently isolated an indole fraction from schizophrenic patients' serum which, when transferred to another person, produced evidence of the disease. This work is still too recent for adequate evaluation.

Other investigators have shown that in schizophrenia the whole range of biochemical and endocrine functions tend to be outside, above or below, the normal range and that, with recovery, the endocrine status tends to return to normal limits.

At one time it was believed that gonadal atrophy was a feature of schizophrenia but nowadays this is usually found to be secondary to chronic disease and inanition, rather than a causative factor.

Dopaminergic Mechanism in Schizophrenia

The activation of adenylate cyclase by dopamine in the corpus striatum is inhibited by neuroleptics and this effect correlates highly with antipsychotic efficacy for a wide range of drugs. Although there is a high correlation between the blockade of dopamine receptors producing extrapyramidal side effects and their antipsychotic effect, this is by no means perfect. Some drugs such as thioridazine and clozapine have little in the way of extrapyramidal side effects but nevertheless are clinically efficacious in schizophrenia. These drugs, however, have a particular characteristic in that they have a high anticholinergic potency. In other words they have an inbuilt anti-parkinsonian activity. Taking this into account the relationship between dopamine antagonism and therapeutic efficacy becomes even more striking. In the corpus striatum, thioridazine and clozapine have relatively weak effects on dopaminergic transmission but this does not occur in the mesolimbic dopamine system (Nucleus Accumbens) where dopamine blockage correlates well with therapeutic efficacy.

Recent study has shown that only the alpha isomer of a thioxanthene neuroleptic, flupenthixol, is effective in treatment, and this isomer blocks the dopamine receptors, whereas the beta isomer, which is very much less potent as a dopamine antagonist, is no more effective than placebo.

There is considerable evidence which strongly indicates that the antagonism of dopamine receptors, particularly those located within the mesolimbic system and especially the sub group of receptors specifically labelled by butyrophenones, is most probably the critical element in diminishing schizophrenic symptoms. The fact that there is no evidence of increased dopamine turnover in post mortem studies of schizophrenic patients, even when they have been on long term medication, provides no evidence that the dopamine neurones are overactive in schizophrenia. On the other hand approximately 66% of patients with schizophrenia have an increase in the number of dopamine receptors in the brain. This has been shown by special receptor assay techniques. In fact the only change found consistently in the post mortem studies of the schizophrenic brain is an increase in the number of dopamine receptors. Whereas blockade of receptors occurs rapidly with neuroleptic drugs, the therapeutic effect clinically takes at least two weeks, suggesting that blockade of receptors may be necessary only to allow some other change to occur.

Early Mother–Child or Parent–Child Relationships

Some workers have claimed that maternal deprivation is more common in schizophrenics than in the general population and that faulty parental attitudes such as over-protection, rejection by the mother, broken homes, divorce of parents are more common in schizophrenia than in the general population.

It is possible that these influences are non-specific as they may be found in other disorders too, such as childhood asthma and, in any event, if the matter is to be studied only the parents of young schizophrenics can be investigated. Schizophrenia very frequently starts after the age of 30 and may even start in the 60s or 70s.

Social Class

There is an excess of schizophrenic patients in Social Class 5. Forty five per cent of the total number of schizophrenics come from Social Class 5 which has only 18.4% of the total population.

Recent work has shown that this correlation with social class is an effect of the illness rather than a cause. Late paraphrenia or paranoid schizophrenia has a high correlation with social isolation and physical factors.

Extrinsic Factors

A large number of extrinsic factors may serve to precipitate schizophrenia in a person so predisposed. Among these are:

1 Physical illnesses
2 Head injuries
3 Childbirth
4 Alcoholism
5 Social and environmental factors.

Social and environmental factors

A consistent finding of psychiatric epidemiology is the detection of a disproportionate number of schizophrenics in certain districts of large cities. This has been found in many parts of the world with schizophrenics being disproportionately high in the lower social classes.

At first this was believed to be a causal relationship, that is, a poor social circumstance either causes schizophrenia or favours its onset in the predisposed by exposing them to social isolation, economic deprivation, poor health care and education. However, most of the subsequent evidence has shown that the correlation is due to a drift downwards in the social scale as a consequence of the schizophrenic illness.

Current stress and family influences

There is now convincing evidence that current stresses can precipitate or exacerbate schizophrenic illnesses. Carefully controlled studies of successive admissions of acute schizophrenia reveal that schizophrenic patients experience a significantly higher frequency of stressful life events during the three weeks prior to the onset of their symptoms than did a matched group of non-schizophrenic controls. This was true even of independent events which could not have been caused by the patient becoming ill. Brown *et al.* found that the role of stressful life events in triggering the florid onset and reappearance of symptoms operated in those who were predisposed and were experiencing tense and difficult situations.

Hirsch and Leff attempted to replicate in Britain some of the results of Lidz *et al.* and Singer and Wynne in the USA. Their conclusion was that all that could be firmly said was that although families of schizophrenic patients showed greatly increased levels of conflict, distress and disharmony, there is no clear evidence for attributing a causal role to these processes.

These findings indicate the unfairness of blaming families for the development of schizophrenia and for the scapegoating and unsympathetic treatment given to the families of schizophrenics.

However, it is now known that environmental factors relating to the family can influence the course and clinical manifestations of both acute and chronic schizophrenia. For example Brown *et al.* provided convincing evidence that expressed criticism and critical attitudes within the family were often associated with the occurrence of acute relapses. Also the time spent in face to face contact with relatives is important, more than 35 hours a week was the cut off point identified as being indicative of an increased risk of relapse. This is a finding of considerable importance in the management of schizophrenia. Furthermore, another finding of importance in treatment was that those schizophrenics subjected to high levels of critical emotion were the ones that benefited most from neuroleptic drugs in preventing psychiatric crises. Vaughn and Leff independently confirmed these results. They found that 90% of patients diagnosed as suffering from schizophrenia going from hospital to homes with a high level of expressed emotion (EE) without protection from neuroleptic drugs, or controlled levels of face to face contact, would have an acute relapse within nine months, whereas only 50% of those either on medication or with limited levels of family contact did so. These findings indicate that schizophrenia is associated with increased vulnerability in which the mechanisms controlling the arousal of the subject are excessively influenced by external factors.

More recent work by Leff and Vaughn showed that factors governing the onset or relapse of schizophrenia were associated with either a high expressed emotion (EE) or with an independent life event which was potentially stressful, whereas in a depressive neurosis it was a combination of both critical expressed emotion and an independent life event which correlated with its onset.

Homogeneity versus Heterogeneity in Schizophrenia

We have seen that the evidence indicates that a multiplicity of causal factors operates in the causation of schizophrenia. These include genetic and constitutional attributes as predisposing causes and a number of environmental factors which act as precipitating causes. At present it is not possible to classify schizophrenia into subgroups on the basis of specific constellations of causative factors.

The spectrum of psychiatric disorders subsumed under the rubric schizophrenia suggests clinically there is heterogeneity rather than homogeneity. However, in treating schizophrenics we find that clinically similar patients may show quite different responses to specific treatments. It is probable that there are many different subtypes of schizophrenia with characteristic genetic, biochemical and constitutional substrata. At present we are unable to delineate such subtypes with certainty apart from the rare form of periodic catatonia studied so effectively by Gjessing.

It is hoped that further research will help to elucidate meaningful subtypes of schizophrenia which will enable the clinician to decide which treatment is likely to be most efficacious and thus result in even greater proportions of recovery than exist at present.

Conclusion

Schizophrenia is probably a genetically determined biochemical disorder which is influenced by other constitutional attributes. In other words, the genetic predisposition to schizophrenia may be influenced (1) by the genotypic milieu and (2) by the physical constitution of the person and other aspects of human constitution.

Environmental experiences may hinder or help to make the predisposition to schizophrenia; these include unfavourable early experiences, abnormal parental attitudes, physical illness, head injury, intoxications, loss of weight and various psychological stresses.

In other words, the essential cause of schizophrenia appears to be genetic and constitutional but a large variety of factors may act as sufficient causes which make the predisposition manifest in illness at a particular time in a person's life.

Diagnosis

Schneider has listed those symptoms which he regards as being of first rank importance in diagnosing schizophrenia and he claims that if a person with no relevant somatic disease experiences any of them, the diagnosis is schizophrenia.

Schneider's first rank symptoms are:

1 Certain types of auditory hallucinations, i.e. audible thoughts, voices heard arguing and voices giving a running commentary on the patient's actions.
2 Somatic passivity phenomena—the experience of influences playing on the body.

3 Thought withdrawal and other interferences with thought.
4 Diffusion of thought (or thought broadcasting) where the patient experiences his thoughts as being also thought by others.
5 Delusional perceptions.
6 All feelings, impulses (drives) and volitional acts that are experienced by the patient as the work or influence of others.

The diagnosis of schizophrenia depends on the recognition of the anomalies described above in the patient and their evaluation against the general background of the development of the illness and their relationship to other symptoms. In the matter of schizophrenic diagnosis, one swallow does not make a summer and the presence of isolated manifestations such as thought blockage, ideas of reference, in themselves would not necessarily indicate schizophrenia; but if they occur in a setting of a definite change in the patient's personality, in the form of increasing withdrawal and deterioration, their diagnostic significance is much greater.

Any marked change is probably of much greater importance than the presence or absence of a particular sign. Sudden change in religious persuasion or philosophical outlook without adequate preparation, or sudden increase of introversion, may also be danger signals. Patients may show lack of propriety and new fads or mannerisms, particularly if there is less firm contact with reality.

It is very important that schizophrenia be diagnosed in its early stages, before it becomes clearly apparent to medical or even lay people. Schizophrenia often occurs in people of introverted personality; the important things to look for are:

1 A change in this type of personality, which is one of the normal forms of personality, as shown by withdrawal, merging into apathy and blunting of affect.
2 Acute anxiety, panic and perplexity, particularly in unfamiliar surroundings.
3 Inappropriate emotional reactions:
   (a) an increasing tendency to dreaminess;
   (b) fleeting smiles, fatuous laughter; sometimes a knowing smile is highly characteristic.
4 A tendency to think concretely and to take things literally.
5 Increasing ideas of reference and persecution.

6 Revaluation of religious and political beliefs without due preparation.
7 Lack of propriety in behaviour, development of mannerisms.

It must be remembered that, in diagnosing schizophrenia, all these signs of abnormality are particularly important when they appear in the setting of a definite change in personality characterized by a falling off in efficiency, effectiveness and increasing withdrawal.

The Differential Diagnosis of Paranoid States

Although the term paranoid really refers to any form of delusion, by general usage it is now used in the sense of persecutory delusions. Apart from paranoid schizophrenia, paranoid delusions may occur in acute toxic confusional states, and are the product of perplexity, bewilderment, and clouding of consciousness in these states.

The following forms of paranoid states occur in a setting of clear consciousness.

1 *Paranoid personality* Some patients are always extremely sensitive, suspicious, mistrusting and querulous, and at times the mistrust may develop into delusions of persecution which may pass off when the stress of the situation improves. Others may gradually become more suspicious and may have paranoid delusions which are persistent or even permanent. Pathological jealousy is one form of paranoid development. These patients tend to show evidence of schizophrenic symptoms but their morbid jealousy is often persistent and often intractable to treatment.

2 *Paranoid delusions in depressive illness* Here the paranoid delusion is in keeping with the patient's mood and attitude to himself during his illness. The depressed patient tends to be self-depreciatory, to feel guilty, or to feel that he has committed sins and that he deserves to be persecuted or punished. In other words, the paranoid delusions are understandable in terms of the patient's mood and his prevailing attitude to himself.

3 *Hypomanic and manic states* Patients may become angry and suspicious of others who interfere with their plans or thwart them, but they do not usually develop persistent delusions of persecution.

4 *Alcoholic paranoid states* These may be acute or chronic and are regarded as being due to an underlying basis of schizophrenia.

5 *Organic states* with paranoid delusions include epilepsy, myxoedema, dementia and chronic intoxications with substances such as bromides. Acute paranoid states may occur with drugs such as amphetamines, lysergic acid and sometimes with large doses of marijuana.

Prognosis

Schizophrenia is a serious disease. A proportion of patients fail to recover, some only make a partial recovery but many patients can recover fully from attacks of schizophrenia.

The prognosis always has to be assessed in each case on its own merits. Follow-up studies on the outcome of schizophrenia indicate that certain features are helpful prognostic indicators. The following are favourable prognostic indicators:

1 An acute onset of illness
2 Precipitation by environmental or physical factors
3 Well-adjusted, stable previous personality
4 The presence of true affective components in the illness
5 A pyknic (eurymorphic) physique
6 A history of previous attacks from which the patient has made a complete recovery.

Features which indicate a poor prognosis are:

1 Long duration of illness, over two years
2 A gradual onset
3 An unstable, ill-adjusted previous personality
4 An early age of onset
5 Marked leptomorphic physique
6 Absence of clear precipitating factors.

Certain features are of little value such as:

1 Family history
2 Type of symptom.

Follow up studies on hospital patients over a 15 year period reveal that about a quarter of all cases end in severe deterioration, another quarter end showing a marked personality defect, a third quarter end in a mild personality defect and a fourth quarter recover completely, without any residual symptoms or defects. This does not include cases of schizophrenia who have not required admission to hospital and in these it is probable that the prognosis and outcome may be much better.

Treatment of Schizophrenia

General

Social and psychological treatments are important for patients cared for in hospital or in the community.

Hospital patients should be allocated to nurses and frequent discussion groups in the ward are desirable. An active daily regime is essential.

Work therapy and occupational therapy are important in promoting recovery and preventing deterioration.

Physical Methods of Treatment

Insulin coma therapy, which used to be the first line of treatment in schizophrenia, is now largely of historical interest as it has been superseded by the use of new psychotropic drugs.

Electroconvulsive therapy is useful for relieving depressive symptoms and many of the florid manifestations of schizophrenia.

The first drug to be used in the treatment of schizophrenia, in the new series of psychotropic drugs, was reserpine, but there were disadvantages in that it took many weeks to produce its beneficial effects, there were phases of turbulence and sometimes severe depression occurred as a side-effect.

Phenothiazine derivatives and other neuroleptic drugs have now taken pride of place in the drug treatment of schizophrenia. For the acute and disturbed schizophrenic patient, chlorpromazine or thioridazine are the phenothiazines of choice. For inert and apathetic schizophrenics, the piperazine derivatives are to be preferred. Pimozide, a new neuroleptic, is also effective in this type of schizophrenia. Depot preparations, such as fluphenazine enanthate or decanoate, flupenthixol or fluspirilene, have revolutionized the management of schizophrenia in the community. These preparations are given by injections at intervals of two to four weeks and are invaluable when patients are unreliable in taking drugs, or their relatives cannot be entrusted to see that the proper medication is given as prescribed. It is necessary to continue treatment with neuroleptic drugs for a prolonged period, up to two years or longer after the initial treatment.

Treatment with the phenothiazines can be supplemented with electroconvulsive therapy.

With regard to the rehabilitation of the patient after discharge from hospital, it has been found that some schizophrenic patients are unable to tolerate demanding or emotionally intense personal relationships and that some do better in lodgings or hostels than with near relatives.

Early diagnosis and prompt treatment with neuroleptics and, if necessary, supplemented with ECT appears to offer the best prospect for the control of schizophrenia.

The community should be provided with adequate resources and facilities to support the partially disabled schizophrenics in their midst.

Among other things, the general practitioner has to ensure that the patient remains on adequate doses of drugs until the symptoms show a true remission.

Further Reading

Fish, F. (1965) *Schizophrenia.* J. Wright, Bristol.

Forrest, A. and Affleck, J. (1975) *New Perspectives in Schizophrenia.* Churchill, London.

Bleuler, M. (1978) *Schizophrenic Disorders.* Yale University Press.

Wing, J. K. (ed) (1978) *Schizophrenia: Towards a New Synthesis.* Academic Press, London.

WHO. (1979) *Schizophrenia: An International Follow Up Study.* Wiley, Chichester.

Strauss, J. S. (1981) *Schizophrenia.* Plenum, New York.

26

Affective Disorders

Affective disorders are illnesses in which mood change is the primary and dominant feature.

The mood change is relatively fixed and persistent and is associated with characteristic changes in thinking, attitude and behaviour.

The main varieties of mood change are anxiety, depression and hypomania (and mania) and the corresponding disorders are termed anxiety state (anxiety neurosis), depressive state and hypomania (mania if severe).

A comparison of depression, anxiety and hypomania is given in Table 26.1.

Depressive Illness

Definition

A depressive illness is one in which the primary and dominant characteristic is a change in mood consisting of a feeling tone of sadness which may vary from mild despondency to the most abject despair. The change in mood is relatively fixed and persists over a period of days, weeks, months or years. Associated with the change in mood are characteristic changes in behaviour, attitude, thinking, efficiency and physiological functioning.

Depression, as a symptom, may occur in many psychiatric and physical illnesses and is a subsidiary or secondary part of the clinical picture. Depression can be a normal feeling and is characteristic of mourning and grief.

In distinguishing the normal reaction from pathological depression, a quantitative judgment has to be made. If the precipitant seems inadequate, the depression too severe and too long lasting, the condition is regarded as abnormal. In addition, the severity and incapacity in depressive illness differs qualitatively as well as quantitatively from depressed feelings which are a part of normal experience.

Depression in depressive illnesses affects the whole organism: feelings, energy, drive, thinking, bodily functions, personality and interests, and tends to influence every sphere of a person's life.

Appearance and General Behaviour

The patient's appearance provides valuable clues to the diagnosis. Appearance and behaviour will be influenced by the degrees with which anxiety and agitation are concomitant.

In depression with retardation the patient is slow in movements. He has a heavy, tired gait and shows a decrease in bodily movement. He has a rigid, immobile face; sometimes the facial expression may be distressed and sorrowful, reflecting anxiety or despair. Sometimes agitation occurs instead of retardation; the patient is restless, often constantly wringing his hands with an anxious, distressed facial expression.

Mood

The affect in depressive states may vary in intensity from a mild feeling tone of sadness to the most intense, distressing misery. Patients describe their subjective state in such terms as 'feeling ill', 'good for nothing', etc. Sometimes the patient has difficulty in expressing adequately the quality and intensity of his suffering.

Although every patient is aware of a feeling of dejection and sadness, few present this as their main symptom, particularly in the early stages of the illness. More usually they will present with physical

Table 26.1

Feature	Depression	Hypomania	Anxiety
Appearance	Pale, dejected posture. Muscular tone poor.	Looks well. Good complexion and posture.	Tense, strained face. Posture tense, movements awkward.
Speech activity	Under-active unless agitated.	Pressure of talk.	Rapid, high-pitched voice.
Motor activity	Reduced except when agitated.	Pressure of activity.	Restless, over-activity, inability to relax, poorly integrated.
Speed of thinking and decision-making.	Difficult to think and make decisions.	Rapid.	Mild anxiety facilitates. Marked anxiety hinders.
Mood	Sad.	Elated ± irritability.	Anxious, apprehensive, fearful.
Self-valuation	Depreciatory.	Over-values self, confident, even grandiose.	Uncertain, constantly needing reassurance.
Awareness. Response to outside stimuli.	Normal or decreased.	Alert and distractable.	Alert, irritable, jumpy.
Energy	Poor.	Conspicuous.	Fitful. Restless with sudden exhaustion.

symptoms such as lack of energy, bodily pains or loss of weight.

Output of Talk

This may vary from complete muteness to constant chattering. Often a tendency to reiteration and preoccupation with certain topics is a feature. Agitation and importunity are often associated with a greater output of talk.

Thinking

Patients complain of difficulty in thinking. They complain of inability to concentrate, difficulty in formulating their ideas and collecting their thoughts and making decisions.

Difficulty in thinking rather than slowness of thought is the characteristic feature of depressive illness, especially when thinking is directed to an end as in carrying out a particular intellectual task such as grasping and answering a question or deciding on a course of action or dealing with a problem. The end is either not attained or only achieved after a long period of effort.

Retardation

In some patients general slowness of motor activity is marked and in a minority it may be so severe that the patient is in a state of depressive stupor. In stupor, activity is reduced to a minimum and response to stimuli is diminished and facial expression is usually one of fixed despair.

Painful Thoughts

The depressed patient is self-concerned and, however much he dislikes it, he tends to be preoccupied with himself and his difficulties. His thoughts are invariably painful and usually centred around difficulties and liabilities. He is quite unable to count his blessings.

He may blame himself for errors of omission and commission and tends to be self-depreciatory and self-accusatory. He tends to magnify minor misdemeanours of the past and may magnify them to the extent of regarding them as unforgivable sins. He ruminates over his past and is filled with doubts about the correctness and morality of his actions.

Anxiety and Agitation

Some degree of anxiety is usually present. Severe anxiety associated with motor restlessness is termed agitation.

Loss of Interest

The patient finds that he has lost interest and enjoyment in his usual work and recreational activities. This may be a particularly striking change noticeable to the observer, especially in the early stages when other manifestations are not so obvious.

The loss of interest may apply to work, home, family, former hobbies and recreations and sometimes personal hygiene and appearance.

Derealization and Depersonalization

These feelings are often present; the patient complains that the environment appears different (derealization) or that he, himself, feels changed (depersonalization).

Hypochondriasis

Hypochondriacal preoccupation is common and varies in degree from mild concern with health on the one hand to delusions that he has diseases such as cancer, a sexually transmitted disease. The patient may also believe that certain organs and functions have stopped functioning or are absent (nihilistic delusions).

Disorders of Perception

Hallucinations are rare but when they occur are in keeping with the depressed mood. Illusions are not uncommon.

Sleep

Disturbance of sleep is characteristic of depression, early morning waking being the rule in endogenous depression and difficulty in getting off to sleep in milder depressive states associated with anxiety.

Loss of Appetite

This is very characteristic and sometimes weight loss may be dramatic, e.g. the patient may lose up to 12 kg in a matter of weeks.

Diurnal Variation

Most commonly the mood tends to be worse in the mornings. Occasionally patients feel worse towards the latter part of the day; this occurs especially if anxiety is a prominent part of the clinical picture.

Physical Symptoms and Signs

The patient may complain predominantly of physical symptoms such as headaches, vague bodily complaints such as pains, dyspepsia, tight feelings in the chest, giddiness, constipation, urinary frequency, palpitations, dyspnoea, blurred vision, dryness of the mouth and paraesthesiae. In women menstrual functions become disturbed and there may be amenorrhoea. Libido is diminished or lost.

Dexamethasone suppression test

Dexamethasone, which suppresses cortisol levels in the blood, has been found to be abnormal in this respect in depressive patients. The test consists of giving 1 mg of dexamethasone at 2000 hours, and blood samples are taken between 1500 and 1600 hours the following day for the estimation of cortisol. About 70% of depressed patients show an abnormal DST, compared with 11% controls.

However, the test is not specific for depression and abnormal responses occur in a proportion of schizophrenics, abstinent alcoholics, neurotics and patients undergoing prophylactic lithium therapy.

It has been found that a reduction of plasmacortisol below a concentration of 100 nd per ml responded significantly better to antidepressants and ECT.

The tyramine challenge test

The tyramine challenge test consists of giving 125 mg of tyramine hydrochloride (equivalent to 100 mg of tyramine) orally at 0900 hours, immediately after voiding the bladder, and collecting a complete urine sample during the three hour period following the ingestion of tyramine.

Depressed patients excrete significantly lower amounts of urinary tyramine as sulphate following oral administration of tyramine hydrochloride compared with normal subjects.

The test appears to be a reliable trait marker for depression.

Prevalence and Aetiology

Between 35 and 40% of all psychiatric illnesses which come to medical notice are depressive. This was found in inpatient surveys in England and Wales and in surveys of various general practices.

Depressive illnesses are of great social and medical importance in view of their frequency as causes of morbidity, distress, disability and sometimes mortality.

The life time expectancy for developing an attack of depression is between 20% and 30% but only 10%–25% of persons with depression seek professional help or advice.

The life time expectancy for a manic depressive (bipolar affective) disorder is 1–2%. Fifteen per cent of depressive illnesses run a chronic course.

Depression is twice as common in females as in males. Age is the important factor regarding the onset of the first attack of depression. The onset increases towards middle age with a maximum onset in the 55–60 age group. It is quite different from schizophrenia where the rate of onset is highest in the 20–30 age group.

In the lowest social class (Social Class 5, unskilled workers) the rate for depressive illness is about double that in other social classes.

The incidence in first degree relatives of a patient who has a depression is about 12% compared with 1% in the general population.

There is strong evidence that the two forms of manic depressive disorder, i.e., bipolar with recurrent depression and mania and unipolar recurrent depressive illnesses, are genetically different. The morbidity risk among relatives of patients with bipolar affective disorders is considerably higher than that of relatives of patients with unipolar recurrent depressive illnesses. The types of genetic transmission in affective disorders have not yet been fully elucidated, whether dominant, recessive, autosomal or sex linked.

Depressive illnesses are the resultant of the interaction of genetic and constitutional factors on one hand with environmental and other exogenous influences on the other. Those depressive illnesses which are predominantly determined by genetic-constitutional factors are usually referred to as endogenous depressions and are characterized by a typical diurnal variation, being worse in the morning and tending to improve later in the day, and an onset which may occur independently of adverse environmental circumstances. Depressive illnesses which are predominantly a reaction to environmental influences are referred to as reactive depressions and are usually less severe and often fluctuate in severity according to external circumstances.

In a large number of depressive illnesses, however, both endogenous and environmental factors are present. In clinical practice an infinite variety of combinations of these factors are found as shown diagrammatically in Fig. 26.1.

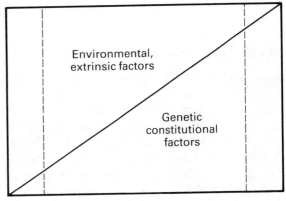

Figure 26.1 *Possible combinations of endogenous and exogenous factors in depressive states.*

Involutional Melancholia (syn. Involutional Depression)

This term is applied to severe psychiatric illnesses which are depressive but often with paranoid and hypochondriacal components, occurring for the first time in the involutional period, i.e. roughly between 45 and 65 years. The personality of patients before the illness is usually characterized by rigidity, ambitiousness, drive, perfectionism, high standards and exaggerated concern with health.

Hypochondriacal ideas are frequent and they vary from concern about health and the decline in physical strength and dexterity, which is common at this time of life, on one extreme, to delusions of a nihilistic and bizarre kind—for example, that the intestines are missing and that the head is empty.

Anxiety, tension and restlessness are common. Disorders of perception are present in the form of illusions which, when they occur, are in keeping with the anxious affect. Hallucinations may also occur but are infrequent; they are often tactile, especially genital in women. Auditory hallucinations can occur but are rare.

Grief Reactions

Grief is a normal reaction to the loss of a loved person, such as a close relative or friend, especially a person who has occupied a key position in the emotional life of the bereft person.

Grief reactions may also occur in response to the loss of a pet and sometimes material things, valuables or even loss of status or reputation.

Normal Grief Reactions

Acute grief reactions in response to the death of a key person, such as a spouse or close relative, constitute a definite syndrome with both physical and psychological manifestations which may appear immediately after bereavement or may be delayed, exaggerated or apparently absent. Immediately following the loss, there may be a period of failure to realize fully that the death has occurred. This can last for a few hours to as long as two weeks and during this time, the bereaved person may experience no distress. Others experience a sense of numbness and inability to appreciate any emotional reactions.

With the realization of the extent of the loss, the full grief reaction appears and is characterized by a variety of mental and bodily changes. These manifestations often decline after two to six weeks and are minimal by six months. However, a proportion of mourners continue to grieve for long periods of time.

The physical distress suffered during grief reactions includes feelings of tightness in the throat, choking feelings, breathlessness, sighing and an empty feeling in the abdomen accompanied by feelings of intense emotional distress. These mani-

festations come on in waves lasting from twenty minutes to half an hour.

Behavioural Changes

A person in a state of grief is often restless and the usual pattern of conduct tends to be disrupted. He may withdraw from social contact and carry out activities aimed at keeping alive the memories of the deceased. Restlessness and continuous aimless movement may persist for as long as a month.

Although many feel an impulse to wander away from home to escape distressing memories and, although revival of memories tends to increase the grief reaction, many mourners seem to be drawn towards the environment associated with the deceased.

Some persons during a grief reaction have the feeling that the dead person is present and they talk to him or otherwise behave as if he were present. It is not uncommon for the bereaved person to forget the loss without realizing it, e.g. will prepare and set the table for tea for the spouse who has been dead for some time.

Another feature of grief reaction is the tendency to search and to look for the deceased person.

Preoccupation with Memories or Image of the Deceased

A very characteristic feature of grief reaction is a preoccupation with the image and memory of the deceased person. This is particularly so during the early months of the grief reaction. The preoccupation with the deceased tends to dominate the thoughts and there is a tendency to idealize the lost person and to overlook his faults.

Emotional Distress

Depression with or without crying, loss of interest in work or leisure, insomnia, anorexia, fatigue, self-neglect, apathy, attacks of panic, guilt feelings and suicidal ideas are frequent features of grief and are aggravated by reminders of the loss. Guilt feelings are common and are accompanied by self-blame for what are considered to be errors of omission or commission. Suicidal thoughts and attempts are a risk in some severely depressed patients.

Disturbance of Perception

Some persons in a grief reaction experience abnormalities of perception which are understandable in the light of their preoccupation with the deceased person. Illusions are frequent—for example, a person in a state of grief hears ill-defined sounds in the house and interprets them as the dead person's footsteps; people in crowds in the street are fleetingly mis-identified as the deceased person.

Sometimes auditory or visual hallucinations occur. These hallucinatory phenomena, which may be visual or auditory and relate to the deceased person, are really pseudo-hallucinations as the person realizes that they have no basis in reality and they are often more comforting than frightening, but they may cause the person who experiences them to fear that he is becoming mentally unbalanced.

Identification

Sometimes a person in a state of grief will take on the personality attributes or even the symptoms experienced by the deceased person in his terminal illness.

Hostility

Intense feelings of hostility may be experienced during a grief reaction. Hostility may be felt towards members of the family, the medical profession, the clergy, hospital authorities, God, etc. Hostility may also show itself as feelings of irritability, resentment and bitterness, with a loss of normal compassion for the sufferings of others and a pervasive feeling of the injustice of their loss.

Atypical and Morbid Grief Reactions

Typical grief reactions occurring as normal phenomena last for less than six months and are usually not of such severity that the mourner stays away from work for longer than two weeks or attempts suicide or isolates himself to such an extent that he is inaccessible to relatives or friends or needs to be referred to a psychiatrist.

Morbid grief reactions may represent distortions of normal grief reactions, for example, a grief reaction may be delayed for months or even for many years. Thus, over-activity may be very marked without any sense of loss. The acquisition of symptoms of the deceased person's illness may be so severe and persistent as to necessitate psychiatric treatment. The feelings of hostility again may be so marked as to disturb interpersonal relationships.

Atypical grief reactions are more common if there is a long delay following the bereavement before grief is experienced. Persistent difficulty in accepting the loss and feelings of guilt and marked hostility are also common features of atypical grief reactions. Certain conditions to which the person is constitutionally predisposed may appear for the first time during the grief reaction, for example, various psychosomatic disorders such as asthma, vasomotor rhinitis, urticaria, migraine, ulcerative colitis etc. A severe agitated depression may be precipitated by bereavement.

Morbidity and Mortality Following Bereavement

There is evidence that bereavement is associated with an increased morbidity risk for psychiatric, psychosomatic and even physical illnesses. There is also evidence that during the second and third years after bereavement, there is a somewhat higher death rate than expected. The mortality rate is higher among males than females and greater among those who had lost a spouse than among other relatives of the deceased. The greatest mortality risk is observed among widowers of whom some one-fifth die in the first year compared with 4% of controls.

Management of Grief Reactions

The duration of the grief reaction will, in part, depend on how successfully the person is able to work through the grief reaction. The grief work involves obtaining freedom from the bonds which tie and imprison the bereft person to the deceased person, and the achievement of readjustment to the environment and the formation of new relationships. Grief is distressing and painful and the patient will do anything to avoid getting emotionally upset and, erroneously, may be encouraged to hide his feelings by his friends or even by his medical advisers. This advice is wrong and tends to prolong the duration of the grief reaction. It is essential for the person to face the fact of bereavement and its discomfort and to deal in memory with the deceased person by discussing the loss with friends, relatives or the physician; this produces relief of distress.

Morbid grief reactions are treated by transference to normal grief reactions which are then more readily resolved.

Care of the Dying Patient

Doctors and others are often uncertain what to say and how to deal with the dying patient. Very often what the dying patient dreads is pain, distress and the inevitable desertion of their responsibilities rather than extinction of life itself. Many dying patients suffer anxiety, depression and other emotional distress which can be relieved by appropriate medication. The important thing is for the doctor to allow and encourage the patient to talk and unburden himself without knowing in advance what answers to give the patient. He should be sensitive to the patient's needs and be led rather than lead. He will then discover what an incurable condition and 'going to die' means to the individual patient, what his personality is like and what he is ready to be told.

Prognosis in Depressive Illness

Prognosis may be considered for the attack and for recurrence.

Prognosis depends on:

1 the inherited predisposition and the evidences of it in constitution and personality
2 the experiences which have moulded the patient and to which he is still exposed and responsive
3 the tendency of an emotional reaction to subside or to continue.

Prognosis therefore depends on heredity, on the environment and on the biological form of the illness.

With regard to heredity, the chances of complete recovery from an attack will be good where a typical affective illness, periodic or solitary, has occurred in one or more of the patient's antecedents. If the patient has always been maladjusted, an attack of depression will increase his difficulties of adjustment and when he recovers from it he will still remain a maladjusted person. Recovery here is, therefore, a qualified one.

If psychological stresses on careful evaluation are important, this may be of some help in prognosis if they can be remedied or are unlikely to recur. Severe depressive illnesses usually subside; mild emotional states tend to persist autonomously.

The most satisfactory outcome occurs when the onset is abrupt, the clinical features are typical of classical depression and the previous personality was healthy and well adjusted or when there is a history of defined previous affective attacks without physical disease. Gross hypochondriacal ideas, nihilistic delusions and admixture of schizophrenic or other anomalous symptoms are unfavourable prognostic indicators.

In fairly well-diagnosed and clear-cut depressive illnesses, it is probable that 95% will recover, 1% will commit suicide and 4% will remain in a state of chronic illness.

Depressive illness in general tends to be self-limiting with a natural tendency to recovery.

Suicide

Suicide is as ancient as man himself and throughout the whole of recorded history, there are references to the act of self-destruction.

Society has viewed suicide from one extreme of outright condemnation to the other extreme of veneration and incorporation into the social cultural system.

Attempted suicide or parasuicide may be defined as an act of self-damage carried out with destructive intent however vague or ambiguous. Both suicide and attempted suicide are symptoms and not diagnoses in their own right. The most common illness in both successful and attempted suicide is depressive illness.

In a series of cases of successful suicide, depressive illnesses were found to constitute 72%, alcoholism 13%, schizophrenia 3%, other psychiatric disorders 5% and no mental illness 7%. In attempted suicide, depressive illnesses account for 50% to 60%. Schizophrenia was found to contribute less than 5% to suicidal attempts. Personality disorders form a considerable proportion of attempted suicides, various observers reporting from 15% to 45%, the suicidal attempt being seen as one of many recurrent episodes of unpredictable and abnormal behaviour in the life history of the person.

Many patients with personality disorders are alcoholics or are drug dependent and there is a positive correlation between alcoholism and drug dependence, and attempted suicide and successful suicide. A small group of people who successfully commit suicide and those who attempt suicide exhibit little or no psychiatric abnormality. In these cases, it is considered that the underlying pathology is social rather than psychogenic. It is important to realize that in clinical practice the aetiology of suicide is multifactorial with personality attributes, social factors and psychiatric disorder producing cumulative effects.

It is commonly believed that people who fail in their suicidal attempts have not really intended to kill themselves and that they are at no extra risk of suicide in the future. This is untrue and people who make one suicide attempt have a significantly higher suicide rate than average.

The degree of intent associated with a suicidal attempt ranges from those who act on impulse with no real wish to die, to those who seriously hope for a fatal outcome. In between, there are people whose attitude to death is more ambivalent and who acted in a mood of depressive indifference as to whether they lived or died. Impulsive acts of less serious intent tend to be the pattern with patients with personality disorders, while premeditated attempts with a strong wish to die are found in endogenous depressive illnesses. Serious, determined suicidal attempts are correlated with males and higher age, whereas suicidal gestures tend to be associated with females and younger age groups. Successful suicide is more common in men than women and reaches its peak incidence in later life.

Another dangerous belief is that those who threaten suicide do not carry it out. It has been found that between 70% and 80% of successful suicides had communicated their suicidal intent which had been ignored.

The methods used in suicidal attempts in general differ from those in fatal suicide acts. Fatal suicide acts are more violent in their form than those used in the non-fatal act—for example jumping from tall buildings or onto railway tracks, hanging, drowning, cutting or shooting.

In attempted suicide, drug overdosage is the commonest method employed. In both suicides and attempted suicides, more women than men take drug overdoses, whilst more violent methods are favoured by men.

High Risk Groups

A number of high risk groups can be identified according to several criteria including age, social class, profession, state of mental and physical health, alcohol and drug intake.

The elderly are a group at excess suicidal risk, elderly men being particularly vulnerable. Retirement from work as well as reducing social contacts and loss of earnings, or decrease in earnings, means loss of status in the eyes of the community and a loss of purpose in the individual which may lead to feelings of uselessness and depression. In addition, ill health, decrease in mental and physical ability, will further increase the problems associated with the elderly. Physical ill health is an important precipitating event in cases of attempted suicide and suicide.

Social Factors

Various studies have shown that the incidence of suicide depends on the extent to which people are integrated with society and controlled by it. If its members share the norms and values of the society, they are protected against suicide and conversely, a loss of domestic, occupational and religious ties promotes it.

The socially isolated are demonstrably more prone to suicide. A large series of studies of the suicide rates of immigrants demonstrate that they are all higher than the rates of their countries of origin. It has also been shown that there are many more suicides in persons who have recently moved house. Moving house, particularly in middle aged or elderly people, tends to isolate insofar as there are fewer links with their family and with their neighbourhood.

Both attempted suicide and suicide are common in communities where rapid social and population changes are taking place. Urban rates are higher than those of rural areas, partly because those who move to cities from country areas tend to be more restless and unstable people in general. The main factor is probably social isolation, and certain groups are more likely to be isolated, and therefore more suicide prone. These include divorced persons and widows and widowers.

Social class and profession is positively correlated with suicide. The professional, administrative and executive classes have a higher suicide rate than those in skilled or partly skilled occupations, whereas the unskilled have a suicide rate intermediate between these two groups, apart from those over 65 years of age who have the highest suicide rate of all. Doctors, dentists and university students have suicide rates far exceeding those of the corresponding age groups in the general population.

Personal crises may be important precipitants of suicidal attempts. Recent bereavement has been found to be the most prominent precipitating stress. Bereavement may lead to depressive states and as a part of a grief reaction, it may result in moving house; this illustrates interaction of psychiatric disorders, social isolation and psychosocial stress in suicide. Suicidal attempts have often been made in the course of acute interpersonal conflicts, for example, married women who have made a suicidal attempt after an acute domestic quarrel occurring in a chronically poor marital situation. Some suicidal attempts are an appeal for help by a person in a desperate situation. These are largely people with some instability of personality who find themselves in an intolerable personal crisis or conflict. In some of these instances, the suicidal attempt may in fact turn out to be fatal.

Interaction of Factors in Suicide

One may consider three important factors in determining suicidal attempts and suicide:

1 psychological predisposition
2 social predisposition
3 personal crises and stressful events.

Psychological predispositions can be clearly identified according to leading authorities in some 90% of suicides. Not all depressive illnesses result in suicide and it is possible that other factors, including personality attributes as well as social factors, may contribute to suicide. For example, the correlation between moving house and suicide may be associated, particularly in people who have moved house more than once which may be associated with an unstable or very social personality. Similarly, frequent previous suicidal attempts, alcoholism and conflicts with the law all attest to personality instability.

Social predisposition and social isolation are particularly important. Moving house diminishes the

person's bond with his family, neighbours and work mates.

Among personal crises and stresses which are important are bereavement, money and legal problems, and illness in the family.

In summary, one can say that in comparison with their fellow men and women, suicides have fewer family and domestic responsibilities, obtain less support from their occupational group and are more often strangers in their neighbourhood. Exclusion from membership of social groups predisposes to a suicide. Mental disorder, notably depressive illness, is a major determinant.

Suicide can best be understood as an interaction of a person's psychological attributes, his social stresses, particularly the degree to which he is isolated, and his capacity to cope with adversity and life's stresses.

Unusual Aspects of Depression

It has been stated that depressive illness is the most frequently missed diagnosis in the whole of medicine. The reason for this is that depression does not always present itself in the classical form with which we are familiar. It may appear in a variety of different forms and is almost protean in its clinical manifestations. The presenting complaints can be a variety of physical symptoms and it may take unusual forms which are referred to as atypical depression. Another reason is that the patient may not complain to the doctor in a way which provides clues about the underlying disorder, e.g. he may not tell the doctor 'I feel depressed or unhappy' but he will tell him that he feels unwell, that he is easily tired, that he has lost interest or that he is unable to concentrate and he may focus his complaints on bodily symptoms which may mislead the physician if this is the main or presenting clinical feature. Sometimes patients do not recognize, acknowledge or communicate the fact that they have a lowering of mood.

Classification

The time honoured dichotomous classification of depression into neurotic versus psychotic or reactive versus endogenous is of limited value for research and indeed for clinical practice. A more useful classiication is to divide affective disorders into two groups:

1 *Primary affective disorders* which are divisible into unipolar and bipolar varieties. These two main sub-groups of primary affective disorders differ in gen-tical predisposition, age and sex distribution, in biochemical and physiological attributes and some-imes in response to treatment.

2 *Secondary affective disorders* Depression may be secondary to other psychiatric illnesses or may be associated with various physical disorders and causes.

a) *Schizophrenia* Depression often occurs in schizophrenia and this sometimes leads to errors in diagnosis. It may usher in the schizophrenic illness and be the main part of the clinical picture before typical schizophrenic symptoms become apparent. This often occurs in post partum schizophrenia.

Depression may exist concurrently with clear cut schizophrenic symptoms, when it is designated a schizo-affective disorder. Depression may constitute a part of natural history of schizophrenia, particularly when recovery is taking place and the patient is developing insight into the nature of the illness from which he is recovering. This is probably the most frequent basis for depression in recovery from schizophrenia but occasionally depression may be induced pharmacologically by long acting neuroleptics such as the phenothiazine and butyrophenone varieties.

b) *Dementia* Depression may form a significant part of the clinical picture in patients suffering from dementia. Pre-senile dementia, particularly the Alzheimer's variety, may be ushered in by depression and it is only later when the intellectual and cognitive deficits become apparent that the true diagnosis is made.

Depressive illnesses may present a clinical picture very similar to dementia and it is a very important diagnostic exercise to ascertain whether the apparent dementia which occurs in an old person who is depressed is in fact entirely or mainly due to the depressive illness and not to an underlying organic dementing process.

Physical Disorders

Depression can occur in any medical or surgical illness as a reaction to the threat inherent in the illness or to the associated disability, pain and distress.

In coronary care units a common sequence of events is that patients at first are relieved or even elated to realize that they have escaped a life threatening attack. Some patients may even be mildly hypomanic. This, however, is usually short lived and is followed by anxiety as the patient faces the reality of his situation and its inherent threat. In the third phase there is usually depression which can be severe and may constitute a greater source of disability and distress than the myocardial lesion itself.

Depression may form a major part of a patient's symptoms in neoplastic disease and in any terminal illness. Depression may follow infections, especially viral, and may persist for weeks or months after the initial infective stage has passed.

Depression may commonly occur with endocrine disorders, such as Cushing's syndrome and many patients are depressed with high blood cortisol level.

Hypothyroidism is frequently associated with depression, which may also occur with thyrotoxicosis and nutritional deficiency. Lack of the vitamin B complex especially can produce a classical picture of depression.

Similarly depression may occur in multiple sclerosis. Some, but not all, patients with anorexia nervosa and bulimia nervosa may suffer from an underlying or accompanying depression. Severe depression may be brought about by drugs. Reserpine is notorious in this respect and can induce a severe depression with suicidal tendencies and may need ECT for its resolution.

Other antihypertensive drugs such as methyldopa and the beta blockers can also cause depression.

Childhood Depression

At one time depressive illnesses were thought to contribute little to child psychiatry. However, research and clinical observation in recent years have revealed that depression is not uncommon in children but it may show itself in a variety of ways which are not obviously due to an underlying depression.

Depression may be manifested in behavioural disorders such as rebelliousness, aggressiveness, truancy and stealing. Depression may interfere with scholastic performance and achievement and it may result in school refusal. It may be manifested by the appearance of nocturnal enuresis or encopresis or other physical symptoms such as loss of appetite and weight.

Adolescence

A depressive illness during adolescence often shows itself by 'acting out' behaviour of an anti-social or rebellious kind. Sometimes it may take the form of risk-taking behaviour which may reach dangerous proportions. This may apply to motor vehicle driving, excessive alcohol consumption and drug abuse.

Depression in Middle Age

There is an increased risk of developing endogenous as well as other forms of depression during middle age. This is a time in life when mental and physical abilities are beginning to decline and these become the focus of complaints and patients can often become very concerned about their bodily functions. Many of the presenting symptoms are somatic and hypochondriacal preoccupation is characteristic.

Depression in Old Age

Depression in old age tends to feature hypochondriacal symptoms and preoccupations. It may also manifest itself as a 'pseudodementia' because difficulty in remembering, concentration and thinking is quite common in depression. It is very important to attempt to determine whether the apparent dementia is due, or could be due, to depression because this is eminently treatable. Psychometric tests are usually not helpful in distinguishing the memory and intellectual difficulties associated with depression from those due to dementia.

Varieties of Depression

Anxious Depression

A number of research workers have found that the presence of marked anxiety in a depressed patient may provide a useful way of identifying a group of

depressions with a predictable treatment response. Patients with anxious depression, usually middle aged with high scores of psychic and somatic anxiety, depersonalization, obsessional symptoms and fatigue, are also moderately or severely depressed.

Anxiety must be distinguished from agitation that is motor restlessness. Agitation tends to occur most frequently in severe depressives.

Atypical Depression

A group of atypical depressions was described by West and Dally (1959) which responded to monoamine oxidase inhibitors. They showed a syndrome including a long illness, phobic and generalized anxiety, fatigue, evening worsening, hysterical symptoms, absence of self-reproach, morning worsening and early wakening and sometimes an impression of life-long inadequate personality although on close examination the pre-morbid personality is not found to be neurotic.

The second variety of atypical depression was described by Pollitt in 1965 in which the patient shows a reversed functional shift, e.g. depression is worse in the evening, insomnia is of the early rather than the late kind or there is increased sleep, increased appetite and weight. All of these are in the opposite direction to the physiological changes said to characterize endogenous depression.

The third meaning of atypical depression is that of non-endogenous depression in general which carries a wider meaning than that usually applied to a specific subgroup.

Another variety has been termed the hysteroid dysphoric depression in which the mood fluctuates widely, the patient shows hysterical tendencies and can react markedly to any emotional upset with sudden depression, pallor and striking changes in physical appearance.

There are many varieties of atypical depression and the important thing is to describe and define the main features outlined above.

There is evidence that the monoamine oxidase inhibitors are of value in anxious depressed patients and in the above forms of atypical depression, but it should be pointed out that tricyclic and other antidepressants in other patients are also effective in relieving anxiety and depression.

Masked Depression

This term is applied when the underlying depressive illness is masked, usually by physical symptoms of various kinds. They may be bodily pains, atypical facial pains, atypical bodily pains, sometimes pains affecting regions of the body such as the forequarter, the hindquarter or the upper half. This is quite different from neurological anaesthesia and also from typical hysterical anaesthesia.

The patient may present with a weight loss as a predominant feature associated with other bodily symptoms of depression. The term 'masked depression' really means a missed depression and the clinician should always look for underlying features indicative of depression behind the physical presenting symptoms.

Depressive Equivalent

This term is applied to disorders, usually physical, which have a reciprocal relationship with depressive illnesses. A patient may exhibit clear cut depression at one time and later, on recovery from depression, develops a physical disorder which when resolved is replaced by depression. It has been reported that in some patients, meralgia parasthetica, which is a condition affecting the lateral cutaneous nerve of the thigh, may exhibit a reciprocal relationship with depression. Similar reciprocal relationships have been described in psychosomatic disorders such as asthma, urticaria and vasomotor rhinitis: when the psychiatric disorder (depression) is present, the psychosomatic disorder is in abeyance and vice versa.

This reciprocal relationship between depression and affective disorders and psychosomatic disorders occurs in a small number of patients, but in the large majority psychiatric and psychosomatic disorders tend to vary concurrently in the same direction rather than exhibiting a reciprocal relationship.

Grief Reactions

Grief reactions occur not only in response to the loss of a key person, that is a person who has shared a very important emotional relationship with the bereaved person, but can also occur with the loss of a pet or the loss of a limb. The manifestations of grief reactions often lead to errors in diagnosis.

A typical grief reaction is fairly easy to diagnose and normally follows the bereavement fairly quickly. It is accompanied by waves of distress and self blame for errors of omission or commission the person believes he has committed. Self blame and identification occur in normal grief reactions. The grief reaction may be pathological or morbid if it is unduly delayed or very severe. Any of the manifestations which occur in normal grief reaction may be greatly intensified and may lead to difficulties in diagnosis. For example, it is quite normal during grief to feel angry with fate, with God, with religion, with the medical profession or hospitals, to feel anger, resentment and hostility because a loved one on whom the person strongly depended for support has been lost. Prolonged and severe hostility may be the predominant feature in some grief reactions which may persist in severe form for many months or even years. Similarly, identification with the dead person may be very marked and persistent. This often leads to medical investigations with no evidence of organic disease and because of the time interval between the death and the development of the symptoms, doctors do not always realize that there could be a link between them. Also certain symptoms can be misleading, e.g. pseudo-hallucinations. The bereft person hears the deceased person talking to them or sees them in shadows or whenever the stimuli are ambiguous. These are not true hallucinations because although the voices can be heard, the person realizes they do not exist in reality and this is why they are termed pseudo-hallucinations. The person may engage in searching activity, persistently looking for the dead person hoping he or she is there. All these can be understood as part of a grief reaction in which the person is trying to regain a person they loved by incorporating their symptoms or mannerisms, hearing them talking or seeing them or continually looking for them. Sometimes a grief reaction may precipitate a typical endogenous depression, just as a variety of psychosomatic disorders may have their onset and association with bereavement.

Anxiety and Depression

Both anxiety states and depressive illnesses are common. The life time expectancy for a depressive illness is between 8 and 20%. For the bipolar variety it is about 2% but in a survey of women in South London George Brown found it was very much more prevalent. These are depressions of mild severity in which the patient probably does not consult a doctor.

When anxiety and depression occur together it is important to be able ascertain whether it is really a depressive illness with anxiety symptoms or whether it is an anxiety state. Many features are common to both anxiety and depression such as autonomic symptoms like palpitations, sweating and tremors. The distinguishing features are those which occur exclusively in a depressive illness. A marked persistent severe loss of interest or loss of energy is indicative of depression. Anxiety states usually are associated with adequate energy and with a sudden development of exhaustion, but persistent fatigue or lack of energy is typical of depression.

Depression can cause a decrease in sexual desire and libido. Anxiety does not affect sex drive; in men it may affect erectile potency or may cause premature ejaculation. In women it may cause dyspareunia or vaginismus. Anxiety can cause sexual difficulties but if the main problem is a decrease or extinction of the sex drive this is indicative of depression. If there is a marked loss of weight, this is also more in keeping with depression.

In many textbooks, features which are used to distinguish depressive illnesses from anxiety states include markers of severe depression such as guilt feelings, retardation, suicidal thoughts, preparations or attempts. In clinical practice there is no problem in diagnosis if the patient exhibits these symptoms, but in mild cases of depression they might not be obvious. For example if the patient is asked, 'Do you ever feel life is not worth living?' he might admit that he often does. He may have considered what preparations to make for suicide or he may have made attempts. This occurs in the more severe depressions. In the milder depressions he may state that he often feels that life is hardly worth it and would not mind very much if he did not wake in the morning or if he were knocked over by a car and killed. In other words it is a form of passiveness which is indicative of the depression. Similarly guilt feelings may not be obvious in the milder depressions but may take the form of self depreciation, feeling unworthy or unloved and somehow that the patient is to blame for his problems, including his illness. This does not amount to a delusion of guilt but it is a mild form of self depreciation.

Common features of depression are finding every thing difficult, even everyday tasks; difficulty in con centration, even with reading the newspaper or watching the television. The diagnostic decision or whether the illness is primarily a depressive illness or an anxiety state is important because treatment is different.

In the treatment of anxiety, the range of anti-anxiety compounds includes the benzodiazepines small doses of neuroleptics and beta-blockers, all of which may provide some relief in anxiety but will not help a depressive illness. Beta-blockers may make it worse. With the criteria described, it should be possible to come to a decision about the illness but sometimes in clinical practice this is very difficult and if uncertain, the clinician should give the benefit of the doubt to depression and treat with anti-depressants as this is more likely to help the patient. If the patient appears clinically to be suffering from an anxiety state but actually there is an underlying depression, the benzodiazepines, neuroleptics and beta-blockers will not help but antidepressants will.

Principles of Management

One must constantly keep in mind that depressive illness causes disability and suffering.

The degree of disability will depend on the severity of the depression and persons with the greatest drive, productivity and creativeness may become completely ineffective during a depressive illness. Such effects are temporary, the patient reverting to his normal state with recovery from his illness.

It is important for the patient to accept the fact that depression does impose great difficulties in coping with everyday tasks and it is better for him to accept this rather than to make desperate efforts to carry on despite his symptoms, as this increases his burden because of the resulting frustration, anxiety and disappointment. He should be encouraged to do what he finds he is able to do during his illness but exhortations that he should pull himself together are absurd, the patient himself realizing that if this were possible he would be the first person to do so.

It is important for those dealing with depressive illnesses to be friendly, to show interest and to give support. This is helpful in all types of depression. In severe depressions the effects of this may not be noticeable; nevertheless, it is important in all depressions and is appreciated by the patient and he will remember it with gratitude later.

It is important not to urge patients to try to undertake normal responsibilities, particularly when they are severely depressed, as they are quite unable to do so at that stage. As they improve they will automatically find it easier to do things. This is the time when encouragement, if needed, will help the patient to return to normal activities, to work and social pursuits.

The general practitioner should also realize the importance of keeping the family informed about the nature of the illness so that they can be more understanding and not add to the patient's burden and frustration. Depressive illnesses, as they affect a person's warmth in his relationships and sometimes bring out the worst traits in his personality, are treated with great intolerance by the family, which does not provide the conditions conducive to the patient's improvement and rehabilitation.

If the depression is sufficiently severe to prevent him from working, this usually indicates that the illness is at least of moderate severity and may be severe. This criterion indicates the need for some active medical treatment.

The severity of the illness as well as the possible risk of suicide, social factors such as home conditions and the ability of the family to look after the patient, will influence the decision whether a patient ought to be treated in hospital or not. Severely depressed patients, particularly those with suicidal pre-occupations or intentions should, of course, be treated in hospital.

A further important point in management is to be able to assess the importance of what the patients say. They will often tell you that 'I am depressed because I foolishly did this or that when I was a child or in my teens' or they attribute the depression to something more recent which they feel guilty about; or they may say that they are depressed because of pressure of work or the attitude of their superiors or the attitude of their family, or that they find the work too much for them. All these, in fact, may be symptoms of depression and the things they believe have brought on the illness may be just the effects of the illness rather than the cause.

Another mistake, which is unfortunately only too frequently carried out, is to advise a severely depressed patient to take a cruise or a holiday, as this usually not only has no beneficial results but also the illness prevents him enjoying himself wherever he is. If a patient says that he feels that life is not worth living and he would be glad if he were run over by a bus or if he did not wake up, or if he has feelings that he would like to take an overdose or gas himself, this should not be dismissed but should be assessed in the light of the patient's general condition.

The risk of suicide is usually associated with the intensity of suffering experienced by the patient and is often linked up with feelings of unworthiness, self depreciation and guilt. The patient feels that he is no good, that life offers nothing for him and that he is unwanted. Elderly depressed patients, when they are socially isolated, carry a greater risk of suicide.

It is important to remember, too, that the risk of a successful suicidal attempt may be present in the early part of the illness, before the danger has been recognized or sufficiently assessed, and again when the patient starts recovering from a severe depression, because during the depth of his depression he may be unable to put his suicidal wish into action but on relief of the retardation he may then put his wishes into effect.

Drug Treatment

1 *Central nervous stimulants* These are of limited value in the treatment of depression. The amphetamine drugs and allied drugs such as methylphenidate have a possible place only in the management of mild depressive states but have serious disadvantages and unpleasant side effects and are of no value in severe depressive states.

They are mostly of value when the depression is limited to one part of the day, for example the early morning, and amphetamines may tide the patient over this period.

Amphetamines are drugs of addiction and with a very high dosage psychotic states can occur.

2 *Antidepressants* The discovery of antidepressant drugs in the mid-1950s has been a major advance in psychiatric treatment (see Chapter 39). They are of three main classes:

(a) The monoamine oxidase inhibitor drugs (see Table 39.7, p. 256).
(b) Drugs similar in chemical structure to phenothiazine and collectively referred to as the tri-

cyclic antidepressants; these include imipramine, amitriptyline, nortriptyline, desipramine.

(c) New generation antidepressants.

Monoamine Oxidase Inhibitors (MAOI)

The quickest acting of the MAOI drugs is tranylcypromine (Parnate) which has a direct stimulant action on the central nervous system as well as its more prolonged action in inhibiting the enzyme monoamine oxidase. It has also a marked tendency to produce side effects which are referred to below.

Isocarboxazid (Marplan) is the safest MAOI drug but usually takes about three weeks to produce its clinical effects.

Phenelzine (Nardil) and nialamide (Niamid) have a greater tendency to produce side effects than isocarboxazid (Marplan), but probably less so than tranylcypromine (Parnate).

The full effect of MAOI drugs is usually achieved by the end of three weeks' medication and if no significant improvement has occurred by the end of this time it is unnecessary and unwise to continue it further.

Precautions It has been shown that certain foods and beverages which contain tyramine may cause severe reactions in patients on MAOI drugs. The reaction usually consists of an intense headache starting at the back of the head and then extending to the front, associated with an elevation in blood pressure which fluctuates in severity. The severity of the symptoms often suggests a subarachnoid haemorrhage, which has in fact occurred in some patients. Foods to avoid are cheese, Marmite, broad bean pods, certain wine like red Chianti and strong beers.

Care has to be exercised with sympathomimetic amines such as amphetamine and ephedrine as sometimes a rise in blood pressure with headaches may result. Drugs like pethidine and other narcotics are potentiated and must be avoided, and it is also important to remember that the MAOI potentiate the effects of sedatives, phenothiazines and alcohol.

If after MAOI therapy it is proposed to try a tricyclic antidepressant, an interval of 14 days must elapse in view of the possibilities of adverse interaction. Some experienced psychiatrists successfully combine antidepressants but this is unwise in general practice.

Tricyclic Antidepressants

The starting dose for most tricyclic antidepressants is 25 mg t.d.s. increasing to 50 mg t.d.s. after a week. In elderly patients a smaller dose must be given, 10 mg t.d.s. increasing to 20 mg t.d.s., because of the risk of producing states of confusion or delirium.

Amitriptyline and trimipramine are of value in depressive states associated with anxiety or agitation, and the full daily dose can be given at night to promote sleep and to minimize the occurrence of undue sedation and side effects during the day.

Nortriptyline, protriptyline and desipramine are of value in depressive states associated with apathy and lack of energy and drive.

Administration for four weeks is generally sufficient, and if there is little or no improvement in that time, or at the most five weeks, the drugs should be discontinued as further improvement is unlikely to occur.

If monoamine oxidase inhibitors (MAOI) are given after one of the tricyclic antidepressants, a period of four to seven days should elapse before introducing them.

The New Generation Antidepressants

Following the discovery of the monoamine oxidase inhibitors and the tricyclic antidepressants, research endeavours were directed toward the discovery of newer antidepressants, different in chemical structure and pharmacological effects, in the hope of discovering compounds with greater efficacy and safety. These constitute the second generation antidepressants, as shown in Table 39.6.

Maprotiline is a rapidly acting antidepressant with a relatively low incidence of anticholinergic side effects. It acts exclusively as a noradrenalin reuptake inhibitor.

Mianserin is notable for its lack of anticholinergic side effects with little or no cardiotoxic actions, and very little epileptogenic activity.

Viloxazine has less sedative and anticholinergic side effects than the tricyclic antidepressants, but tends to cause nausea and sometimes vomiting.

Trazodone is an effective antidepressant with also marked anti-anxiety effects. It is also relatively free from anticholinergic side effects.

Mianserin, maprotiline and trazodone can be conveniently given in the full daily dose at night. This ends to promote sleep and minimizes daytime sedation.

Flupenthixol, in small doses, has been an effective antidepressant in some patients.

L tryptophan is a precursor for serotonin and has an antidepressant action in its own right, but it can also be given with monoamine oxidase inhibitors or tricyclic antidepressants, such as clomipramine.

Indications for Tranquillizers, Tranquillo-Sedatives and Sedatives

Patients exhibiting marked anxiety and agitation in addition to depression may need drugs in this class as well as antidepressants. It is important to realize that tranquillizers, or tranquillo-sedatives such as chlordiazepoxide (Librium) and diazepam (Valium), and sedatives such as barbiturates do not significantly influence the degree of depression but are mainly effective in relieving associated anxiety and tension.

The MAOI drugs are mainly of value in depressions of mild or moderate severity and more in atypical than the typical endogenous depressions. In cases of severe depression none of the antidepressants is as effective as electroconvulsive therapy which may be given as an outpatient or as an inpatient depending on the needs of the case.

Electroconvulsive Therapy (ECT)

This remains the most effective treatment available for severe depressive illness (see Chapter 40).

Other Physical Methods of Treatment

Another treatment sometimes used for depressive states is continuous narcosis, in which narcotics and sedatives are given to induce sleep for up to 18 hours a day. This method sometimes shortens a depressive illness. Patients with depressive states developing after prolonged stress and associated with marked loss of weight often benefit from modified insulin therapy. This treatment consists of giving gradually increasing intramuscular doses of insulin to induce hypoglycaemia. In contrast to the insulin coma treatment for schizophrenia, the hypoglycaemia is terminated by glucose administration before it deepens sufficiently to cause loss of consciousness.

When all other methods of treatment have failed, prefrontal leucotomy by one of its modern modifications may have to be considered for patients with long-standing depression associated with marked emotional tension. The best results are obtained in patients with good previous personality and whose social and home circumstances are favourable for successful resettlement and rehabilitation after the operation.

Hypomania and Mania

The clinical manifestations of hypomania and mania are the antithesis of those seen in depressive states.

Hypomania is characterized, as in other affective disorders, by a fixed change in mood which here is one of excitement and elation. The patient is optimistic, confident and has a general feeling of well being and sometimes marked euphoria.

The determination of the onset of hypomania may be difficult. It is essential to know the previous personality of the patient and the ways in which his hypomanic state differs from his normal behaviour.

Patients show very marked pressure of activity which affects thinking, speech and general activity. Patients usually talk a great deal and sometimes talk may be almost incessant. Pressure of talk and physical activity (psychomotor over-activity) is characteristic. The talk is replete with details and is circumstantial and easily influenced in trend and content by the patient's distractability to any stimuli he may encounter. In fact any stimulus or any association can influence content of speech.

In contrast to schizophrenia, hypomanic and manic states show flight of ideas, the patients going from one subject to another, such flights of ideas being determined by their inner pressure and by the patients' circumstantiality and by associations they form with what they say or with external stimuli. Nevertheless, they tend to reach the goal, though it may take a long time with a great deal of circumstantiality in speech on the way.

Hypomanic patients frequently make puns based on sounds, clang associations or other stimuli.

Ceaseless activity is the rule but the activity is easily distractable and patients change from one activity to another before finishing the task already started.

Mood is one of elation which is often infectious, a feature which distinguishes the elated state of hypomania from the elated state sometimes found in schizophrenia.

In schizophrenia there is a characteristic glass wall between the observer and the patient and difficulty in establishing rapport. One may be tempted to laugh *at* some of the things the schizophrenic patient says but, with the hypomanic, one will laugh *with* them. Their enthusiasm, wit and good humour have an infectious quality.

They are over-confident, lack reserve and feel that no obstacle is too great for them to overcome. They are often productive in ideas but often are unable to record them because they are too much in a hurry or too distractable.

Hypomanic patients are alert, notice many things. This, together with the increased drive and distractability, makes them go off tangentially in speech and actions but this is quite different from the disconnected speech and behaviour found in schizophrenia.

Hypomanics are expansive, friendly, and interfering as they like to manage other people's affairs and are often a nuisance to others. They have little or no insight into their condition; they feel very fit and their ideas and plans are presented with enthusiasm and are often convincing to others.

The following are the usual difficulties that persons with hypomania and mania get into:

1 They spend a great deal of money, buy unnecessary things or enter into unwise legal agreements in business. They will sometimes issue cheques which cannot be met.
2 They often drink excessively or indulge in excessive or unwise sexual activity leading to venereal disease or pregnancy.
3 When thwarted they tend to become angry or even violent.

Such disturbances of behaviour and social difficulties bring the patient into conflict with society and, as a result, to medical attention. Sometimes treatment has to be arranged compulsorily, e.g. when the patient is unwilling to accept treatment voluntarily and when behaviour or circumstances make admission necessary.

In the most severe forms, i.e. acute mania and delirious mania, all the above features are shown in greater degree and severity with greater psychomotor activity and distractability and greater tendency to be involved in problems of social behaviour. Grandiose tendencies may take the form of delusions, e.g. delusions of great physical or intellectual strength and prowess or sometimes delusions of grandeur regarding possessions, birth and personal beauty.

The extreme form is delirious mania, in which the psychomotor activity is so great that the patient's speech is incoherent and he is continually restless leading eventually to exhaustion. There is a risk of a terminal pneumonia supervening on such a state of physical exhaustion.

Illustrative Examples

The following are pen sketches of two typical patients with attacks of hypomania.

1 A lady aged 48; gets up early in the morning, is very cheerful, talkative, noisy, keeps singing in the bath and gets on with the housework quickly. She has completed the housework and has got her husband and family out of the house by 8 o'clock in the morning. She then dresses in her brightest clothes, puts on excessive make-up—slaps on plenty of lipstick and daubs on excessive eye shadow—and then goes visiting her friends to whom she talks incessantly, making jokes, puns and tries to manage their affairs, persisting to a degree which makes her a nuisance.

She will spend a great deal of money in buying flamboyant new clothes and hats which she does not need or cannot afford and in buying things for her family and friends. She is tireless, talking incessantly with great circumstantiality until the early hours of the morning.

2 A male patient aged 56 with an attack of hypomania: he gets up early in the morning with a great deal of energy, is very active, singing in the bath, talking, a great deal of slapping people on the back, making jokes and puns. He may start decorating his house, e.g. he may start painting the front door and before finishing he will start dismantling his car and then start digging the garden, at the same time talking with rapidity to anyone nearby, giving advice and often interfering with their affairs.

He feels very fit, wants to be doing everything at once and is readily distracted by any external stimulus.

He will tend to go off buying things, things that he does not need or cannot afford; he may change his car unnecessarily or buy new outfits of clothes. He is excessively generous, giving away money by cheques that cannot be met. If anybody thwarts him he will get angry, even violent. He may go off to the local pub and drink excessively, standing everyone drinks, incessantly talking and making puns. He makes rash promises to do things for people and feels that nothing is impossible for him to achieve. Such a state of over-activity and drive continues through the day and until the early morning, as he regards going to sleep as a waste of time.

Treatment of Hypomania and Mania

General Management

The hypomanic or manic patient very rarely realizes or admits that he is in any way unwell, as he feels euphoric, energetic and over-confident. The risks are that he may get into difficulties by over-spending, excessive drinking or due to heightened sexual activities.

Admission to hospital will depend on the severity of the hypomania or mania and on the patient's social behaviour. In very severe states of mania admission becomes imperative, due to the fact that ceaseless over-activity carries the risk of exhaustion which may endanger the patient's life due to the development of intercurrent infections.

Drug Treatment

The introduction of the new major tranquillizing drugs (see Chapter 39) such as chlorpromazine brought a new hope that these drugs would be effective in hypomania and mania. However, although these drugs help many patients, there are some who, even on extremely high doses of chlor-promazine, continue to be hyperactive and to present problems of management.

The newer drugs in the butyrophenone series, such as haloperidol, have proved to be more useful in the treatment of mania. Haloperidol is given in doses of up to 10 mg–30 mg daily.

Haloperidol carries a high risk of producing Parkinsonism but this can be controlled by the concurrent administration of benzhexol, benztropine mesylate or orphenadrine.

Lithium is also used in the treatment of mania. It is essential that the blood level should be determined regularly and that an adequate sodium chloride and fluid intake is ensured.

Surprisingly, ECT is effective and necessary in some patients. ECT given 3–5 times a week will sometimes terminate an attack of mania. It should be pointed out that the use of ECT for mania is not a matter on which there is general agreement.

In conclusion it can be said that the more potent major tranquillizers such as haloperidol at present offer the best means for the control and management of attacks of hypomania and mania and that extra-pyramidal drugs need to be given concurrently.

There is no evidence that medication fundamentally shortens the course of the illness, so that medication has to be given for a sufficient time for the attack to run its course.

Anxiety States

Anxiety is a normal emotion which in moderate degree can be a helpful force by increasing effort and alertness. In excess anxiety impairs effectiveness and is a handicap.

The term anxiety state refers to a disorder in which anxiety is the primary and dominant part of the clinical picture, with the mood change being relatively fixed and persistent and of such a degree as to affect well being, efficiency and normal adjustment.

Anxiety states vary in severity and duration. Thus they may be acute and mild or acute and severe or chronic mild or severe. The prevalence of anxiety states in the United Kingdom has been variously given as 2–5% of the total population and 7–16% of psychiatric patients.

Anxiety is a common feature of many clinical states and may be found in any medical and surgical condition. It may form a prominent feature of many psychiatric illnesses. It is frequently found in depressive illnesses and in its most severe form in agitated depressive states. It is also found in obsessional states and is an essential feature of phobic conditions. Anxiety also occurs in acute toxic confusional states and may occur in any form of dementia particularly when the sufferer has to attempt tasks which are at or beyond the limits of his capacity. It is not infrequent in mentally handicapped patients when they try to undertake tasks difficult for them. It may occur in any form of schizophrenia and is very marked in the form known as pseudo-neurotic schizophrenia, and contrary to popular belief anxiety may be present in conversion hysteria.

Anxiety may be an integral part of epileptic phenomena particularly of the temporal lobe variety.

The Biological Significance of Anxiety

Throughout the animal kingdom, an animal in danger shows all the bodily and behavioural manifestations of anxiety.

Cannon has shown that, during such situations, the body becomes mobilized for action either for fight or flight and that the mechanisms involved include the autonomic nervous system, the locomotor system and other changes throughout the body which serve to increase the organism's ability to deal with the threat by action. The sympathetic part of the nervous system is predominantly involved but certain aspects of parasympathetic activity come into action, i.e. those subserving the need for total mobilization for activity, e.g. the sacral parasympathetic causing evacuation of the bladder and bowel.

Various changes which occur alert the animal, increase awareness and responsivity to various stimuli and serve to bring about more effective blood supply to the muscles of locomotion, where it is most urgently needed during an emergency. The rate of respiration is increased to cope with the increased demands for oxygen by the muscles, heart rate is increased to pump the blood round to the muscles where it is needed. The blood vessels to muscles and heart tend to be dilated whereas the arterioles to the skin and digestive tract, where food and oxygen are not urgently needed, are diminished, so that there is a redistribution of blood supply to the vital organs of circulation and locomotion. Muscular tone is increased so that the animal can go into action without delay. Dilatation of the pupils and increased alertness in response to stimuli also help the organism in being effectively aware of the environment.

In some animals, pilo-erection makes the animal look more fierce. In man, anxiety just inconveniently produces goose pimples without serving any obvious beneficial effect, biologically or otherwise.

Clinical Features of Anxiety States

General Appearance and Behaviour

A person with an anxiety state has a tense, anxious, apprehensive attitude and demeanour. Increased muscular tension is shown in his facial expression, posture and his difficulty in relaxing. Characteristically he sits on the edge of the chair during an interview and jumps at any sudden noise.

When muscular tension is marked, tremors of the hands, knees and sometimes other parts of the body are noticeable. Palpebral fissures tend to be wide and pupils dilated; the mouth tends to be dry so that the patient can be observed licking his lips and moistening his tongue.

Mood

The patient is in a constant state of worry and usually looks apprehensively ahead, anticipating problems and crossing his bridges before reaching them, fearing that dangers and catastrophes lie awaiting him around the corner. He is apprehensive about his health, family, finances, about his abilities and other aspects of his life. He seeks constant reassurance. His thoughts are concerned with worries for the present and the future. Speech is often rapid and may exhibit stammering or hesitancy.

Bodily Concomitants of Anxiety

These are to be seen as changes in locomotor system, sudomotor system and the autonomic nervous system control of functions of various organs and systems. An understanding of the physiological basis of these will enable one to understand the patient's symptoms and to be in a better position to explain and reassure him effectively.

1 Muscular system

Increased tension of the voluntary musculature is characteristic of anxiety states and has been referred to already. Symptoms directly referable to increased muscular tension include tremors, aches and pains in various muscles of the body—for example, pain in the back, limbs, neck and side of the head. One type of headache is due to increased tension of the scalp muscles.

A useful diagnostic test is that the pains arising from increased muscular tension disappear with a small quantity of intravenous 10% sodium amytal; i.e. one or two cc injected intravenously slowly. The pain will go long before there is any interference with the patient's consciousness and when the patient develops feelings of relaxation. Sodium amytal in this dosage has no analgesic effect and produces this reaction by relief of anxiety, tension and, concomitantly, reduction of muscular tension.

2 Cardiovascular System
Tachycardia and the subjective experience of increased rapidity and forcefulness of heart beat, palpitations, are common effects of anxiety. The patient often becomes worried about this and develops fears of heart disease which further increases his anxiety thus creating a vicious circle. Precordial pain is frequent which, again, the patient tends to assume is evidence of heart disease, but precordial pain in young people is invariably due to psychogenic factors. It has its origin in the intercostal and pectoral muscles and, if it were necessary for this to be proved, an injection of local anaesthetic into these muscles would immediately abolish the pain.

Blood pressure is often increased, systolic pressure being mainly affected, and it usually soon returns to normal. During physical examination initial readings tend to be much higher than subsequent readings, which provides evidence of the effect of anxiety and apprehension on level of blood pressure.

Pallor and cold, blue extremities are evidence of vasoconstriction in the arteries supplying the skin.

3 Respiratory System
Anxious patients tend to have rapid, shallow breathing, sometimes frequent sighing and, in general, to show poor effort tolerance—much poorer effort tolerance than is characteristic of their normal states.

4 Gastro-intestinal System
Decrease of salivary secretion gives rise to characteristic dryness of the mouth. Epigastric tremulousness, nausea, dyspepsia, bowel urgency, frequency or diarrhoea are common.

In some patients, anxiety and tension produce spasm of the large bowel, giving rise to constipation.

It should be noted that, in some people, anxiety makes them eat more because eating gives them relief of tension and may serve as a substitute for love and affection. As a rule appetite is diminished in anxiety states.

5 Sudomotor System
Increased sweating in anxiety states is typically emotional in distribution, i.e. from the palms, the axillae and forehead. The cold, moist palm is typical of a person suffering from an anxiety state, in contrast to the warm, moist palm of a patient suffering from thyrotoxicosis.

Aetiology

The principle of multiple aetiological factors can be clearly seen in the genesis of anxiety states. Aetiological factors may be conveniently considered as (a) extrinsic or environmental and (b) intrinsic or constitutional, or they may be classified into (1) predisposing factors and (2) precipitating factors.

Genetic and Constitutional Predisposing Factors

It was demonstrated in World War II that a person's constitution determined the degree of environmental stress that he could cope with before developing a psychiatric illness, such as an anxiety state. The constitutional predisposition included genetic factors, probably a number of genes of small effect.

Genetic factors may be manifested in a number of ways:

1 by determining the predisposition to breakdown
2 determining, in part, personality type and stability
3 determining physiological features such as autonomic imbalance and, possibly, certain neuro-endocrine mechanisms which may be important.

Genetic factors cannot be considered in isolation because parents and siblings with anxiety states or other psychiatric disorders may also exert a direct influence on the person and influence his personality disposition and may cause him to develop certain traits of personality which are conducive to the development of anxiety and distress, the tendency to be very sensitive, the tendency to be timid, apprehensive and unassertive and the tendency to emotional instability over minor frustrations. It has been suggested that people of introverted personality tend to develop conditioned responses more readily and tend to learn anxiety reactions more rapidly than extraverted persons.

Physical Factors

These include fatigue, exhaustion and infections, particularly virus infections which may leave depression and anxiety persisting for many weeks after the physical aspects of the infection have passed off.

Endocrine Factors

In hyperthyroidism, anxiety is a common feature. Similarly, changes in the hormonal balance of the body which occur at puberty, following childbirth and at the menopause may be associated with emotional lability and increased tendency to anxiety.

In some women, the various psychophysical changes comprising the premenstrual tension syndrome are particularly associated with development of anxiety and tension.

It should be remembered, too, that certain addicts develop very marked anxiety as a part of the withdrawal effects of the drugs. Originally, people may take barbiturates for the relief of anxiety but, if they take a sufficiently high dose over a long period of time, they become physically dependent and when the drug level of the barbiturate decreases, they develop marked anxiety which leads to the taking of further barbiturates, thus creating a marked vicious circle and increasing the problems of addiction.

Similarly, increased anxiety can follow the intake of alcohol and, again, one can get alcoholism developing as a part of this mechanism.

Psychological Factors

Psychosocial stresses may be acute and severe or may be prolonged. Every person has his breaking point. Some people are more vulnerable to certain stresses—for example, financial or marital—whereas others are mainly affected by threats to their status and prestige. Severe stresses include accidents, frightening experiences, bereavement, prolonged stresses relating to interpersonal problems, to marital, financial and occupational worries and conflicts.

Stresses tend to have a cumulative effect and sometimes the experience of a series of stresses or prolonged stress combined, perhaps, with infections or fatigue may be the culminating point which leads to the development of an anxiety state.

Conflicts relating to any sphere of a person's life may be associated with anxiety. Desires related to instinctive drives and the conflicts imposed by the person's standards or the requirements of society or, indeed, conflicts about any wish can lead to the development of anxiety.

Anxiety and tension may become a part of the life pattern of successful business men. They live in a constant state of tension and over-activity and are unable to relax. Some remain well for years without much rest or recreation. Others become increasingly fatigued and depressed and ultimately break down with a psychiatric or psychosomatic disorder.

In some persons, the relief of pressure of work, such as holidays or weekends, leads to increased anxiety unless they are able to channel their energies into substitutive activities.

The Occurrence of Anxiety and Other Psychiatric, Physical and Psychosomatic Disorders

Anxiety may occur in practically all psychiatric disorders but here it is a part and not the main and predominant and primary component of the clinical picture.

For example:

1 *Schizophrenia* Anxiety may be prominent in many forms of schizophrenia; the diagnosis will rest on the discovery of features which are indicative of schizophrenia.

One type of schizophrenia, referred to as pseudoneurotic schizophrenia, may cause difficulties in diagnosis. Here the anxiety is overwhelming. It is a state of pan-anxiety but careful observation will illustrate deterioration of personality, emotional incongruity and other features which indicate the true nature of the disorder.

2 *Depressive States* Anxiety is a frequent component in depressive illnesses. In those illnesses which are a reaction to environmental difficulty, anxiety is particularly prominent but it may also occur in endogenous depressions and is particularly intense in agitated depressions.

In patients developing anxiety for the first time

after the age of 40, in the absence of any organic disease, one should bear in mind the possibility that this may, in fact, be a depressive state in which the main manifestation to the observer is anxiety.

Anxiety occurs in acute organic states such as delirium; also in cases of organic dementia, including senile dementia and arteriosclerotic dementia, and is related to the emotional lability of those patients and also to the difficulties of adjustment which the dementia imposes on them.

3 *Post-concussional syndromes* are often associated with anxiety and irritability.

4 Anxiety symptoms are common in all psychosomatic disorders and in almost all physical disorders, depending on a variety of factors including the patient's reaction to the illness and the threat which it presents to him.

Prognosis

This will depend on the strength of the predisposing factors and the personality of the patient, his habitual modes of reaction, the role played by organic and endocrine factors in predisposition and the extent to which they can be modified and, finally, the severity and nature of the stresses and the extent to which these can be modified.

Factors of good prognosis are an acute onset, short duration of symptoms, stable personality, good work record and good general previous adjustment. Factors of poor prognosis are family history of neurosis, neurotic traits in childhood, poor work record and other evidence of difficulties of adjustment, unstable personality and the extent to which various vicious circles have developed in the perpetuation of symptoms, such as worry about somatic effects of anxiety and, in the case of phobias, avoiding situations which were previously associated with phobias.

Treatment

The steps in treatment include:

1 first of all, taking a full history
2 thorough physical examination
3 discussion, explanation and positive reassurance
4 general support and management, giving further explanation, encouragement and guidance in coping with their problems (see Chapter 37)

5 social measures dealing with problems of work and home, as far as they can be modified
6 symptomatic treatment—the use of anti-anxiety drugs to relieve symptoms and to encourage resumption of normal activities (see Chapter 34)
7 psychotherapy if indicated and according to the needs of the case, e.g.
   (a) shorter supportive
   (b) prolonged and intensive psychotherapy
   (c) group therapy.

General Strategy of Treatment

In the treatment and management of anxiety states, investigation is an integral part of treatment. The first step in treatment is the taking of the history in which the patient is allowed to talk about his past and present problems and life situations freely with minimal interruption from the doctor. The interview enables both the physician and the patient to see what factors in the environment, in interpersonal relationships or in the patient's own conflicts, may have contributed towards the development of his anxiety state. It also enables the physician to develop rapport with the patient and can be the beginning and the foundation of a good doctor–patient relationship.

Physical examination can also be an important part of treatment. If there is no evidence of physical disease the nature of the patient's symptoms must be explained to him in terms suitable to his intelligence, education and personality and it must always be remembered that a negative reassurance is not enough. It does not usually satisfy the patient to be told there is no physical basis for his symptoms. This must be accompanied by a positive explanation of the nature and basis of his symptoms in terms which he can understand. The physician can also help him to understand the relationship between life events and stresses in the development of his illness, and can help him either to cope or to modify circumstances if this is feasible.

If anxiety is mild and causing minimal incapacity or suffering there may be no need for pharmacotherapy. If the anxiety state is sufficiently severe to interfere with well being and adjustment and to cause considerable incapacity, pharmacotherapy will need to be considered along with other methods of treatment.

Pharmacotherapy of Anxiety States

It is proposed to present an evaluation of available pharmacotherapeutic agents for the treatment of anxiety.

1 Barbiturates

The disadvantages, limitations and hazards of barbiturates have become increasingly realized in recent years. Barbiturates act widely on the central nervous system and have a general depressant action on the cortex, the reticular system and other parts of the CNS. Barbiturates tend to cause difficulty in thinking and to produce dysarthria and ataxia. With prolonged barbiturate medication patients appear to show a falling off in standards of general behaviour and reliability and tend to experience unexplained accidents due to their ataxia. There are many other more serious disadvantages, for example, when barbiturates are taken in an overdose there is a high risk of fatality because of their marked depressant action on the respiratory and vasomotor centres. Their addictive potential is high, leading to physical as well as psychological dependence. When physical dependence develops patients in fact suffer from a barbiturate-induced anxiety which appears when the barbiturate blood level falls and further quantities of barbiturates have to be taken in order to be relieved of distressing anxiety. If supplies of barbiturates are cut off completely, intense anxiety develops followed after an interval by a major epileptic fit or a cardiovascular collapse which can be fatal, or a delirium similar to delirium tremens.

Although effective as hypnotics, barbiturates tend to produce a 'hangover' the following day. They also tend to suppress REM sleep which is a disadvantage as dreaming probably has important functions in maintaining mental health and well being. A further disadvantage of barbiturates is that they induce enzyme activity in the liver, thereby interfering with the efficacy of other drugs such as tricyclic antidepressants. Nowadays barbiturates have no place in the management of anxiety states either as daytime sedatives or as hypnotics.

2 Carbamates

The carbamates were precursors of the benzodiazepines and include the drugs meprobamate and tybamate.

Meprobamate has a high degree of addictive potential. Physical dependence on meprobamate causes an abstinence syndrome, consisting of insomnia, vomiting, tremors, muscle twitches, anxiety headache, ataxia, convulsions and a toxic confusional state resembling delirium tremens. Meprobamate when used in the treatment of anxiety states should only be given for short periods in view of its high addictive potential.

Tybamate appears to have less addictive potential than meprobamate but both drugs are far less effective than the benzodiazepines in the treatment and management of anxiety.

3 Chlormezanone

Chlormezanone has been used as an anti-anxiety agent and is reported to be of benefit in conditions associated with muscle spasm. It has also been promoted for inducing sleep.

4 Chlormethiazole

This is a very useful compound for treating alcoholic withdrawal. It is also an effective anti-anxiety agent and anti-epileptic but is addictive and must be given only for strictly limited periods.

5 Beta adrenergic receptor blocking drugs

Turner and Granville Grossman carried out the first double blind control trial of a beta-blocking drug in the treatment of anxiety at St Bartholomew's Hospital in 1966. This pioneering work has only been adequately recognized in recent years. The consensus of opinion is that beta receptor blocking drugs have a place in the management of anxiety particularly in patients who suffer from marked concomitant somatic symptoms of anxiety such as palpitations, tachycardia and tremors. There are many other symptoms associated with anxiety, including lactate-induced anxiety, which are not significantly affected by beta-blockers. Beta receptor blocking drugs have also been used in the prophylactic treatment of migraine and also in the treatment of situational anxiety, such as examination anxiety, stage fright in actors and musicians and severe anxiety associated with motor vehicle driving tests. The advantages in situational anxiety is that beta-blockers such as oxprenolol, given about half an hour before the anxiety evoking occasion, can relieve anxiety and its bodily concomitants including tremor without significantly affecting concentration, reaction time and mental clarity.

6 Neuroleptics

The phenothiazines and rauwolfia alkaloids were the first neuroleptic agents to be introduced into psychiatric treatment. When chlorpromazine was first introduced it promised to be a potentially valuable drug in the treatment of anxiety. Rees and Lambert (1955) carried out a double blind control trial of chlorpromazine on 100 patients suffering from anxiety states and found that although it produced some relief of anxiety its side effects seriously limited its use.

Other neuroleptic drugs have since been used in low doses to minimize side effects. These include phenothiazines such as trifluoperazine, fluphenazine, and thioridazine. These are less effective than the benzodiazepines but have an advantage in that they are free from risk of physical dependence. Other neuroleptics such as haloperidol and pimozide have also been used in low doses in the management of anxiety. Thioxanthene derivatives have been used in the treatment of anxiety, for example, flupenthixol has been found to be valuable in low doses in the management of anxiety, and in moderate doses for depressive illness. Oxypertine, first introduced for the treatment of schizophrenia, has been found in a double blind control study to be useful in the management of anxiety.

In summary, neuroleptics in low doses can have a place in the management of anxiety although they cannot compete with the benzodiazepines. They have certain advantages, particularly lack of addictive potential, and they may also be useful in the management of patients coming off addictive drugs.

7 Tricyclic antidepressants

There is a wide range of tricyclic antidepressants available and they can be subdivided according to the main target action. Certain members have sedative properties, including amitriptyline and trimipramine. These are the drugs of choice for depressive states associated with severe anxiety or agitation, and it is convenient for the entire daily dose of these drugs to be given at night. This promotes sleep, the anticholinergic side effects cause less distress and the patient, although receiving benefit from the antidepressant action, remains more alert during daytime. The demethylated derivatives such as nortriptyline and protriptyline are much

more stimulating and are not useful in the management of anxiety as they tend to increase drive, alertness and arousal. There are others which possess both anxiolytic and antidepressant effects such as clomipramine, a very effective antidepressant useful in the treatment of anxiety, phobias and obsessional symptoms.

The role of a tricyclic antidepressant is that it is helpful when anxiety accompanies a depressive illness.

8 Monoamine oxidase inhibitors (MAOI)

These have a place in the management of some patients with anxiety states, that is, patients with intractable anxiety and phobic states which fail to respond to other methods of treatment. Despite the practical disadvantages of using these drugs, i.e. the need for dietary precautions and caution with the use of other medicaments, they do have a place in this narrowly defined group.

9 Benzodiazepines

The barbiturates have been virtually replaced in the treatment of anxiety by the benzodiazepine series of drugs which offer many clinical and pharmacological advantages. The benzodiazepines affect the limbic system and the reflex pathways governing muscle tension, and have comparatively little effect on the cerebral cortex. They therefore are free from the risk of producing the difficulties in thinking and impairment of judgment which is frequently found with barbiturates. Overdoses are relatively safe and there is no tendency to induce enzyme activity in the liver. The suppression of dreaming activity is much less than barbiturates. There is a risk of psychological and physical dependence.

Biofeedback

In recent years biofeedback techniques have been used to treat anxiety and related symptoms due to increased muscle tension. For example attempts have been made to train patients suffering from anxiety to control their alpha waves. This method appears to have limited application and its efficacy has yet to be established. However, there is some evidence of biofeedback techniques that are useful in the relief of tension headaches.

Behaviour Therapy

Various methods used in behaviour therapy may be useful in the treatment of certain states associated with anxiety and phobias. Systematic desensitization can be used for the treatment of phobias and also for anxiety associated with obsessional states and psychosexual problems. Implosion therapy and flooding achieve results more rapidly than systematic desensitization.

Phobias

A phobia may be defined as an irrational or morbid fear in relation to a thing, situation or stimulus which normally would not evoke such fear.

A phobic reaction is a form of fear which is out of proportion to the danger of the situation, cannot be explained, is beyond voluntary control and tends to lead to avoidance of the feared situation or stimulus. Certain fears, however, cannot be avoided by escape from the stimulus, e.g. fears of disease, death or one's own harmful impulses. The patient experiencing a phobic reaction can experience all the distressing mental and bodily concomitants of anxiety. Many patients become preoccupied with the possibility of encountering the phobic object or situation and suffer greatly as a result of such anxious apprehension. They may also become afraid of the experience of anxiety, i.e. they become phobophobic, a mechanism which intensifies the distress and disability associated with phobias.

Characteristically, because of the unpleasantness of the emotion of anxiety, the patient will tend to arrange his life to avoid the phobic stimulus, thereby greatly restricting his daily activities.

Varieties of phobic states:

agora-claustrophobias
social phobias
animal phobias
other specific phobias
illness phobias
obsessional phobias

Agoraphobia is one of the commonest phobic disorders seen in clinical practice.

About 75% of patients are women and the onset usually is between 15 years and 35 years. They tend to show generalized anxiety as well as phobic fear reactions. They may also be depressed and have obsessional symptoms or depersonalization. They have fears of going out alone, or going into crowded or enclosed places. They do not show any increased tendency to condition easily and do not respond well to desensitization therapy.

Social phobias These again are most common in women and have their onset between 15 years and 30 years. They have fears of social situations and activities, e.g. eating, drinking, writing or reading in company.

Animal phobias are less common and differ from the above in having their origin in childhood and usually being a monosymptomatic fear of a single animal species. There is usually no general anxiety. The large majority of sufferers are women. On psychological testing they condition rapidly and extinguish slowly. They respond well to systematic desensitization.

Other specific phobias such as for thunderstorms, heights, winds, darkness, etc. are usually monosymptomatic phobias with no generalized anxiety or associated symptoms such as depression or depersonalization. They respond well to systematic desensitization.

Illness phobias These patients are preoccupied with fears of disease like cancer, heart disease, venereal disease, death, etc. The symptoms superficially resemble obsessional symptoms but do not include the tendency to resist the preoccupation.

Obsessional fears fulfil the criteria for obsessional symptoms in that they are associated with a subjective feeling of compulsion which patients try to resist but cannot get rid of although they may realize that they are irrational. Examples are fears of harming people, fears of contamination leading to compulsive handwashing.

Treatment

In recent years advances in the treatment of phobias have occurred by the use of various forms of behaviour therapy especially systematic desensitization and implosion (flooding therapy). For details of these methods see Chapter 38.

Further Reading

West, E. D. and Dally, P. J. (1959) Effects of iproniazid in depressive syndromes. *British Medical Journal*, **1**, 1491–1499.

Pollit, J. (1965) *Depression and Its Treatment.* Heinemann, London.

Watts, C. A. H. (1965) *Depressive Disorders in the Community.* J. Wright, Bristol.

Marks, I. M. (1969) *Fears and Phobias.* Heinemann, London.

Hinton, J. (1971) *Dying.* Penguin, Harmondsworth.

Brown, G. W. and Harris, T. (1978) *Social Origins of Depression.* Tavistock, London.

Garfield, C. A. (1978) *Psychosocial Care of the Dying Patient.* McGraw Hill, New York.

Paykel, E. S. and Coppen, A. E. (1979) *Psychopharmacology of Affective Disorders.* Oxford University Press, Oxford.

Arieti, S. and Bemporad, J. (1980) *Severe and Mild Depression.* Tavistock, London.

27

Hysteria

Hysteria is defined as a disorder in which the patient develops symptoms and signs of illness (mental, physical or both) for some real or imagined gain without being fully aware of the underlying motive.

Frequently the term hysteria is misapplied to histrionic or uncontrolled behaviour, whereas it should be reserved for psychogenic illnesses having a motive of gain.

Hysteria is protean in manifestation and may simulate any disease.

The mental mechanism underlying the formation of hysterical symptoms is a process of dissociation whereby certain dynamically important experiences (usually psychic traumata) become separated from the mainstream of consciousness in predisposed individuals under conditions of stress. The development of the hysterical symptom usually enables the patient to escape from a difficult situation. It is on account of the gain resulting from the illness that hysteria has been confused with malingering.

A malingerer is a person who claims he has symptoms when he knows he has none, whereas the hysteric has genuine symptoms.

Forms of Hysterical Reaction

The varied manifestations of hysteria can be conveniently classified into three main groups.

1 *Dysmnesic*
   (a) Amnesia
   (b) Fugues
   (c) Somnambulism
   (d) Twilight states

2 *Conversion symptoms*
   (a) Motor, e.g. paralysis, paresis, tremors, rigidity, abnormal gait, ataxia, fits.

   (b) Sensory general—anaesthesia, paraesthesia, hyperalgesia and pains.
   Sensory special—visual difficulties, blindness, deafness, loss of taste, loss of smell.
   (c) Visceral, e.g. vomiting, retention of urine, constipation.

3 *Quasi-psychotic state.* Ganser syndrome.

4 *Hysterical superadditions to physical diseases.* Hysterical prolongation of illness and certain iatrogenic disorders.

It should be noted that all hysterical manifestations involve functions which are under the control or the influence of volition. This applies to the voluntary muscles concerned with vomiting, retention of urine and dyschezia. A great deal of confusion occurs because some authorities describe as hysteria symptoms which are the bodily manifestations of emotional tension mediated by the autonomic nervous system.

Dysmnesic

These forms of hysteria include amnesia, fugues, somnambulism, hysterical fits, multiple personality.

1 *Hysterical amnesia* may cover a short period of a person's life or may cover a large part of it or even the whole of it. Amnesia may or may not be associated with loss of personal identity. Amnesia usually occurs to escape from intolerable anxiety and distress about some problem or difficulty or situation in which the patient finds himself.

Amnesia is sometimes claimed as a defence when the patient has committed a criminal offence, but hysterical amnesia is not accepted in law as mental illness and therefore the patient is held to be responsible quite irrespective of the presence of amnesia.

As a deterrent during World War II and to avoid epidemics of amnesia, notices were sometimes put up that any soldier losing his memory would be dealt with disciplinarily in the same way as he would if he lost any other part of his equipment.

2 *Fugues* Fugue is a state of wandering, with amnesia for the period during which the wandering occurred. Again, the fugue is usually determined by a need to get away from some intolerable situation.

It should be noted that fugues may be of three kinds:

(a) hysterical; (b) as a manifestation of a depressive illness in which the patient is extremely distressed, wanders around, sometimes contemplating suicide and, because he does not register clearly what is happening to him, he is unable to remember the events which occurred during the period of wandering; (c) manifestations of organic mental states, for example post-epileptic phenomenon, or wandering in a state of confusion.

3 *Hysterical fits* Hysterical fits may sometimes create confusion in diagnosis because of superficial similarities to grand mal epilepsy, but the following features will serve to distinguish between them.

Hysterical fits never occur when the person is alone and usually occur in reaction to a situation which is emotionally important.

Epileptic fits, on the other hand, can occur during sleep and come on out of the blue without being necessarily related to what has happened immediately before in the patient's experience; they may occur in dangerous situations such as in crossing a busy street, near the fire or when the person is in dangerous situations such as working at heights or whilst swimming in the sea. All these situations are dangers with epileptic fits.

There is no real loss of consciousness as in epilepsy, no sequence of tonic and clonic phases, no tongue-biting and no incontinence. Hysterical fits consist of purposive movements of both the limbs including struggling, fighting, scratching, clawing.

Thus, if during a fit the patient gives evidence of any purposeful movements, such as fighting or resisting or talking spontaneously, answering questions or deliberately attacking or biting, this indicates that the patient is not unconscious, that the cerebral cortex is acting and therefore it is not epileptic. Hysterical fits can go on for much longer than a single major epileptic fit.

Conversion Symptoms

1 *Hysterical motor conversion symptoms* These may consist of paresis or paralysis of limbs, or other parts of the body. They never involve single muscles but movements and conform to the patient's idea of the form of the symptoms.

Hysterical gaits tend to be bizarre and are not similar to any organic neurological gait. Similarly, hysterical weakness; when the patient is asked to contract the muscles of the limb, contraction of both agonist and antagonist will occur.

2 *Sensory conversion symptoms* Special senses e.g. hysterical blindness, hysterical deafness, hysterical anosmia, hysterical loss of taste will occur for some special reason which determines the selection of the particular sense modality to be affected. Sometimes it may be the patient's weak point, for example myopia may be the determinant of the development of hysterical blindness in certain traumatic situations when the stress is sufficiently severe, or deafness may be determined by the occupation of the person, for example a telephonist, or it may be determined by a desire not to hear.

3 *General sensation* The most common hysterical symptom affecting general sensation is anaesthesia of the skin; this corresponds to the patient's idea of anaesthesia and is usually of a glove and stocking distribution and stops at one of the joints, wrist joint, elbow joint or shoulder joint and is quite different from the distribution or loss of sensation due to any affection of the sensory nerves.

Quasi-psychotic State

This usually takes the form of hysterical pseudo-dementia or Ganser syndrome, which is characterized by tendency to give approximate answers. The answers are incorrect, but near enough to show that the patient has the mental capacity to work out the correct answer, and behaviour again corresponds to the patient's concept of what mental illness is. This condition most commonly occurs in penal institutions.

Hysterical Superadditions to Physical Diseases

Hysterical superadditions can occur in any physical disease for motives of gain, such as gaining attention and sympathy. Any illness may similarly be prolonged by hysterical mechanism. Some iatrogenic illness are hysterical and brought about by suggestion.

Aetiology

At one time it was believed that genetic factors played an important role in the predisposition to hysteria, but twin studies have thrown considerable doubt on this and hysteria is nowadays regarded as a reaction to environmental problems in which the patient's personality plays an important part in determining the mode of reaction. Environmental circumstances determine the time of development of hysterical symptoms. A specific type of hysterical personality has been described which is characterized by the need to exaggerate, the need to be in the centre of attention and to give an impression to the outside world of being better than one is, of tending to manipulate people and situations for some personal need, to have shallow emotional reactions which are often demonstrative and dramatic and histrionic, a tendency to be untruthful and to exaggerate statements and claims. Many patients feel they have been deprived of affection from an early age and have an intense need for affection and approval which it is very difficult to satisfy. When they do get the attention and approval which they need, they test the person who gives it to such an extent that very often this produces a withdrawal of affection. Hysteria may be regarded as a protective mechanism to safeguard the person from the stress and strains of life and anxiety which are difficult to tolerate.

Diagnosis

The diagnosis of hysteria must not be made on negative grounds, that is merely the absence of organic diseases to account for the symptoms. It must be made on positive grounds in relationship to the patient's personality, to the situation in which it occurs and the gain which the patient derives from it. This gain need not be a real gain in the eyes of other people, but it may be a gain only from the patient's point of view. It should be noted that hysterical symptoms affect functions which come under conscious control and that they serve some personal gain to the patient. The reactions which are subserved by the autonomic nervous system and which may be biologically purposeful should not be confused with hysteria, because these are outside the conscious control unless this has been acquired by special biofeedback learning. Therefore, one cannot get hysterical pylorospasm or hysterical nystagmus or tachycardia.

Hysterical symptoms may be superadded on organic conditions, for example, disseminated sclerosis or physical injuries or any organic condition or neurological state.

Hysterical symptoms appearing for the first time in older people suggest the need to investigate carefully for an organic basis.

Treatment of Hysteria

It should be borne in mind that hysterics are suggestible and respond readily to harmful as well as beneficial suggestions. They usually crave attention but the more attention paid to their symptoms the more implicit will be the suggestion that these are serious and the longer will they tend to persist.

The hysterical symptom should as far as possible be ignored and no notice taken of any worsening of the symptom, but the slightest improvement should be encouraged. The patient must be persuaded by those with whom he is in contact to carry on living as normally as possible. Keeping a patient with hysterical symptoms in bed or helping a patient with a hysterical gait to walk only serves to impress the patient that he is ill and needs support. Every effort must be made to make the patient assume responsibility for his functional recovery, and the more active part he can be made to play in treatment the better.

The general rule in management is firmness and, what is even more important, it must be consistent firmness.

Sometimes symptoms will disappear if they are completely ignored, but it is sometimes necessary to tackle the symptom actively in order to prevent habituation and incapacity due to the symptom, and early removal makes it possible to bring the patient to face his problems and be guided to a more salutary solution.

The best method undoubtedly is to produce full functional recovery in one session. It is, therefore, important for the physician to allow himself ample time for the therapeutic session and to be prepared to carry on with his treatment until full functional recovery is achieved.

The following procedures are useful tactical aids to some patients: (a) hypnosis. (b) intravenous barbiturate narcosis.

Both of these will help to elicit further information about the psychopathology of the disorder, as well as increasing the patient's suggestibility to beneficial persuasion.

When the patient has recovered from his symptom he will often become more anxious because now he has to face his problems more directly. It is now necessary to discuss with the patient his reactions to life's difficulties. The hysteric tends to give in readily and retreat into illness in the face of difficulties, and the patient must be guided in dealing with the problems which precipitated his illness in a more satisfactory manner.

Hysterics tend to attempt things beyond their capabilities in order to impress people. They must be encouraged to accept their limitations and work within the limits of their abilities, and at the same time to learn to gain satisfaction from whatever assets they possess.

Further Reading

Abse, D. W. (1966) *Hysteria*. J. Wright, Bristol.

28
Obsessional States

Obsessions can occur in many psychiatric disorders or they may constitute the entire illness which is then referred to as an Obsessional State.

Definitions

An obsession is a content of consciousness, that is, an idea, an impulse to action or an emotional state which, when it appears, is accompanied by a subjective feeling of compulsion which the patient tries to resist but cannot get rid of. The most important diagnostic features are the feeling of compulsion accompanied by a tendency to resist, the latter being the most important criterion of all. Obsessional symptoms may or may not appear to be nonsensical to the patient. They are characteristically alien to the patient, but in spite of this he always recognizes that they arise from him. The realization that the obsessional idea, feeling or impulse to action is irrational is less important as a diagnostic criterion. The tendency to resist the obsession is the most important and characteristic feature. Obsessional thoughts tend to be recurrent and often associated with a great deal of anxiety and distress. In some patients the obsessional symptoms and the associated distress can occupy most of their daily lives. In others, the obsessional symptoms come on intermittently with intervals of comparative freedom.

The term **compulsion** is applied to an obsessional impulse to carry out certain acts, such as having to do things in a certain way, or to repeat them a certain number of times, to touch various objects, to carry out cleansing operations by repeated washing, and so on.

Obsessional Personality

It is important to differentiate obsessional traits of personality from obsessional symptoms. The obsessional personality is characterized by overconscientiousness, meticulousness, tidiness, reliability; by being parsimonious and persevering, and by a tendency to pay a great deal of attention to detail. The obsessional person often tends to be rigid, to dislike changes in his plans or daily routines and to be generally cautious and timid in his outlook. These are common traits of personality, many of which are socially desirable insofar as they are conducive to reliable work and socially acceptable behaviour. If they become very marked and develop the features of compulsion and resistance, they then become obsessional symptoms. It should be noted that the obsessional personality is very common in the normal population and is found in association with anxiety states, depressive illnesses and a variety of psychosomatic disorders, and although it is correlated to some degree with obsessional illness, it is by no means always present in those who develop obsessional illnesses. Various surveys have shown that about one-third of obsessional states are free from previous obsessional traits of personality.

The **anankastic personality** is a term which denotes certain personality characteristics which include obsessional traits. The anankastic personality is characterized by a strong sense of personal insecurity, associated with excessive caution and conscientiousness. The essential traits are timidity, rigidity often with extreme self-control and excessive tendency to doubt.

Differential Diagnosis of Obsessional Symptoms

Obsessional symptoms must not be confused with the following.

Habit patterns are learned reactions of behaviour which we carry out easily and automatically. There is no feeling of compulsion or a tendency to resist.

Habit spasms or tics are involuntary movements which are not necessarily accompanied by feelings of compulsion or tendencies to resist.

Rituals are certain acts based on superstitious beliefs which are carried out to ward off dangers or misfortune. They are carried out deliberately and, although there may be varying degrees of compulsion to carry out such acts, there is no tendency to resist. Certain types of behaviour of children, such as avoiding walking on the lines of the pavement, are usually carried out deliberately without exhibiting any tendency to resist them.

Any of the above could become obsessional symptoms if they were accompanied by a feeling of compulsion associated with a tendency to resist, but normally they do not have these features.

Autochthonous ideas in schizophrenia appear with an overwhelming feeling of compulsion or conviction, but they are accepted with conviction and there is no question of any resistance.

Stereotyped patterns of behaviour in schizophrenia are also disconnected forms of behaviour which are carried out without subjective feelings of compulsion and without any tendency to resist.

Varieties of Obsessional Symptoms

Obsessional Thoughts

Obsessional thoughts, ideas, words or mental images appear in consciousness against the person's will and despite resistance. John Bunyan suffered very greatly from obsessional thoughts relating to religion. The obsessional thoughts are distressing and repetitive and mental images may take the form of distressing or horrible scenes, sexual images which the patient tries to resist but cannot get rid of and all are associated with emotional distress.

Obsessional Ruminations

Here the patient is compelled to ruminate over questions which have no ready answer, such as 'Who created God?' 'What is the purpose of life?' etc. These recurring thoughts distress the patient. John Bunyan, for example, suffered from ruminations about God.

Obsessional Doubts

These often relate to whether certain actions have been carried out, such as putting a letter in a pillar-box, turning off the electric light switch, turning off gas taps and water taps.

Obsessional Vacillations

These may occur when there is a choice of two alternatives, even when it is unimportant which one is chosen, such as deciding which of two suits to wear to work.

Obsessional Phobias

It should be remembered that the majority of phobias are not obsessional. They are learned phenomena whereby a fear becomes attached to some object or situation. A phobia is an irrational fear of such things. Some phobias may be obsessional and in this instance they have the characteristics of obsessional symptoms in that they are accompanied by repetitive feelings of compulsion associated with resistance and emotional distress.

Compulsive Actions

Motor activities of an obsessional kind are referred to as compulsions. Compulsions are an irrational impulse to perform some form of action. Examples of obsessional compulsions are tendencies to carry out acts a certain number of times, such as switching off electric lights, undressing and dressing, the tendency to count things and do things by numbers, the tendency to carry out certain activities like washing and cleaning repetitively.

One of my soldier patients during the war had a compulsion to part his hair exactly in the middle. In the morning he spent half an hour in an attempt to get it right, first parting it to the left of the middle line and then to the right of the middle line until eventually it was more or less correct but never completely to his satisfaction. He had a compulsion to do things four times; on going to bed he would have to undress and dress four times and similarly on getting up. He had a compulsion to touch things four times. All this made his life very complicated and difficult; he also always had to start doing things on the right, the right hand or the right foot, but customary procedure in the Army is 'by the left quick march' and this used to put him off for the rest of the day.

Patients with obsessional states have varying degrees of anxiety, tension and distress and may have secondary depression.

It has been found that about one fifth of obsessive-compulsive states have depressive symptoms and one eighth symptoms of anxiety.

Obsessions as Parts of Other Illnesses

Obsessional symptoms may occur in many psychiatric illnesses, e.g.:

1 *Schizophrenia* It is probable that the occurrence of obsessional illness in schizophrenia represents the occurrence of two disorders rather than a single illness. There is some evidence that persistent obsessional symptoms may inhibit the development of schizophrenia. Sometimes obsessional symptoms may merge into those of schizophrenia. Ominous signs are the development of a loss of anxiety and concern about the illness and a decrease in tendency to resist.

2 *Depressive states* It has been estimated that some 20% of patients with depressive illness have obsessive-compulsive symptoms, and a third have obsessive-compulsive traits of personality. These figures are even higher in patients suffering from depression during the involutional period. It is also noteworthy that patients with an obsessive-compulsive illness may develop a typical depression as a secondary reaction. Another association is the tendency for obsessional symptoms to appear only during attacks of depressive illness, and in this situation the obsessional symptoms usually resolve with recovery from the attack of depression, whether this occurs spontaneously or as a result of treatment by drugs or other means.

3 *Organic brain diseases* The occurrence of obsessional symptoms in organic brain disorders has aroused a great deal of interest and speculation. In encephalitis lethargica, sometimes patients develop obsessional symptoms having previously been free from the disorder.

Sometimes obsessional symptoms occur only when the patient develops oculogyric crises. It is interesting that some metallic poisons, particularly those which produce extrapyramidal symptoms, may also produce obsessional symptoms—for instance, manganese poisoning.

Natural History and Prognosis

The illness may come on in attacks and episodes with intervening periods of freedom, or they may last for longer periods with exacerbation, and during the intervening periods the symptoms may be less distressing to the patient, although they are still present. Environmental stresses may act as precipitants in some patients. The illness may show spontaneous recovery and when this takes place it is more likely in the early years of the illness. In those patients in whom the obsessional illness has gone on for many years, five years or longer, the probability of spontaneous recovery or complete recovery in response to treatment decreases.

About one half of the patients develop their main illness before the age of twenty, and only 4% start after the age of 35 years.

Studies of the outcome of obsessional states give different figures for the degree of recovery, ranging from 25% to 50% over a follow-up period of five to ten years. The prognosis is, on the whole, favourable for obsessional states which develop as part of a depressive illness, as they disappear with recovery from depression. A relatively early age of onset tends to carry a poor prognosis. A marked obsessional premorbid personality and severity of clinical picture on first admission are also regarded as unfavourable prognostic factors.

Social Aspects Most authorities find that the families of obsessional patients have a significantly higher incidence of obsessional disorders than the corresponding control groups, whilst there is evidence that genetic factors predispose to the illness. There is also evidence that a strict tyrannical upbringing with insistence on rectitude, obedience, and cleanliness may also be contributory. It has been found that patients are often ill for many years before being referred for outpatient or inpatient treatment. They form a small proportion of patients admitted to hospital, between 2% and 3%.

Relationship to Obsessional Personality

The obsessional personality is described as being meticulous, conscientious, orderly and punctilious. These are clean, punctual people paying a great deal of attention to detail and being trustworthy, reliable and tending to take their work home in their minds at night.

They are precise, careful, cautious, pedantic and conservative. They dislike change and get very disturbed if their plans have to be altered. They become creatures of habit, rigid, unadaptable people. As employees they are appreciated, the salt of the earth, dependable and will work at their best without supervision. They set themselves very high standards and tend to be anxious.

Obsessional personalities are common in the community and are not necessarily related to obsessional illness. Some of them can develop obsessional states but there are many patients with obsessional states who do not have this type of personality before the illness.

Obsessional personalities are of importance in predisposition to the development of anxiety states and various psychosomatic disorders.

Psychopathology

According to psychoanalytic theory obsessive compulsive illnesses are associated with conflicts and regression at the anal-sadistic phase of psychosexual development. In favour of this is the frequency with which patients are preoccupied with aggression or dirt, either in their personality or in their symptoms. The mental mechanism underlying an obsession involves a conflict between drives which seek expression such as sex drives, self-assertion, aggressive drives on one hand, and the controlling forces on the other. This conflict is dealt with by displacement and substitution into an obsessional symptom, and sometimes the obsessional symptom may symbolize the nature of the conflict; for example, the handwashing compulsion may symbolize the getting rid of dirt, this is resolving guilt feelings about sexual problems.

Proponents of the learning theory suggest that certain phobias and obsessional symptoms may involve learning mechanisms, particularly as the obsession is associated with anxiety. As a compulsive act relieves the anxiety this will produce a reinforcement which will be conducive to its perpetuation and eventually, because of its capacity for reducing anxiety it becomes fixed by learning as a pattern of behaviour.

General Management of Obsessional Disorders

Associated anxiety and tension can be relieved by appropriate tranquillo-sedative drugs. These will help to make the patient's life more bearable and will make it easier for him to learn to adjust himself to his illness. Many patients will recover on a simple regime of his kind.

If the obsessional symptoms are part of a depressive illness, the treatment is that of the depression, either by antidepressant drugs or, if severe, by electroconvulsive therapy. Psychotherapy is of more value in explaining the psychopathology and genesis of symptoms than effecting improvement. Obsessional states are notoriously resistant to psychotherapeutic approaches because of the strength of the patient's defences and the rigidity of his personality. Hallucinogenic drugs such as lysergic acid and phencyclidine have been used to make the patient more accessible to psychotherapy.

The Treatment of Phobic and Obsessional States

The treatment of phobias and obsessional symptoms has been revolutionized by the introduction of new techniques of behaviour therapy. In addition behaviour therapy may be combined with pharmacological methods of treatment. Specific phobias, including morbid fears of animals such as dogs or spiders, or defined events, such as heights or thunder storms, can effectively be treated with systematic desensitization which involves a gradual exposure in increasing intensity to the phobic situation, usually with a state of relaxation induced to prevent the evocation of anxiety. Flooding, which involves a more rapid, intense exposure to the phobic stimulus, is useful in the treatment of general phobias including agoraphobia.

The common feature of systematic desensitization and flooding is that there is either a gradual or a sudden exposure to the stimulus which enables the patient to adapt to it.

Compulsions, often related to cleaning activities, avoidance, repetition or checking, usually result in a reduction of anxiety and subjectively they are considered to avoid disasters or ill fortune. For example, hand washing can be treated by behaviour therapy involving contact with the feared contaminant and prevention of washing. This has been termed apotrepic therapy because apotrepic means turning away or dissuading. Flooding associated with modelling, in which the therapist carries out the contact with the phobic stimulus or object, can also be carried out with response prevention. Other workers have shown that deliberate contamination and allowing washing to take place is also quite as effective as that achieved by response prevention.

Obsessional slowness has been treated by behavioural techniques including prompting and pacing by the therapist, and also shaping, which is achieved by graduating the tasks and giving reward in the form of praise or approval when they are achieved.

Obsessional ruminations are not helped by systematic desensitization; they are more effectively treated by thought stopping. The thought stopping technique requires the patient to think his obsessive thoughts deliberately, the therapist then makes a sudden loud (aversive) noise and shouts 'Stop'. This appears to interrupt the induced rumination and the patient is then taught to shout 'Stop' each time he deliberately produces his distressing thoughts. After some practice he whispers 'Stop' and eventually uses a subvocal command. The technique of paradoxical intention is in some ways similar. Six sessions of instructions in deliberately magnifying and exaggerating obsessional ideas have been found to produce a marked decrease in the occurrence of obtrusive unwanted thoughts.

Psychotropic drugs have also been used either alone or in combination with behaviour therapy for the treatment of phobias and obsessional symptoms. Clomipramine, a tricyclic antidepressant, may be given intravenously in doses of 300–375 mg daily for 15 days or may be given orally in a daily dose of 400 mg. Favourable reports have been made on the use of clomipramine both in the treatment of obsessional thoughts and ruminations, certainly when they are based on a depressive illness, but even sometimes when there is no associated depression. Monoamine oxidase inhibitors have been used in association with systematic desensitization in severe phobias, including agoraphobia. Systematic desensitization techniques can be facilitated by inducing relaxation by giving small doses of methohexitone, propanidid or diazepam intravenously. For single phobias prolonged exposure by flooding techniques is most effective but some patients may need preliminary exposure in fantasy. Agoraphobias respond well to monoamine oxidase inhibitors combined with flooding. Social phobias respond well to a combination of monoamine oxidase inhibitors and systematic desensitization. Compulsions respond well to exposure with or without response prevention and are helped by training in assertiveness. Obsessional ruminations may be helped by tricyclic antidepressants or electroconvulsive therapy when associated with a depressive illness. In other instances, thought stoppage and paradoxical intention usually is efficacious. Psychosurgery may be indicated in intractable severe obsessional and phobic states with a high level of free floating anxiety. The following improved methods of psychosurgery have been successfully applied in such cases:

1 *Subcordate tractotomy* using yttrium seeds. This method interrupts the connections between the agranular cortex to the cingulate posterior orbital and amygdaloid regions

2 *Limbic leucotomy* Three lesions are produced by cryogenic probes, one in the lower median quadrant of the frontal lobe, and two pairs of cingulate lesions.

3 *Bimedial leucotomy*.

When psychosurgery is used, active postoperative rehabilitation is of paramount importance, and postoperative behaviour therapy can provide additional benefit.

29

Psychopathic Disorders

The term psychopathic personality is emotionally charged and has been overworked, abused and ill-used. It is sometimes employed as a term of abuse for one's political or religious opponents and the term tends to engender hostile attitudes on the part of society.

Although many definitions have been given, the consensus of opinion is that the psychopath's behaviour shows a lack of social responsibility, of consideration for others and of prudence and foresight. A convenient definition is that a psychopath is a person who, from an early age, shows abnormality of character marked by episodes of antisocial behaviour and tendencies to act on impulse to satisfy the need of the moment, without giving due regard to the consequences of such action.

The psychopath's persistent antisocial mode of conduct ranges from inefficiency and lack of interest in any form of occupation, to pathological lying, swindling, slandering, alcoholism, drug addiction, sexual offences and violent actions with little motivation and an entire absence of self-restraint.

If the term is to have any real value, it should be applied to antisocial or criminal behaviour only after the strict exclusion of intellectual defect, psychosis, neurosis, cerebral injury or disease.

The characteristics of psychopathy are immaturity, self-centredness, little or no regard for the rights or convenience of others; the immediate satisfaction of desires is imperative. If frustrated, the psychopath tends to act violently without any feeling of guilt.

The Mental Health Act (1983) describes psychopathic disorders as persistent disorders or disability of mind (whether or not including significant impairment of intelligence) which result in abnormally aggressive or seriously irresponsible conduct on the part of the person concerned.

The various definitions applied to psychopathic personality have four common features:

1 *Excluding cause* viz. the condition does not amount to mental defect, he is not insane or psycho-neurotic; whether or not the person is of low intelligence, it is independent of subnormality and mental illness.
2 *Time factor* The abnormality exists throughout life or from a comparatively early age and is usually recurrent, episodic or persistent.
3 *Description of behaviour* viz. antisocial, unable to accept social requirements on account of abnormal peculiarities of impulse, temperament or character; conduct is abnormally aggressive or irresponsible.
4 *Personality characteristics* which have been described as part of psychopathy are marked ego-centricity, lack of sincerity, lack of feeling and lack of guilt. In practice, one sees many psychopaths who possess these attributes quite clearly in certain circumstances.

The differentiation between aggressive and inadequate psychopaths is not satisfactory, as one form may turn into the other.

Scott classifies psychopaths as follows:

1 *Persons trained to antisocial standards* These are persons who behave as they were taught to behave and do what is normal in their families or districts. The offender has learned this behaviour consistently and will not feel guilt about doing what he was taught to do. His family or circle will not be critical. The offence is strictly goal-motivated, intended as a means to material gain or the acquisition of prestige. The observer can easily find sympathy and find it

possible to identify himself with the offender and his setting.

Treatment requirement is retraining.

2 *Reparative behaviour* Here the offence is part of an intelligently, laboriously and often consciously worked out policy, aimed at the adjustment of the individual to difficulties in his environment and to personal handicaps which that environment has produced in him, e.g. compensations for feelings of inadequacy, inferiority.

The offender is identified with his pattern of mis-behaviour and his even proud of it. The offence is goal-motivated.

Treatment is retraining.

3 *The untrained offender* Here there are no steady standards of behaviour provided in early life. The adult is, therefore, without standards and weak in character. Conduct difficulties show themselves diffusely and from early childhood.

4 *Rigid fixations* Here learning has broken down and has been replaced by a fixed, maladaptive pattern of response. The crime is stereotyped, non-adaptive and non-goal-directed, which persists unaltered despite long periods in a controlled environment and is utterly unimproved by severe punishment.

The offender dissociates himself from his behaviour but may be genuinely remorseful and anxious about it. He is bewildered about it.

The offence is stereotyped. It brings nothing but relief from immediate tension. The observer cannot feel sympathy with the offender.

Punishment is useless.

Aetiology

Studies of the degree of concordance of criminality in pairs of uniovular and binovular twins show that personality is dependent, to some extent, upon hereditary factors but that the environment may largely control the expression of the personality disposition.

Neuroses and psychopathic states are multi-factorially determined.

Studies of the relationships between rates of juvenile crime and social disturbances conclude that there appears to be something particularly significant in social disturbances occurring in the fourth and fifth year of a child's life.

Constitutional attributes found in psychopaths also favour genetic factors, such as mesomorphic body build and abnormalities in the electro-encephalogram which are correlated with aggressiveness.

The evidence regarding aetiology is conflicting and we are not yet in a position to make dogmatic statements as to the relative importance of inherited and environmental factors, except to say that it is the interaction of both rather than either one or the other which is important.

The Management and Treatment of Psychopathy

Psychopaths notoriously lack persistence and determination and, even when they present themselves for treatment, they often want a magical cure and are prepared to do very little themselves to help. Very often they only seek treatment when they are in difficulties with the law or with their families.

Individual psychotherapy over a period of years, if the patient cooperates, may occasionally help to achieve a better adjustment.

Drug Treatment

In some aggressive psychopaths with marked aggressive outbursts, amphetamines given with phenytoin sodium have been found to be helpful, particularly if there is evidence of cerebral dysrhythmia.

Major tranquillizers and tranquillo-sedatives are of limited value in psychopathy itself and although one of the phenothiazines (Pericyazine) has been claimed to be helpful in the management of behaviour disturbances in psychopaths, these claims have yet to be substantiated.

Group Therapy

Group therapy is often a preferable method of dealing with psychopaths and group therapy in a special hospital such as that at Belmont, Surrey, is particularly promising.

It is generally agreed that psychopaths admitted to psychiatric hospitals are probably better treated as a group in separate wards or units because of their tendency to act out their behaviour. It is interesting that patients with psychiatric illnesses such as depression or schizophrenia do not usually regard psychopaths as being ill. Psychopaths, in turn, very often manipulate people and situations and create a great many difficulties in the running of the ward or hospital.

In a proportion of psychopaths there is a tendency for greater maturity with greater normality and better adjustment to occur in middle life, but this is not invariably so.

Further Reading

Craft, M. (1966) *Psychopathic Disorders and Their Assessment*. Pergamon Press, Oxford.

30

Sexual Disorders

These disorders may be conveniently discussed as follows:

1 Disorders of heterosexual functioning, e.g. impotence and frigidity.
2 Disorders in which the aim of sexual activity deviates from the normal, e.g. homosexuality, exhibitionism, transvestism, etc.

Heterosexual Dysfunctions in Men

Sexual disability in men may take various forms such as:

1 Absence of sexual desire for the sexual partner or absence of sexual desire in general
2 Inability to procure erection
3 Inability to sustain erection
4 Inability to ejaculate in spite of well sustained erection
5 Premature ejaculation

The sexual act involves a chain of reflexes and anything which interferes with this chain can give rise to any of the above dysfunctions. The large majority of cases of the above forms of impotence are psychogenic. The most common cause of interference is anxiety.

One frequent situation which has been traditionally associated with impotence is the honeymoon. Both partners are tired, excited, anxious and self-conscious, and some are ignorant and inexperienced. Not infrequently these factors combine to render a man impotent on this occasion.

On the next occasion, he approaches the sexual situation with anxiety which, in itself, is sufficient to render him impotent or cause him to ejaculate prematurely. After this, secondary anxiety increases

in snowball fashion until the man is convinced that he is abnormal or congenitally impotent.

Masturbation anxiety is possibly quite a common factor, but any form of anxiety or depression can produce impotence.

The following are other causes of impotence. Some men unconsciously identify their sexual partner with their mother or sister and the incest taboo asserts itself and they are impotent with their wives but may be potent with prostitutes or other women. Other men associate the sexual act with aggression and violence; they have a very marked fear of violence and this may be another mechanism.

The above forms of impotence, particularly those due to general anxiety, are common.

Ejaculatory impotence, that is incapacity to ejaculate even when aroused and with erection, is much rarer. There are many reasons for this, some are very deep-seated such as fears of pregnancy, or difficulty in giving.

Another type is the professional man's impotence, the hard working professional man works all day and in the evening until the early hours of the morning and he virtually has no energy left over for love-making.

Any drugs which produce marked stimulation of the sympathetic nervous system can lead to impotence. This applies to the monoamine oxidase inhibiting drugs and amphetamines. In cases of impotence due to depression, mild doses of these drugs may in fact help by relieving the depression and therefore permitting libido to become enhanced, but large doses or prolonged medication will tend to have the opposite effect by stimulating sympathetic activity and thus interfering with the sacral parasympathetic which subserves vasodilation.

Heterosexual Dysfunctions in Women

Disturbances in heterosexual activity in women may be classified as follows:

1 Frigidity
2 Vaginismus
3 Dyspareunia

Frigidity is lack of sexual feeling in women and may vary in degree from an intense feeling of revulsion to any sexual advance to varying sexual arousal without orgasm.

Frigidity may be primary or secondary.

Primary frigidity is when the woman has never experienced an orgasm and may be partial or complete.

Secondary frigidity is when a woman has experienced orgasm in the past but is unable to do so now. It may also be partial or complete.

Complete primary frigidity may be due to anatomical defects, physiological deficiency in endocrine glands, viz. in pituitary-ovarian functions, or may be psychological.

Partial primary frigidity may be due to ignorance, fear, or to feelings of hostility. These women have lacked sexual instruction from their parents and very often their partners are ignorant of their needs and of sexual techniques.

In secondary frigidity, physical causes may sometimes contribute by causing dyspareunia. Physiological factors are sometimes responsible during lactation.

Psychological factors include:

1 Fears of pregnancy
2 Inadequate stimulation due to coitus interruptus or the partner being weakly potent or suffering from premature ejaculation
3 In professional women who are financially and socially emancipated, it becomes an emotional problem of dependency versus independency
4 Depression or anxiety symptoms may also be a contributory factor

Vaginismus

Vaginismus is an involuntary spasm of the vaginal muscles, always psychogenic in origin. It is usually an automatic fear or anxiety reaction, sometimes coming on after painful experiences during intercourse.

In some women, it is a difficulty in accepting the full female role and is a manifestation of psychosexual immaturity.

Treatment by systematic desensitization with or without the use of vaginal dilators achieves good results.

Homosexuality

Definition

The term homosexual is applied to sexual relationships whether overt or psychic between individuals of the same sex. It is derived from the Greek 'homo' meaning the same, rather than the Latin for man. It denotes the sameness of the two individuals involved in the sexual relationship and is the antithesis of the word heterosexual.

It has been shown that there is a continuous gradation among members of the general population between exclusively heterosexual and exclusively homosexual behaviour.

Kinsey (1948) proposed a very useful heterosexual–homosexual rating scale:

0 Exclusively heterosexual with no homosexual tendencies
1 Predominantly heterosexual and only incidentally homosexual
2 Predominantly heterosexual but with more than incidental homosexuality
3 Equally heterosexual and homosexual
4 Predominantly homosexual but more than incidentally heterosexual
5 Predominantly homosexual but incidentally heterosexual
6 Exclusively homosexual

Surveys in the United States have revealed that 3–4% of males and 1% of females are exclusively homosexual.

It must be remembered that homosexuality can occur in apparently normal, stable persons free from psychiatric symptoms and who are otherwise socially well-adjusted.

It can also occur in unstable personalities, persons with neurosis, psychopathy, mental subnormality, psychosis and organic mental states.

Aetiology

Different authorities emphasize the importance of one or more of the following:

1 Genetic factors
2 Constitutional predisposition
3 Conditioning factors
4 Psychodynamic mechanisms
5 The influence of physiological and hormonal factors

Twin studies provide some evidence that homosexuality may be genetically determined, but only in a proportion of patients. Studies of endocrine factors have been, on the whole, inconclusive.

With regard to personality, it must be remembered that masculinity and femininity is not an 'all or nothing' affair, because persons of each sex may show varying proportions of both. One may get extremely masculine females and extremely feminine males.

Surveys reveal that homosexuals who have come to psychiatric care or who have come to the notice of Courts of Law tend to have a higher incidence of neurotic or schizoid types of personality but, on the whole, only showed minor differences from normals.

The following classes of homosexuals may be described:

1 Adolescents and emotionally immature adults, who go through a phase in which they are uncomfortably aware of their attraction to both sexes and are in a quandary which they cannot solve. They usually respond well to supportive psychiatric treatment.
2 Markedly abnormal personalities with marked effeminacy who often solicit and not infrequently become homosexual prostitutes, preferring the chase to the actual sexual contact.
3 The inadequate, dull person who has never experienced loving relationships with anyone, and who is usually very socially isolated.
4 The resentful, antisocial person who often has a long record of Court appearances.
5 Homosexuality in relatively normal, intact personalities.
6 Latent, well-compensated homosexuals. These may be intelligent, married and have children.
7 Homosexuality occurring along with serious mental disability such as psychopathy, psychosis or organic brain damage. These patients are apt to injure victims in a way that none of the other would contemplate, nor do they take only predisposed victims.

Some authorities believe that parental influences may play an important role in the causation of homosexuality. Some implicate a maternal attitude of excessive strictness and perfectionism; others implicate father-deprivation at a time when awareness of homosexual attraction is not abnormal as a phase of development.

Treatment may be by psychotherapy or by behaviour therapy.

Psychotherapy can help some homosexuals who are burdened by guilt, neurotic difficulties or intolerable sexual tension, and also those persons who request help in order to fortify them in restraining overt behaviour likely to involve them in trouble with the law.

It is the view of most practising psychiatrists that no cure can be offered to complete homosexuals with a Kinsey rating of 6. A great deal can be done to make the homosexual a more happy, well-adjusted and effective person.

Aversion therapy may be applied, either using apomorphine injections to produce vomiting or an electrical current to produce a painful stimulus. Whenever nausea, vomiting or pain are felt the patients are confronted with photographs of nude or near nude men whom they find attractive. This is repeated until a marked aversion develops. Sometimes a substitution of photographs of sexually attractive women are presented, accompanied by injections of testosterone propionate.

It is difficult to evaluate the role of aversion therapy. It is important to realize that in many patients the goal of treatment has to be realistic and must be limited. Many patients cannot and have no wish to change their homosexuality. If they can be helped to be relieved of psychiatric symptoms and to adjust reasonably well in work and society a worthwhile result is achieved.

Behaviour therapy, consisting of systematic desensitization of fears relating to approaching females, is also effective and sometimes more acceptable in some forms of male homosexuality.

Transvestism and Transexualism

Transvestism is the impulse to wear the clothing of the opposite sex. Transexualism is the term given to escribe the wish to change the anatomical sex.

Transvestites proper are defined as those men who obtain sexual gratification from dressing as women. In transvestism the clothes or the wearing of them may provide an end in itself, as they are usually endowed with sexual significance and the act of wearing them may provide the sole form of sexual expression. Many transvestites lack sexual drives and state that they feel mainly more contented and more comfortable while wearing female attire. The onset of transvestism and transexualism is usually before 12 years of age. It occurs in all social classes and in men and women.

Aversion therapy has proved effective in treating transvestism and may need to be supplemented by vocational, social and psychotherapeutic guidance to help readjustment.

Transexualism is more difficult to treat and the result of surgical treatment attempting to make the person appear more like the opposite sex has, on the whole, been disappointing.

General Principles in the Management of Psychosexual Disorders

The first requirement is a physical examination and a full psychiatric history with an assessment of the patient's personality and present mental state.

Masters and Johnson have elaborated very effective techniques for dealing with psychosexual problems. They point out that psychosexual problems frequently reflect other areas of disharmony or misunderstanding in the marriage. The marital relationship is treated as a whole with the emphasis that sexual function is a part of this relationship. The couple, together with a male and female therapist, meet at a round table session to clarify, discuss and work through problems. Specific exercises are prescribed for the couple to help them with their particular sexual difficulty. Experience has revealed that most forms of sexual inadequacy involve a lack of information, or misinformation, and fear of performance. Couples are specifically prohibited from any sexual play other than that prescribed by the therapist. In the beginning, exercises are usually devoted to increasing sensual awareness to touch, sight, sound and smell, and the couples learn to give and receive bodily pleasure without the pressure of performance. A very important element is that they simultaneously learn to communicate bodily in a mutually satisfactory way and that sexual foreplay is as important as intercourse. Genital stimulation is later added to general bodily stimulation. The plan is to start an educational process to diminish fears of performance felt by both sexes and to facilitate communication between the couple, both in sexual and non-sexual spheres.

Further Reading

Kinsey, A. C., Pomeroy, W. G. and Martin, C. (1948) *Sexual Behaviour in the Human Male*. Sanderson, Philadelphia.

Comfort, A. (1963) *Sex in Society*. Duckworth, London.

Masters, W. H. and Johnson, V. E. (1966) *The Human Sexual Response*. Little, Brown, Boston.

Dominion, J. (1968) *Marital Breakdown*. Penguin Books, Harmondsworth.

Masters, W. H. and Johnson, V. E. (1970) *Human Sexual Inadequacy*. Churchill Livingstone, Edinburgh.

Kaplan, H. S. (1974) *The New Sex Therapy*. Brunner/Mazel, New York.

Trimmer, E. J. (1978) *Basic Sexual Medicine; A Textbook of Sexual Medicine and an Introduction to Sexual Counselling Techniques*. Heinemann, London.

Bancroft, J. (1985) *Human Sexuality and Its Problems*. Churchill Livingstone, Edinburgh.

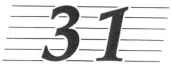

Chemical Dependence

Alcoholism

Alcoholism is a disease in an individual who has, over a long period of time, consumed large amounts of alcohol.

The disease is characterized by:

1 A pathological desire for alcohol after ingestion of small quantities which act as a trigger dose
2 Black-outs during intoxication with alcohol
3 Physical dependence on alcohol after withdrawal following a drinking bout

These are the cardinal symptoms of alcoholism. Heavy consumers who do not present these cardinal symptoms, or only exhibit one of them, are simply called alcohol abusers and this group cannot be clearly demarcated from the average normal consumer.

Types of Alcoholism

Jellinek has subdivided alcoholism into the following types:

1 *Alpha alcoholism* Excessive and inappropriate drinking without loss of control or ability to abstain.
2 *Beta alcoholism* Excessive and inappropriate drinking without clear psychological or physical dependence but with physical complications such as cirrhosis, neuritis or gastritis.
3 *Gamma alcoholism* Characterized by physical dependence, tolerance, and inability to control drinking, with a progressive course.
4 *Delta alcoholism* This type occurs in wine-consuming countries and is characterized by inability to abstain, tolerance, withdrawal symptoms, but the quantity consumed can be controlled.

5 *Epsilon alcoholism* Intermittent or spree drinking.

The prevalence of alcoholism is difficult to assess reliably for a variety of reasons.

The Department of Health and Social Security, in 1976, estimated that there were 500 000 people in England and Wales with a serious drinking problem. This must be regarded as a minimum figure. In recent years there has been a change in the distribution of people with alcohol dependence problems in that there has been a substantial increase in younger age groups and also in women.

It should be noted that the term alcoholic is reserved for the individual in whom alcohol has induced mental and physical changes.

Aetiology

Social Factors

Social pressures, economic trends and cultural attitudes all exert some influence on the pattern of drinking and, indirectly, the incidence of alcoholism.

Psychological Factors

There is no typical pre-alcoholic personality. What usually happens is that a proportion of all regular users of alcohol become occasional excessive drinkers during periods of stress or when depressed and, as a result of this, a smaller proportion become constant drinkers. Some of these, in turn, may eventually become alcoholics. Finally, a small group again, lose control and become addictive alcoholics.

In the pre-alcoholic phase, alcohol is taken to provide relief. This becomes more regular and tolerance is increased. The prodromal phase follows and is marked by black-outs in which the drinker, after a moderate intake of alcohol, may show no signs of intoxication and be able to carry out acts requiring skill and co-ordination, of which he subsequently has no recollection.

The prodromal phase advances with additional secret drinking, preparation for social gatherings with alcohol and periods of avid drinking followed by guilt feelings. At this point, the person avoids reference to alcohol in his talk and has more frequent black-outs.

The crucial phase is ushered in by a loss of control, in which the ingestion of even a small quantity of alcohol sets up a compulsive demand for more, which ceases only when his stomach or nervous system calls a halt.

In the subsequent chronic phase, prolonged periods of intoxication with absence from work make their appearance and there is a deterioration in ethical attitudes.

Psychiatric Disorders Associated with Alcoholism

Delirium Tremens

In the early stages, which may last some weeks, the patient is tense, anxious, jumpy and suffers from terrifying illusions and hallucinations at night. As a rule, the onset is sudden.

The features of delirium tremens are: disorientation, hallucinations of vision, equilibrium, sensation and hearing. The visual hallucinations are often quite frightening as are vestibular sensations of rocking and flying. Illusions are quite common, i.e. misinterpretation of cutaneous sensations, the patient believing that insects are crawling over him.

Clinical signs include ataxia, coarse tremor, jerkiness of speech and writing, active deep reflexes, sweating, rapid pulse, increased tension, albuminuria and pyrexia. Epileptic attacks occur in 10%. Insomnia is highly characteristic.

The usual course is that, before the end of the first week, a crisis occurs during which the patient falls into a deep sleep to awaken clear in mind.

Fatal cases are usually those having pneumonia or when a delirium passes into a coma, the latter being due to polioencephalitis haemorrhagica superior.

Sometimes the delirium passes into a chronic Korsakov state.

Acute Alcoholic Hallucinosis

In this condition, auditory hallucinations—the voices are often abusive, threatening—occur during relatively clear consciousness. At the onset there is increased acuity of hearing with noises in the head and poorly differentiated hallucinations such as banging, shouts, bells, and screams. Many voices may be heard and identified and as a rule are not attributed to bystanders. The patient is frightened and is usually glad to seek refuge in a hospital or police station.

Sometimes delusions develop as a secondary development of the hallucinations.

Usually a full recovery in three or four weeks takes place but sometimes insight is never regained; delusions may persist and the condition can develop into a fairly typical paranoid schizophrenic illness.

Acute alcoholic hallucinosis may be a sequel to delirium tremens. A characteristic feature is the hearing of abusive voices which talk about the patient in the third person and experienced as occurring above the patient's head.

Chronic Alcoholic Delusional States

Chronic alcoholics often become suspicious and paranoid in disposition but sometimes they may develop delusions of jealousy, which start when the patient is drunk but may continue when he is sober.

Most frequently the man accuses his wife of adultery with neighbours and he attempts to extort a confession from her. Undoubtedly his diminishing sexual potency, his sexual maladjustment, his bad conscience and his wife's inevitable aversion to him when drunk, play a part in the development of delusions of jealousy. However, delusions of jealousy may develop also in abstinent men in late middle life.

Korsakov's Syndrome

Alcohol is only one of many causes of Korsakov's syndrome. It is most frequently seen in middle-aged alcoholics. The features are:

1 Grossly disturbed memory
2 Fabrications to cover gaps in recall
3 Disorientation in space and time
4 Clear consciousness
5 Poor judgment

6 Apathy, varying from empty euphoria to irritability

7 Polyneuritis is common but not invariable

Pathologically, there are degenerative changes in the periventricular and periaqueductal grey matter, mammillary bodies and dorso-medial nucleus of the thalamus.

The distribution of lesions is identical with Wernicke's encephalopathy and it has been suggested that both Korsakov's psychosis and Wernicke's encephalopathy are due to thiamine deficiency, differences in symptomatology depending on the acuteness of the underlying disease process.

Wernicke's Encephalopathy

Alcohol is one of the most common causes of this condition. Occular changes are constant; horizontal nystagmus is more common than vertical nystagmus. External rectus paralysis is an early sign. Ataxia with wide, reeling gait. There is lack of interest and lack of initiative but full consciousness in the early stages. There is difficulty in attention.

Marchiafava's Disease

This is characterized by demyelination of the corpus callosum and optic tracts. The clinical picture is one of acute confusion and hallucinations and outbursts of excitement.

Pathological Intoxication

Some people react severely to alcohol, even in small amounts. They may react with sudden violence which is similar to an epileptic automatism, ending in a deep sleep with complete amnesia.

EEG studies show that the condition is correlated with psychomotor epilepsy. In these patients the alcohol acts as a stimulus in small doses, producing a theta activity of six cycles per second in the temporal regions.

Chronic Dementia

This may be the end result of prolonged alcoholism and may follow any of the above syndromes.

Treatment of Alcoholism

The first step in treatment is medical assessment of the patient's condition; whether he suffers from any known physical disorders which may complicate alcoholism, particularly cirrhosis of the liver and organic brain syndromes. The next step is psychiatric assessment, including the role played by his personality make-up; whether the patient drinks for pleasure mainly or as a defence mechanism to relieve emotional distress due to emotional problems; whether he is suffering from psychiatric disorders such as a depressive state or anxiety state or the syndromes specially associated with alcoholism. It is then necessary to assess the patient's social relationships at work, with his family and friends. The patient's adjustment in these spheres will have an important bearing on his rehabilitation after treatment.

Acute alcoholic intoxication needs hospital treatment and skilled nursing.

Detoxification

The principles of detoxification include the following:

1 To minimize distress, adverse effects and dangers of withdrawal. These include severe anxiety, epileptic fits, delirium and cardiovascular disturbances.

2 Detoxification is an important first step in treatment but of much greater importance is the management and after-care following detoxification.

In order to relieve anxiety and to counteract the possibility of epileptic fits, chlormethiazole in doses of 1000 to 4000 mg daily may be given for a period not exceeding 7 to 10 days, otherwise there is a risk of dependence. An alternative is carbamazepine which also has anti-anxiety, anti-depression and anti-epileptic properties. It is given in doses ranging from 400 to 1600 mg a day and is free from risk of dependence. Anti-histamines, such as promethazine may be given to counteract any allergic reactions and to relieve anxiety and promote sleep.

In view of the fact that alcoholics have neglected their dietary intake and may have impaired absorption of food stuffs and vitamins it is often desirable to give parenteral injections of high potency vitamins.

either intravenously or intramuscularly for a period of ten days.

The above medications are given on a gradually reducing regime with the aim of stopping all drugs in about ten days.

It is undesirable to prescribe addictive drugs, such as benzodiazepines, barbiturates and similar hypnosedatives either for the relief of anxiety or for promotion of sleep, unless given for a very limited period (7–10 days). On the whole they are best avoided.

Long term treatment may involve specific therapeutic measures, such as aversion therapy with apomorphine or treatment with disulfiram.

Supportive psychotherapy is important and social therapy, particularly the help of Alcoholics Anonymous, can make all the difference between success and failure in long term treatment.

Aversion Therapy

Apomorphine is the most commonly used agent for aversion treatment of alcoholism. It is a powerful emetic and each injection induces nausea and vomiting. The patient is allowed to drink his favourite drink and the injection is then given. Sometimes the aversion gradually diminishes and a booster course may be necessary at intervals of six months or a year, depending on the patient.

Antabuse Treatment

Antabuse (disulfiram) interferes with the metabolism of alcohol causing an increase in the level of blood acetaldehyde. This causes unpleasant reactions which make it difficult to continue drinking. The patient on Antabuse, on taking a small quantity of alcohol, has distressing symptoms including flushing, sweating, dyspnoea, headache, tachycardia, drowsiness, falling blood pressure, nausea and vomiting. If the fall in blood pressure is rapid, the patient may develop a peripheral circulatory collapse.

Antabuse is given 800 mg the first day, 600 mg the second day, 400 mg the third day, and 200 mg the fourth and fifth days. A test of the reaction to alcohol is carried out on the fourth day in order to demonstrate to the patient what will happen to him if he attempts to drink. The test dose of alcohol is the equivalent of 15 cc of alcohol as given in whisky, wine, beer or other drink to which the patient is addicted. After this, a maintenance dosage, usually 100 mg to 200 mg daily is given.

Antabuse is of value in the management of the alcoholic who genuinely wishes to overcome his addiction and who requires an additional prop to help him to overcome any craving that might develop particularly when confronted with difficult situations, disappointments, or the temptation to be involved in various social events. If there is a relative who can supervise the administration of Antabuse, this greatly enhances the effectiveness of the treatment.

It is essential that the alcoholic must abstain from the use of alcohol absolutely and permanently and, as it usually takes a number of years for marked dependency on alcohol to develop, it may take some years before he is completely free from this dependency. The physician must bear this in mind and help the patient in shifting his dependency through better interpersonal relationships, new interests and satisfying achievements as a substitute for alcoholic indulgence.

If the patient joins Alcoholics Anonymous, this is extremely valuable in helping him to withstand the temptation to revert to alcohol.

Drug Dependence

Drug addiction may be defined as a state of periodic or persistent intoxication, detrimental to the individual, to society or both and is characterized by the following features:

1 A strong drive, need or compulsion to continue taking the drug
2 The development of tolerance, with a tendency to increase the dose to produce desired effects
3 Physical and emotional dependence

Physical dependence results from an altered physiological state, which necessitates continued administration of the drug in order to prevent the appearance of a characteristic series of symptoms referred to as the abstinence syndrome or withdrawal state.

The term drug habituation has been applied to the person who has a strong drive or need or compulsion to continue taking the drug on which he is emotionally dependent, but he does not develop the withdrawal state characteristic of addiction.

The World Health Organization has suggested

that the term drug dependence should be applied to both drug addiction, drug habituation and all types of drug abuse.

Drug dependence is defined as a state arising from repeated administration of a drug on a periodic or continuous basis. Its characteristics will vary with the agent involved.

Individuals may become dependent on a wide variety of chemical substances, with a diversity of pharmacodynamic effects ranging from stimulation to depression. All such drugs have at least one effect in common, in that they are capable of creating a state of mind in certain individuals which is termed psychic dependence. This is a psychic drive which requires periodic or chronic administration of the drug either for pleasure or to avoid discomfort.

True drug addiction is associated with physical dependence, which is an adaptive state characterized by intense physical disturbance when the administration of the drug is stopped or its action is counteracted by a specific antagonist.

Many of the drugs causing physical dependence also include tolerance, which is an adaptive state characterized by diminished response to the same quantity of drug or requiring a larger dose to produce the same pharmacodynamic effect.

Drug dependence and drug abuse can occur without the development of tolerance.

Harmful Effects

All addictive drugs have powerful actions on the central nervous system and their harmful, adverse and detrimental effects are related to neurological and behavioural changes as shown in Fig. 31.1.

The nature of the effects varies according to the class of drug; dependence may be emotional or physical or both. All addictive and dependence-producing drugs create emotional dependence, that is to say the drug has to be taken as a means of coping with life's stresses and to produce various effects desired by the person on his emotions, drives, perceptual powers, conflicts and problems.

Physical dependence varies in type and severity according to the class of drugs. It is marked with opiate drugs and less marked with drugs such as marihuana and amphetamines.

The features of drug dependence are characteristic for each generic group of drugs as follows: morphine and allied drugs, barbiturates, alcohol, cocaine, amphetamines, hallucinogens and cannabis.

1 *Opiates and their synthetic equivalents* If morphine and other opium derivatives and their synthetic equivalents are given over a period of months, striking changes occur in the central nervous system. Reflexes are originally depressed but later become hyperactive and an increase in the dose of the drug is required to depress the reflexes as tolerance to the drug is established and, also, because of the greater degree of over-activity produced by the usual dose if the administraton of the drug is delayed.

This hyper-irritability which occurs during drug dependence affects multineuronal arcs at all levels of the central nervous system, from the spinal cord to the cerebral cortex.

Physical dependence is a real physiological disturbance, largely independent of psychological influence.

The characteristics of dependence on this group of drugs include a strong psychic dependence, manifesting itself as an overwhelming drive or compulsion to continue taking the drug and to obtain it by any means for pleasure or to avoid discomfort.

There is a development of tolerance which requires an increase in dose to maintain the initial pharmacodynamic effect.

The early development of physical dependence increases in intensity, paralleling the increase in dosage. This necessitates a continuation of drug administration in order to prevent the appearance of the symptoms and signs of withdrawal. Withdrawal of the drug or the administration of a specific antagonist precipitates a definite characteristic and self-limiting abstinence syndrome.

The abstinence syndrome with morphine appears within a few hours of the last dose, reaching its peak in 24 to 48 hours and subsides spontaneously most often within 10 days.

The first signs are development of anxiety, restlessness and feelings of tension, followed by frequent yawning, profuse sweating, running of the nose and eyes, dilatation of the pupils, trembling, goose flesh, diarrhoea and cramps. These symptoms increase in intensity for the first 24 hours and twitching of muscles occurs, together with vomiting, loss of appetite, inability to sleep and increase in respiratory rate.

The effects are predominantly parasympathetic but sympathetic over-activity also occurs, such as

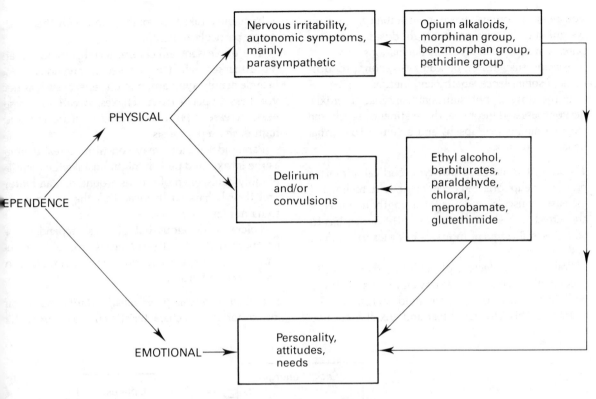

Figure 31.1 *Drug dependence.*

rise in body temperature, respiratory rate and systolic blood pressure.

All substances in this category possess, in varying degree, a capacity to induce physical dependence. They are mutually interchangeable, in that substitution of one for the other will maintain tolerance and physical dependence and prevent the appearance of abstinence phenomena.

Withdrawal effects appear more rapidly with heroin and, although present with methadone, they are very much less severe.

Pethidine addiction is particularly associated with doctors and nurses. Tolerance is not as marked as with other drugs in this class and is not as complete. Large doses of pethidine produce muscle twitching, tremors, confusion, hallucinations and even convulsions. Inability to work is greater than with morphine addiction.

2 Barbiturates and drugs like meprobamate, glutethimide, chloral, paraldehyde, chlordiazepoxide and other tranquillosedatives These give rise to a pattern of subjective and objective effects which resemble that with alcohol. For example, symptoms of intoxication include ataxia, dysarthria, impairment of mental function, loss of emotional control, confusion, poor judgment and, occasionally, a delirium. Withdrawal of the drug is characterized by an abstinence syndrome, which is entirely different from that following the withdrawal of opiates and the opiate group of drugs.

The signs occurring most consistently in the usual order of appearance include anxiety, involuntary twitching of muscle, intention tremor of hands and fingers, progressive weakness, dizziness, distortions in visual perception, nausea, vomiting, insomnia, weight loss and a precipitous drop in blood pressure on standing or even on sitting.

Other effects which may be hazardous to life may occur including hyperpyrexia, grand mal convulsions and/or delirium resembling alcoholic delirium tremens.

Abrupt withdrawal is hazardous because of the serious effects and the difficulty in controlling them.

3 Amphetamines Chronic intoxication with amphetamines shows the following features: anorexia, nervousness, insomnia, tremor, irritability, loss of weight and, in sufficiently high doses, a schizophrenic-like psychosis with hallucinations.

Abrupt suspension of administration produces marked somnolence, apathy and inertia.

If the dose is not sufficient to cause anorexia, nervousness and insomnia, the abstinence syndrome may be minimal or absent and a return to normal behaviour occurs.

4 *Cocaine* Cocaine is a powerful cortical stimulant producing euphoria and excitement, with feelings of increased muscular and mental strength. Its pleasurable effect is of short duration and the addict has to take doses at frequent intervals in order to produce sustained effects.

Following the feeling of euphoria, there usually occur marked feelings of anxiety and fear, sometimes with hallucinations and paranoid delusions. To counteract this associated fear and anxiety, cocaine

is frequently taken in combination with the opiate drugs, particularly heroin.

The unpleasant effects produced by cocaine are more marked when it is taken intravenously and include mainly sympathomimetic effects such as nervousness, hyper-reactive reflexes, sweating, hoarseness, increase in pulse rate, blood pressure and, with high doses, a psychosis.

Paranoid delusions may constitute a real danger as the intoxicated person might mistake the identity of individuals, even of friends around him and interpret their behaviour to mean that they were going to harm him.

Tolerance develops but physical dependence is not marked. Psychic dependence is sufficient in some patients to rate cocaine only second in order of preference to heroin.

5 *Cannabis sativa (marihuana)* Marihuana is an intoxicant and its characteristic effects occur within

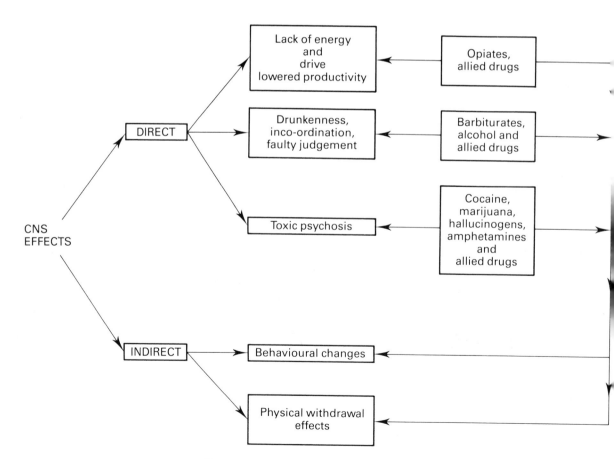

Figure 31.2 *Harmful effects of addictive drugs.*

few minutes when it is smoked but, after ingestion by mouth, half an hour to an hour may elapse before the appearance of symptoms. The effect of an oral dose may last from five to twelve hours.

The effects are a feeling of power with distortions of time, space, kinaesthetic and body image perceptions which are usually regarded as pleasurable. Mild inebriation takes place immediately following smoking, a voracious appetite for food occurs which is just the reverse of the effects induced by opiate drugs.

Marihuana diminishes inhibitions, increases suggestibility and increases auditory sensitivity.

The drug is misleading and particularly dangerous because it does not appear on the surface to be addictive, as its withdrawal produces no clear abstinence syndrome in the majority of people.

Psychic dependence can be marked and addicts, when deprived of the drug, have a strong desire to consume it whenever it is available but those who are mildly addicted can take it or reject it at will. In many parts of the world, though, it is often the first step to heroin addiction, particularly among teenagers and young people, who first of all become habituated to marihuana and then pass to heroin or cocaine mixed with heroin.

6 *Glue sniffing* During recent years there has been a marked increase in the inhalation of industrial solvents to produce feelings of intoxication. The following solvents are involved: toluene, benzene, acetone, ethyl acetate, diethyl ether and hexane. Probably the most commonly used is aeroplane glue, which contains toluene. The acute effects are similar to alcoholic intoxication, and ataxia and dysarthria are common. Hallucinations occasionally occur, and some solvents produce long-lasting neurological damage.

The Prevalence of Drug Dependence and Drug Addiction

It is notoriously difficult to obtain accurate figures of the prevalence of drug addiction and there are many obvious reasons for this. A further complicating factor is the relationship between the prevalence of drug usage and the actual incidence of drug addiction and drug dependence.

The number of known addicts to narcotics in Great Britain increased from 199 in 1947, 1549 in 1971 and 5869 in 1984.

The pattern of addiction is changing, for example, the number of known heroin addicts has increased

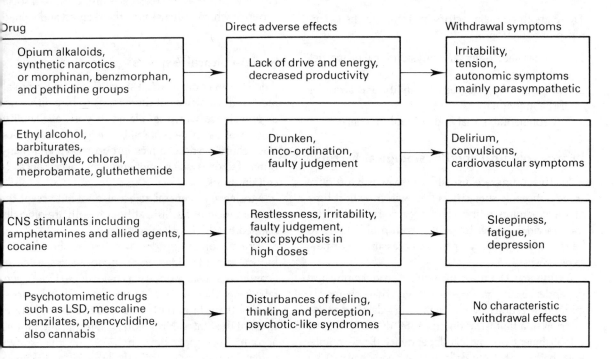

Drug	Direct adverse effects	Withdrawal symptoms
Opium alkaloids, synthetic narcotics or morphinan, benzmorphan, and pethidine groups	Lack of drive and energy, decreased productivity	Irritability, tension, autonomic symptoms mainly parasympathetic
Ethyl alcohol, barbiturates, paraldehyde, chloral, meprobamate, gluthethemide	Drunken, inco-ordination, faulty judgement	Delirium, convulsions, cardiovascular symptoms
CNS stimulants including amphetamines and allied agents, cocaine	Restlessness, irritability, faulty judgement, toxic psychosis in high doses	Sleepiness, fatigue, depression
Psychotomimetic drugs such as LSD, mescaline benzilates, phencyclidine, also cannabis	Disturbances of feeling, thinking and perception, psychotic-like syndromes	No characteristic withdrawal effects

Figure 31.3

from 68 in 1959 to 237 in 1963, and to 959 in 1971, and there are now more addicts to heroin than to any other narcotic drug. Forty-five new cases of heroin addition were reported during 1971.

Whereas in the past about a third of the known heroin addicts started their addiction in the course of medical treatment, about 94% of the present known addicts started their addiction in other ways.

The age distribution has also changed, with an increasing number below the age of 20 years and the great majority of new addicts belonging to this younger age group.

The number of cocaine addicts has also increased from 30 in 1959 to 171 in 1963, and to 178 in 1971. Nearly all of these also take heroin or methadone.

It has been estimated that in the United Kingdom in 1965 the number of patients on regular dependent use of barbiturates was 100 000, and on dependent use of amphetamines, 80 000, but since 1965 other synthetic stimulants such as methylphenidate have tended to be abused in place of the amphetamines.

Marihuana smoking has also become more prevalent in recent years among teenagers and young adults.

Factors Concerned in Addiction

There are three main factors operating in the occurrence of addiction:

1 The pharmacological and physiological properties of the drug
2 The personality, degree of stability and attitudes of the individual
3 Environmental, social and cultural influences

Pharmacological and Physiological Factors

Addictive drugs are usually those which produce some noticeable subjective effect within a short time of their administration. The effects are desired by the individual either to escape from problems or to be relieved of anxiety or to gain pleasurable or new experiences.

With regard to the drugs which produce physical dependence, it has been shown that there are minimum requirements regarding daily dosage, interval of administration and total duration for the establishment of physical dependence. For example, with barbiturates the daily intake needs to be 0.5 g at six to eight hourly intervals for four to six months.

Personality

Addicts show the whole range of personality characteristics from the normal to the neurotic, psychotic, psychopathic and sexually deviant.

Although many addicts show marked personality disorders with emotional instability, immaturity and impulsiveness and, although these undoubtedly increase vulnerability to addiction, these traits are also quite common in non-addicts. It is also clear that a number of addicts were previously normal, stable, well-adjusted persons.

It is also important to bear in mind the harmful effects of drug dependence and addiction on the person's behaviour and interpersonal relationships. The behaviour changes, the falling off of reliability and efficiency, the need for deception and the measures needed to obtain drugs to counteract abstinence syndromes can all exert adverse effects on the person's disposition and personality, but these are not necessarily permanent, as follow-up studies of addicts have shown.

The drug addict is a person with certain personality characteristics, who happens to have selected this way of coping with his problems for a variety of reasons of which he is usually unaware. Not the least of these reasons is his access to a social group in which drug use is both practised and valued.

Social-cultural Aspects

Addicts can come from all social classes and from all races and countries but there tends to be a difference in prevalence which is related to cost, availability, degree of social acceptability, religion, economics, class consciousness, ethics, group mores and many other factors which influence the acceptance of certain drugs.

Moslems, in general, reject alcohol but accept the consumption of hashish, although both are officially banned by the Moslem religion.

Oriental opium-producing countries show a much higher rate of addiction than do others, such as Scandinavia. Many observers have noted that Orientals keep their opium habits under much closer control than do non-Orientals. In the United States three of the States, New York, California and Illinois, account for approximately 77% of the known addicts, most coming from the large cities. Of these 25% of known addicts are native-born whites

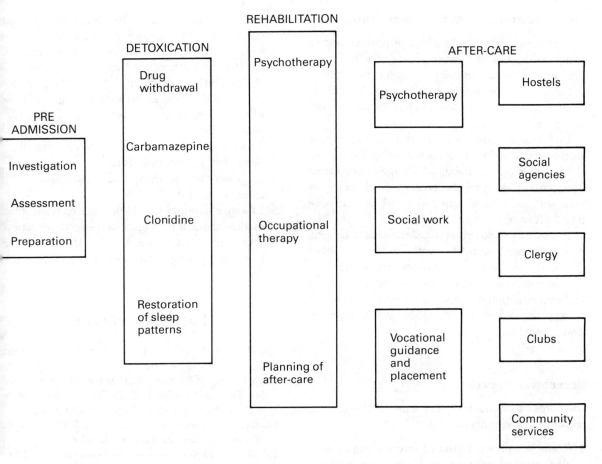

Figure 31.4 *Stages in treatment of drug addiction.*

Negroes, Puerto Ricans, Cubans and Mexicans make up the rest.

In the post war period, in New York in particular, there has been a marked increase in the use of narcotics by teenagers and young adults and one of the few intensive epidemiological studies on narcotics addiction has been carried out by Chein (1956) in New York. His group consisted of boys aged 16 to 21 years who, during a four-year period, had come to the attention of some official agency connected with narcotics. It was found that the districts in which teenage drug usage flourished were usually the most overcrowded, underprivileged areas, with the lowest income, lowest level of education and highest incidence of breakdown of family life. Round about the age of 16 was found to be a particularly susceptible time and it was thought that at this age there was no major institution playing a controlling role or strongly involved with their lives. The control group who had had opportunities but had not become drug addicts differed from the addicted group, in that there was a greater availability of information on the dangers and effects of drug usage and also that the attitudes of significant adults were such as to disapprove and lessen the tendency to drug addition.

It may also be said that the use of drugs creates a fraternal spirit which may lead to social organization which, in turn, is reinforced by the rejection of the addict by society. Further strengthening occurs by economic and psychological factors. The prohibitions placed on the use of drugs may, to some extent, make the consumption more attractive to youngsters.

Detoxification of Opiate Dependence

The principles here are to alleviate distress and to minimize the risk of adverse effects of withdrawal. Carbamazepine is a useful preparation for treating withdrawal from opiate substances. It relieves anxiety and depression, is anti-epileptic and is non-addictive.

Clonidine is used to counteract the adrenergic storm which may occur during the withdrawal phase. It is effective but has the disadvantage of producing hypotension. A synthetic analogue, lofexidine, is used with success and is free from risk of increasing blood pressure.

Acupuncture and neural stimulation are also useful adjuncts in the treatment of withdrawal from opiate drugs. It has been demonstrated that both acupuncture and neural stimulation cause a release of endorphins within the central nervous system which is the probable basis for their value in treating withdrawal symptoms.

Preventive Aspects

Measures which could help in the prevention of drug addiction are as follows:

1 *Research* is urgently needed into the personality attributes and environmental factors conducive to addiction.
2 *Legal measures* such as making the unauthorized possession of drugs illegal would help to control traffic in drugs. In the United Kingdom new regulations in 1968 confined the right to prescribe heroin and cocaine to addicts for their addiction to licensed doctors working mainly in hospital clinics. The Misuse of Drugs Acts (1971) provides among other things, methods for the rapid and effective control of overprescribing of controlled drugs.
3 *Medical measures* would include care in prescribing dependency producing drugs.
4 *Early diagnosis*, treatment and rehabilitation of the addict is needed.
5 *Educative measures* should provide relevant information about the dangers and effects of various drugs with a view to influencing the attitudes of teenagers, young adults and society generally to drug usage.

Further Reading

Kessel, N. and Walton, H. (1965) *Alcoholism*. Penguin Books, Harmondsworth.

Royal College of Psychiatrists. (1979) *Alcohol and Alcoholism. The Report of a Special Committee of the Royal College of Psychiatrists*. Tavistock Publications, London.

Camberwell Council on Alcoholism. (1980) *Women and Alcohol*. Tavistock Publications, London.

Jaffe, J. *et al.* (1980) *Addictions—Issues and Answers*. Harper & Row, New York.

Murray, R., Ghodse, H., Harris, C., Williams, D., and Williams, P. (eds) (1981) *Misuse of Psychotropic Drugs*. Gaskell Books, Ashford, Kent.

32
Mental Handicap

Mental handicap is the general term now used to describe retarded intellectual and cognitive development (which is usually also associated with social and emotional retardation). It should be distinguished from the term 'mental impairment', as defined in the Mental Health Act 1983 (see Chapter 35), which implies mental handicap **and** either a serious behaviour disorder or seriously irresponsible conduct. Only a few mentally handicapped people also suffer from mental impairment and they come under the provisions of the Act.

Mental handicap varies in severity and may exist from birth or an early age, or result from accident or illness later in life. About 5% of all babies are born mentally handicapped; some suffer from physical malformations and have a high mortality rate. Between 1 and 4% of all school age children are handicapped.

Intelligence tests are a convenient measure of intellectual level but may be unreliable in mentally handicapped people, depending on the motivation of the person and the particular test used. It is preferable to describe all facets of the individual, not only his intellect.

However, a useful informal grading of handicap is:

1 *Slight* IQ between 50 and 70. Under the Mental Health Act 1983 this includes the mentally impaired (formerly 'mentally subnormal').
2 *Moderate* IQ of 30 to 50. Under the 1983 Act this includes **some** severely mentally impaired patients (formerly 'severely subnormal').
3 *Severe* IQ below 30. Under the 1983 Act this includes the severely mentally impaired (formerly also 'severely subnormal').

Slightly Handicapped Patients

This group comprises by far the largest proportion of mentally handicapped patients. The intelligence quotient may range from 50 to 70 and the upper level merges into the lower range of the normal frequency distribution of intelligence.

The intelligence quotient is not the best guide to mental handicap because psychological, educational and social factors operate in a fairly direct manner in producing the important problems associated with slight impairment of intelligence.

This group is mostly derived from the lower end of the normal frequency distribution curve of intelligence and is multifactorially determined, as is normal intelligence.

Whilst saying this, it is also important to remember that all diseases and factors which cause gross mental disorder may operate in attenuated form to produce mild degrees of mental handicap.

Clinical features

Mentally handicapped children tend to be slower, to lack in alertness, curiosity and spontaneity compared with the normal child. They are inert and passive, easily fooled, credulous and easily led into delinquent, criminal or other forms of undesirable behaviour. They are easy dupes for the schemes of others.

Thinking tends to be concrete, as the ability to handle concepts and abstract modes of thinking is limited.

Children just below the normal intelligence range may show no obvious signs of mental handicap but are often late in passing the milestones of development. If they attend an ordinary school, they fail to make progress and often need to be transferred to special classes or to special schools.

In the case of well-to-do families, mentally handicapped children are often looked after in private schools.

After leaving school, they may settle down to a job of a simple, routine nature, providing it is within the limits of their mental capacity and providing they are relatively stable.

It must be emphasized that level of intelligence *per se* is not the most important criterion in mental handicap. Intelligence quotient gives a guide as to the upper limits that the person can achieve, but it does not provide an index of the person's capacity to adjust to society.

In all mentally handicapped people, aspects other than intelligence need to be assessed, such as emotional stability, impulsiveness and social behaviour, which are far more important deciding factors as to whether action for care, supervision and control is needed.

At school, mentally handicapped children are often a disturbing element; their behaviour tending to be antisocial, impulsive, unreliable and unpredictable.

After leaving school, they often have poor work records and change jobs unduly frequently. They may become delinquent, and, as a result, be sent to approved schools, Borstal or prison.

Moderately Handicapped Patients

The intelligence quotient of this group ranges from 30–50. These people may be incapable of earning their living and fending for themselves in society but they can be taught to look after themselves, to wash, dress and feed themselves. They are incapable of learning in ordinary schools and are appropriately dealt with at occupation centres and, later, may be found in a sheltered workshop.

Severely Handicapped Patients

This group includes patients with an intelligence quotient below 30. The lower in the scale the patient is placed with regard to intellectual endowment, the greater the frequency for anatomical and physiological abnormalities to be found; e.g. disproportionate and stunted growth of the head, limbs and body are frequent. Neurological phenomena,

e.g. hemiplegia and diplegia, frequently occur and epileptic fits occur in about half the patients. Expectation of life is limited; some die in the first two years of life and a large number die before reaching adult life. The most common causes of death are intercurrent infections (e.g. pneumonia), the development of circulatory failure or death due to epilepsy, usually in status epilepticus.

Recognition of Mental Handicap in Infancy and Childhood

The following are some useful landmarks of development in the normal child for comparison with suspected mentally handicapped children:

1 Smiling in response to the mother's overtures at 6 weeks
2 Grasping at an object when placed in the hand at 3 months
3 Ability to reach for an object and get it at 5 months
4 Ability to lift head from the supine when lying on a firm surface at 6 months
5 Walking when held with hands at 9 or 10 months
6 Walking without support at 13 to 15 months

Speech

1 6 months able to say 'mum, mum'
2 8 to 9 months, 'Da, da, da', 'Ma, ma, ma'
3 10 to 11 months able to say one or two words with meaning

Other Useful Pointers

1 Turning head to a sound at 3 months
2 Playing games, such as peep-bo at 6 months
3 Chewing at 6 months
4 Imitate parents coughing, putting tongue out, knocking on the table at 6 to 9 months
5 Wave hand good-bye at 10 months
6 Feeding self with a cup and placing it back on the table without help at 15 months

Taking the history, questions about the delivery and the condition of the baby immediately after birth and during the first two or three weeks are important, e.g. whether delivery was difficult and whether birth asphyxia, twitching, convulsions, drowsiness, sucking difficulties, birth injuries, etc., were present.

Table 32.1 Aetiological classification of mental handicap

Polygenic or multifactorial	Single recessive	Single dominant	Chromosome abnormalities	Embryopathy	Birth	Infancy and childhood
Moderate and severe handicap	Phenylketonuria	Tuberous sclerosis	Down's syndrome (Mongolism)	Rubella	Cerebral haemorrhage and other damage	Cretinism
	Galactosaemia			Syphilis		Kernicterus
'Mental Impairment' Mental Health Act 1983	Hurler's disease	Some late infantile varieties of Tay-Sach's	Trisomy XXX syndrome	Toxoplasmosis		Cerebral palsy
IQ 50–70	Tay-Sach's disease (infantile type)		Klinefelter's syndrome (XXY)	Kernicterus	Excessive oxygen to premature babies	Encephalitis
				Teratogenic		Trauma
Social and psychological factors also important	Craniostenosis		Turner's syndrome (XO)			Schizophrenia
	Microcephaly		Patau's syndrome Cri-du-chat syndrome			Nephrogenic diabetes insipidus
	Laurence-Moon-Biedl syndrome		Edward's syndrome			

Causation of Mental Handicap

Mental handicap may be largely genetically determined or it may be due to factors operating during pregnancy, at birth or during infancy and childhood.

An aetiological classification of different forms of mental handicap is shown in Table 32.1.

Genetic Factors

Genetic and environmental factors interact in the production of mental handicap.

The following genetic mechanisms play a role in the pathogenesis of some forms of mental handicap:

1 Major single gene mutation
2 Chromosomal abnormalities
3 Multifactorial (polygenic) inheritance

Pregnancy

Certain infections of the mother may damage the foetus, e.g. German measles, syphilis, toxoplasmosis.

Certain drugs can act as teratogenic agents when given during pregnancy.

Birth

Prolonged or difficult birth, instrumental delivery, etc., giving rise to anoxia in the baby, or excessive oxygen to premature babies.

Infancy and Childhood

Any disease, trauma or metabolic disturbance which interferes with growth or damages the central nervous system can cause mental handicap.

Mental Handicap due to the Action of a Single Mutant Gene

The forms of mental handicap due to the action of a single gene are seen in Table 32.1.

It has been estimated that single gene inheritance accounts for one-sixtieth of all cases of mental handicap.

Patients afflicted with phenylketonuria, Hurler's disease and tuberous sclerosis are usually severely mentally handicapped.

Mental Handicap due to Chromosomal Abnormalities

Chromosomal aberrations may occur during meiosis as well as during mitosis. The most frequent anomaly is non-dysjunction. This results in an abnormal number of chromosomes in both daughter cells, one having one chromosome too many and the other having one too few. The individual chromosomes are distinguished from each other by the total length, the length of the long arm and the site of its centromere. Human chromosomes are numbered from 1 to 22. The largest pair is No. 1 and the smallest No. 22. They are grouped as follows: A. 1–3, B. 4 and 5, C. 6–12 and X, D. 13–15, E. 16–18, F. 19 and 20, G. 21, 22, and Y.

The following syndromes result in some forms of mental handicap due to chromosomal abnormalities:

1 Klinefelter's syndrome
2 Trisomy X syndrome
3 Down's syndrome

Klinefelter's syndrome and trisomy X syndrome are due to a non-dysjunction of at least one of the sex chromosomes. Down's syndrome is usually due to non-dysjunction of a small autosome. In rare instances the condition is caused by the transmission of a supernumerary autosome which is fused with another autosome by translocation. There appears to be a relationship between older maternal age and the tendency to develop these chromosomal aberrations.

Other autosomal anomalies are:

4 Cri-du-chat syndrome, due to the deletion of the short arm of one of the chromosomes of pair 5. Mental handicap is serious, with microcephaly and hypertelorism and a typical cat-like cry.
5 Patau's syndrome is due to an extra chromosome of the D group. Mental handicap is severe, with microcephaly, eye defects, low-set ears, hare-lip and polydactyly. Brain and heart are often malformed. Death usually occurs in the first few months of life.
6 Edward's syndrome is due to trisomy of group E chromosomes. It occurs more often in females, the ears are low-set and malformed, with micrognathia, flexed and overlapped fingers. Death usually occurs before 3 years.

Biochemical Aspects of Genetical Transmission of Mental Handicap

The genes produce their effects by controlling enzyme systems and by chemical functions in the body. It has been estimated that a biochemical factor plays a role in the aetiology of between 2 and 4% of cases of severe mental handicap.

Normal metabolism occurs through sequential steps, each step being regulated by a specific enzyme. The situation is a steady state, each intermediate product being metabolized as it is formed by the succeeding enzyme in the sequence. It is now known that each enzyme in turn is controlled by one specific gene within the chromosome.

In the case of human inborn errors of metabolism, it appears that clinical manifestations of enzyme defects are most frequently due to toxic effects of excessive accumulation of normal metabolites above the metabolic block, as has been observed in phenylketonuria and galactosaemia.

The following are types of inborn errors of metabolism associated with specific forms of mental handicap:

1 Protein metabolism—phenylketonuria, maple syrup disease, Hartnupp disease
2 Lipid metabolism—amaurotic family idiocy, Gaucher's disease, Neumann–Pick's disease
3 Carbohydrate metabolism—galactosaemia, gargoylism
4 Miscellaneous—Wilson's disease (copper), Toni-Fanconi syndromes (cysteine)

Multifactorial Inheritance

Intelligence is polyfactorially determined and the distribution of intelligence in the normal population is in the form of a normal frequency curve.

About three-quarters of all cases of mental handicap represent the lower extreme of the normal range of intelligence frequency distribution.

Below an IQ of 50 a variety of factors may be found—genetic, environmental, traumatic, inflammatory, etc.—which have caused arrested development of mind.

Clinical Types of Mental Handicap

Recessive Transmission

Phenylketonuria

Phenylketonuria is an inborn error of metabolism occurring at the rate of between 2 and 6 per 10 000 of the British population and transmitted in the recessive manner.

It is an enzyme defect like the majority of hereditary metabolic errors. The enzyme defect is due to a failure of the enzyme system in the liver to convert phenylalanine into tyrosine, with the result that phenylalanine and its products accumulate in the blood and damage various organs, particularly the CNS.

The biochemical disorder in phenylketonuria affects the entire metabolism of the body. For example, patients tend to be fairer than their siblings and are liable to dermatitis. The main effect, however, is on the brain. The level of phenylalanine in the blood becomes high and secondary disturbances of various metabolic processes essential to normal functions in the brain occur.

Patients with phenylketonuria may, however, appear normal and the diagnosis is made on examination of the urine. The metabolites are not usually detectable in urine until the second or third week and sometimes not until the sixth week. The fourth week of life is probably the optimum time for routine testing and the sixth week probably detects more cases. The test is simple and is a modification of the ferricchloride test in which a paper strip (Phenistix) is impregnated with ferricchloride and applied to the wet napkin.

One of the urinary metabolites usually found in this condition is phenylpyruvic acid in large quantities, which makes simple screening tests possible and gives the standard green colour with ferric chloride. Other abnormalities are easily demonstrable by simple paper chromatographic techniques, phenyllactic and phenylacetic acids, phenylalanine, o-hydroxyphenylacetic acid, phenylacetylglutamine, inolylacetic and lactic acids. The urine test is not specific for phenylketonuria and may be positive in histidinaemia; the diagnosis must be confirmed by an estimate of the blood levels of phenylalanine. Screening tests are now possible on all babies by using the bacterial inhibition test of Guthrie.

In recent years there has been considerable interest in the treatment of phenylketonuria by diet in which the quantity of phenylalanine is restricted to the minimum compatible with well-being. Follow-up studies of children who from an early age received this diet correctly, revealed that the majority were of normal intelligence.

In addition, it was clear that the diet produced definite changes in the patient in the direction of normal, e.g. the hair became darker during treatment and fairer when the treatment was relaxed. The level of 5-hydroxytryptamine, which is depressed in the blood if the patient is untreated, also moved towards the normal level. Although isolated cases of untreated phenylketonuria are of normal intelligence, they are rare. The overwhelming number of patients are severely or moderately impaired in intelligence.

Homocystinuria

Homocystinuria is the second most common error of metabolism associated with mental handicap. It is transmitted by a single autosomal recessive gene. The urine contains homocystine and methionine.

The clinical features are ectopia lentis, fine fair hair, thrombo-embolic episodes, head enlargement and a shuffling gait. Treatment is by a methionine-free diet, and the results are encouraging.

Galactosaemia

Here, the genetically determined enzyme defect is a failure in breakdown of lactose with the result that galactose accumulates in the body.

Children are normal at birth but later develop feeding difficulties, enlargement of the liver, jaundice, enlargement of the spleen, hepatic failure, sub-cutaneous haemorrhages, oedema and wasting. Eventually death occurs from hepatic failure or infection.

Severe mental handicap is common.

Treatment is by giving a lactose and galactose free diet, if possible from early infancy. This can lead to considerable improvement in physical and mental state.

Hurler's disease

This is a genetically determined metabolic disorder autosomally recessive.

The biochemical abnormality results in over-production of certain mucopolysaccharides which can be detected in the urine.

Growth is stunted and disproportionate, the skull is malformed, the bridge of the nose is depressed, the tongue protrudes and the neck is short. The liver and spleen are enlarged and corneal clouding and abnormalities of the cardiovascular system sometimes occur.

These patients show behavioural difficulties.

Death usually occurs in childhood from circulatory failure or pneumonia.

An allied sex-linked form is known as Hunter's syndrome.

Amaurotic family idiocy (Tay-Sachs disease, cerebral macular degeneration)

This is a genetically determined disorder of metabolism in which a ganglioside is stored in excessive amounts in the brain cells. There are three forms, the infantile, the early childhood variety and the juvenile form.

The early infantile form is confined more or less to Jewish people. The child is born normal and remains normal up until about six months. Then it becomes listless, apathetic, showing no interest in its surroundings and losing the ground it has gained. It begins to show signs of visual failure which ends in blindness. Later it develops widespread paralysis. The child gradually wastes away and usually dies within two years of the onset. Diagnosis of the disease is revealed by the optic atrophy which causes the blindness and the appearance of a cherry-red spot at the macula.

The early childhood form begins at three years of age after a period of normal development. It is characterized by progressive deterioration in mental growth, spasticity and blindness. The blindness is due to optic atrophy, a reddish brown macula spot being present. The disease is usually fatal within a few years.

The juvenile form starts between 6 and 12 years of age. Visual failure progresses to blindness, optic atrophy is present with a deposit on the retina of a scattered pepper and salt pigment. Ataxia, paresis terminating in hopeless dementia, complete paralysis and death occur. Some late juvenile varieties are dominantly transmitted.

An adult form starts between 15 and 25 years and is slowly progressive, with mental deterioration

and convulsions as early manifestations. There is usually no impairment of vision.

Microcephaly

A small size of head is the distinctive feature. In the adult a small skull is associated with a face of normal size giving a bird-like shape, characteristic of microcephaly.

There are two groups of microcephaly. One is genetically determined, due to a single recessive gene. The other microcephalic disorders accompany a variety of types of mental handicap.

The majority of patients are severely handicapped and about half suffer from epilepsy.

Laurence–Moon–Biedl syndrome

This is characterized by intellectual impairment from infancy which does not usually amount to very severe mental handicap, with retinitis pigmentosa, defective vision, polydactyly of hands and feet, obesity and hypogenitalism. Among relatives, incomplete forms of extra digits, obesity and hypogenitalism, etc, occur.

Single Dominant Transmission

Tuberous sclerosis (epiloia)

This is due to a single dominant gene and it usually causes severe mental handicap. It has been estimated that up to 50% of cases are due to new mutations.

Tuberous sclerosis is characterized by the following features:

1 Severe intellectual impairment
2 Adenoma sebaceum of the face which begin during the second to fourth year of life and have a butterfly distribution on the face
3 Cutaneous naevi, cafe au lait pigmentation, white patches due to absence of pigment
4 Epileptic fits
5 Changes in the bones, osteosclerosis, periosteal thickening
6 Glial nodules appear in the brain causing epilepsy, paralysis, premature puberty and calcification of the overlying skull
7 Rhabdomyomata of the heart which cause heart block and cardiac failure
8 Fibrosis of the lungs
9 Mixed tumours of the kidneys

The majority of patients die young from inter-current infections such as pneumonia or from status epilepticus, cardiac or renal failure.

Chromosomal Abnormalities

Down's syndrome

Down's syndrome was first described by Langdon Down and called 'Mongolism' because of a super-ficial resemblance to Oriental people. Nowadays the term Down's syndrome is used.

Down's syndrome occurs in about one in every 600 live births but the high infant mortality rate reduces its incidence in the general population to one in 1000. Down's syndrome acounts for one-thirtieth of all cases of mental handicap. Most people with Down's syndrome fall into the category of severely mentally handicapped. Few of them have an intelligence quotient above 60.

In 1959 it was found that Down's syndrome was associated with an extra chromosome.

The incidence of Down's syndrome in cousins and the occurrence of trisomy in more than one Down's syndrome sibling when the chromosomes of the parents are normal suggests an underlying genetic mechanism as a cause of non-dysjunction.

If an additional chromosome is present resulting in three matched chromosomes instead of the usual pair, the individual is said to be trisomic for this chromosome. The majority of cases of Down's syndrome are trisomic for one of the two smaller pairs of autosomes.

It is usually considered that trisomy of chromosome 21 is the most common anomaly associated with Down's syndrome.

Other chromosomal abnormalities occur less frequently, e.g. translocation and chromosome mosaicism.

The translocated chromosome is frequently found in Down's syndrome children of phenotypically normal parents. The occurrence of chromosome mosaicism in Down's syndrome may be associated with incomplete manifestation of the syndrome and the ultimate mental development of such patients has varied from normal to severe retardation.

One important advance arising from chromosome studies is that it is possible to explain more clearly differences in the probability of young mothers, who have already given birth to a Down's syndrome child, producing further similarly handicapped off-spring as compared with older mothers. The incidence of Down's syndrome in relationship to maternal age shows two peaks, one being at an earlier age, and this suggests that two mechanisms are involved. In the case of young parents, if the Down's syndrome child has trisomy 21 and the parents have normal chromosomes, the chances of a second Down's syndrome child being born are 1 or 2%, irrespective of maternal age. However, if one of the parents is a carrier of a translocation chromosome, the chances of a second child being born affected are greatly increased, as high as one in three.

The risk of a woman below 25 years of age giving birth to a Down's syndrome child is 1 in 2 300 and is 1 in 100 for women between 40 and 45 years and 1 in 46 for women older than 45.

The trisomy XXX syndrome

This comprises less than 1% of mentally handicapped women. They have three female sex chromosomes instead of the normal two. They are often mentally handicapped but they can produce normal children.

The trisomy XXY (Klinefelter's) syndrome

This occurs in only 1% of male mentally handi-capped. Men with this abnormality may be mentally normal; mental handicap occurs in 17%. These patients have two X chromosomes instead of one, as well as a Y chromosome. Half of the affected men are chromatin positive, i.e. they are genetically female.

They show under-development of genitals with small testicles, scanty pubic hair of female distribution and scanty facial hair, sometimes gynaecomastia, and are infertile.

XYY syndrome

These men are tall and show hypogonadism, neuro-logical effects and bone disease. The original view that XYY syndrome is specifically related to anti-social behaviour is no longer held.

Turner's syndrome (monosomy X)

Here the patient has one X chromosome instead of two. It is characterized by ovarian agenesis, absence of secondary sex characteristics at puberty in girls, small stature, digital anomalies, webbed neck, congenital heart disease, renal anomalies, intellectual impairment and other developmental errors.

Some of these patients may be of normal intelligence.

Embryopathy

Embryopathy is a term given to damage to the foetus by a variety of agents operating before birth. Examples are:

1 *Rubella* Infection of the mother within the first three months of pregnancy with German Measles causes some two-thirds of the children to suffer congenital defects such as congenital cataract or congenital heart defects. Microcephaly, deafness and deaf mutism may all result.

2 *Syphilis* Syphilis, like rubella, is one of the few diseases in which there is good evidence that maternal infection during pregnancy may damage the infant. The risk is high and it has been estimated that a woman with latent syphilis has only one chance in six of bearing a normal child if she is untreated. Transmission of infection probably does not occur until the fifth month of pregnancy which gives a period of grace during which infections discovered by routine ante-natal seriological investigations can be treated.

The effects on the infant are such as to produce well-recognized syndromes such as general paralysis, and meningo-vascular syphilis.

Syphilitic mental disorder is eminently preventable and should disappear. The incidence of this type of mental disorder declined with the decrease in the incidence of syphilis, but with the recent increase, it again becomes a danger.

3 *Toxoplasmosis* This is the result of human infection with toxoplasma gondi. When a pregnant mother suffers from this, the child can be affected and the condition is characterized by encephalomyelitis, cerebral calcification, hydrocephaly and chorio-retinitis, the symptoms being apparent at birth or soon after. The prognosis is very poor and those patients who survive are usually mentally handicapped and epileptic.

4 *Kernicterus* This is due to rhesus incompatibility which results in over-production of bilirubin, which causes brain damage. The striate body, hippocampus,

subthalamic nuclei, cerebellar nuclei and cranial nerve nuclei are particularly prone to become damaged.

Affected infants show clinical features from the second to the sixth day after birth. They are severely jaundiced, have a temperature, vomit, cannot be wakened, show respiratory distress, have twitching limbs and face, rigidity, opisthotonos, and convulsions.

Those who survive show permanent sequelae such as mental handicap.

5 *Teratogenic agents* A number of agents have been recognized as being potentially harmful to the foetus if administered to the mother during pregnancy. These include X-radiation, drugs such as colchicine, physostigmine, quinine, thalidomide and heavy metals such as lead and cobalt. Sex hormones and cortisone may also produce inter-sex abnormalities in children. Hypovitaminosis with A and D may also produce maldevelopment.

Causes Operating at Birth

Prematurity is a possible cause of mental handicap and is sometimes associated with blindness. The administration of oxygen has been considered to be a factor in these patients. Oxygen poisoning is also considered to be a cause of retrolental fibroplasia. Birth trauma can occur with prolonged and difficult labour, high forceps delivery and anything that causes anoxia, such as anaesthesia, protracted labour, twisting of the umbilical cord.

Causes Operating in Infancy and Early Childhood

Head injuries after birth due to accidents can cause impaired development depending on the site and severity of the injury. Poisons, particularly lead poisoning from lead paint scraped off cots, doors, etc., infections, meningitis, including tuberculous meningitis and meningococcal meningitis, if they are not treated with antibiotics or do not respond satisfactorily, can lead to severe mental handicap, as can encephalitis due to virus infection.

This was common in the epidemic of influenza in 1917; it is associated with intellectual impairment, extrapyramidal symptoms, hyperkinesis, personality difficulties, vicious propensities and impulsive behaviour.

Cretinism

This is due to hypothyroidism beginning in foetal life. If failure of thyroid function occurs after a normal infancy it is then referred to as myxoedema. Cretinism is endemic in iodine-deficient areas, the mother will usually have a goitre. If the condition is untreated, there is marked handicap, physical and mental.

The child is apathetic and somnolent, quiet, cries little, has difficulty in feeding due to his torpor and difficulty in sucking due to his enlarged tongue. Constipation is characteristic; the skin is dry and the lips thick, the hands and external genitalia are often eczematous, the tongue large and protruding, the features coarse; the neck is thick with supra-clavicular pads of fat and the abdomen is large, sometimes with an umbilical hernia; the temperature tends to be subnormal and the pulse is slow. Fusion of the epiphyses and dentition are delayed. Anaemia and hypotonia of the muscles may be found.

Diagnosis

Cretinism can usually be diagnosed within the first few months of life. This condition has to be distinguished from Down's syndrome and Hurler's disease and from various other causes of mental handicap.

Down's syndrome is diagnosable at birth. The Down's syndrome person is active, has coarse features, fissured skin and a small, round head, and is not usually constipated. Down's syndrome, unlike cretinism, is associated with chromosomal abnormality.

Distinguishing features of Hurler's disease are enlargement of the liver and spleen, corneal opacities, typical X-ray appearances of the bones and failure to respond to thyroid treatment.

It is important that cretinism be diagnosed as early as possible because if thyroid treatment is delayed mental and physical handicap can be permanent.

A dry thyroid extract in doses of 15–30 mg up to 3 months of age, 30–60 mg at 12 months, rising to 200 mg at 12 years, will usually be adequate to produce normal growth and development. Alternatively, sodium laevothyroxine may be given (100 μg is equivalent to 60 mg of desiccated thyroid extract). Treatment must be continued throughout life. If signs of hyperthyroidism occur, the dose can be reduced.

Cretinism is of particular interest in that it was the first form of mental handicap to respond to treatment.

Cerebral Diplegia ('Cerebral Palsy')

This may result from any process which damages the brain before birth, during birth or within the first few years of life and includes a number of conditions already considered under genetic factors; embryopathy, birth injuries, anoxia at birth, infections, trauma and vascular accidents after birth. Spasticity of the limbs and myotonic twitches often occur.

The term diplegia is not satisfactory as it refers to a paralysis affecting both arms or legs, whereas all varieties of paralysis of the limbs can occur from monoplegia, hemiplegia, paraplegia, triplegia and quadriplegia.

Tendon reflexes are exaggerated and plantar reflexes are usually extensor.

Athetosis occurs in many patients and tremors and choreic movements less frequently.

Epilepsy is common and speech and hearing defects may also be associated with the condition. About three-quarters of the patients show mental handicap. A proportion of patients may have normal or even above normal levels of intelligence.

Prevention

Our knowledge of mental handicap is vastly greater than it was even five years ago but yet it is still trivial. Mental handicap in a large part is due to the action of a large number of separate causes in different individuals. Already advances into the biochemical, genetic and the chromosomal basis of various types of mental handicap have resulted in opportunities both for effective therapy in some cases and prevention in others. For example, in the case of kernicterus, remarkably good results have been obtained by the injection of anti D immunoglobulins immediately after amniocentesis in unsensitized rhesus negative women. It is probable that kernicterus, already a rarity due to exchange transfusion, will be eliminated almost completely in time. Similarly, the early detection of phenylketonuria and its dietary treatment have achieved excellent results which are confirmed by long term follow up. For example 83% of the normal population have IQs over 85 and 67% of treated phenylketonurics have IQs of over 85.

Another new field, which is promising, relates to amniocentesis for prenatal diagnosis and possible selective abortion. In addition to considering the short term effects many of which could be potentially valuable to the family, we need also to consider what the long term effects might be.

Autosomal Recessive Disease

When diagnosed by amniocentesis, selective abortion could result in a reduction in the order of 15–25%. However reproductive compensation will result in a slow rise in the gene frequency in the population ultimately with little change in the incidence of the effect homozygote.

With regard to autosomal dominant conditions, such as tuberous sclerosis and Huntington's chorea, when it becomes possible to detect these disorders by amniocentesis, selective abortion could be of great benefit to the individual family but will not eliminate the recurrence of disease by fresh mutation. Indeed it would be a great disadvantage if we could prevent fresh mutation as this would end much of the possibility of our further evolution.

Chromosomal Abnormalities

These occur at the rate of 2 per thousand live births. With regard to Down's syndrome 3–5% are due to imbalanced translocations and are not age dependent. Therefore it might be worthwhile doing amniocentesis on subsequent pregnancies, but it should be remembered that most of this type of Down's syndrome are sporadic.

With regard to Down's syndrome due to trisomy 21, if amniocentesis was carried out on all women over 35, it would be possible to eliminate 35% of all trisomics with amniocentesis on approximately 8% of the total number of pregnancies. For the remainder the number of amniocenteses would be unacceptably large, particularly as amniocentesis itself carries risks.

The correlation between neural tube defects, such as spina bifida, and the possibility of detecting this by measuring alphafoetal protein is promising.

Amniocentesis is therefore of limited value. When results are positive, selective abortion could be of immense value to the family but in the long term the incidence of these types of mental handicap will not be dramatically changed.

Treatment and Training of the Mental Handicapped

It has been estimated that 8 per 1 000 of the population are mentally handicapped but that, at most, only 2 of these will need admission to hospital.

The majority of mentally handicapped patients, both children and adults, are looked after in their homes most of their lives.

Admission to hospital is determined mainly by behavioural difficulties in the patient or by social factors. For example, the child's behaviour may be so difficult, so destructive and noisy that the family, although they would like to keep him at home, are unable to do so. Social factors such as overcrowding, incompetent parents or complaints by neighbours may also influence the need for admission.

In the case of adults, admission may become necessary when parents die or become unable to look after them.

In recent years there has been an even greater tendency for maintaining mentally handicapped individuals outside hospitals as useful members of the community. Research studies have shown that young moderately handicapped children, who were cared for in small groups which tried to provide a substitute family environment, developed social and verbal abilities more rapidly than a comparable group of children who remained in a large ward of a psychiatric hospital. Recent studies of the learning abilities of mentally handicapped adults have shown that some of them attained the standards necessary for employment in open industry and others became self-supporting in sheltered workshops. Many such patients can live at home or in hostels and travel to work each day.

Patients in the community can attend occupation centres and training centres. Children of school age can receive special education in special schools or special classes.

Nowadays, patients can enter a hospital informally but some have to be admitted compulsorily from home as a result of a Court Order.

In hospital, children are given education and training suitable to their ability and adult patients are given instruction in adult social behaviour and training in various forms of employment. Industrial workshops are utilized by some hospitals, in which patients are employed in repetitive work for outside firms. Physical training, recreations and social activities also form part of the regime of treatment.

Neuroleptics have greatly improved the behaviour of disturbed and destructive mentally impaired patients.

Further Reading

Heaton-Ward, W. A. (1975) *Mental Subnormality: Subnormality and Severe Subnormality*, 4th edn. J. Wright, Bristol.

Owens, G. and Birchenall, P. (1979) *Mental Handicap: The Social Dimensions*. Pitman Medical, London.

Tredgold, R. F. and Soddy, K. (1979) *Mental Retardation*, 12th edn. Bailliere, London.

Wilkin, D. (1979) *Caring for the Mentally Handicapped Child*. Croom Helm, London.

Ellis, R. (ed) (1980) *Inborn Errors of Metabolism*. Croom Helm, London.

Yule, W. and Carr, J. (eds) (1980) *Behaviour Modification for the Mentally Handicapped*. Croom Helm, London.

33
Child Psychiatry

Child psychiatry is of comparatively recent origin. The first Child Guidance Clinic was established in the United States in 1921 and the first Child Guidance Clinic in Great Britain was opened in 1926.

Child Guidance Clinics are run by a team consisting of psychiatrists, psychologists and psychiatric social workers.

The psychiatrist is the head of the team and investigates the medical and clinical aspects. The psychologist measures intelligence, aptitudes, personality and deals with educational problems. The psychiatric social worker investigates the social aspects and serves as liaison with the parents.

Psychiatric disorders of children may be arbitrarily classified as follows:

1 Disturbances of eliminative functions
2 Disturbances of eating
3 Disturbances of sleep
4 Unhealthy behavioural and emotional responses, e.g. aggression, jealousy, lying, stealing, fears, phobias
5 Gratification habits, e.g. thumb-sucking, masturbation, day-dreaming, tension habits such as nail-biting and tics
6 Educational backwardness
7 Speech difficulties
8 Psychosomatic disorders
9 Severe psychiatric disorders, e.g. childhood schizophrenia and manic-depressive illness.

Disturbances in Eliminative Functions

Enuresis

Involuntary micturition is normal in infancy both by night and by day. Daytime control should be acquired in the second year and in the third year a dry bed should be achieved.

In the absence of disease, repeated involuntary micturition occurring after the third year is termed enuresis. If due to organic disease, the description urinary incontinence is applied.

Four stages in the progress of normal control of micturition may be described:

1 The automatic bladder of infancy
2 The small bladder of increasing capacity in which the impulse to void is still uninhibited
3 The bladder which will hold three ounces or more but in which the impulse is still succeeded by micturition
4 The adult functioning bladder in which the contractions are inhibited by cortical activity

The incidence of enuresis is variously estimated as between 5 and 15%. The high figure includes children who are occasional and intermittent bedwetters and the low figure includes only those whose enuresis is unremitting for long periods. In adults the incidence is probably less than 1%.

Enuresis may be:

1 The primary type
2 The acquired type

The primary type is characterized by a failure to develop control by the usual age and the acquired type denotes enuresis developed after the child has acquired normal control.

The child has to pass through the stage of automatic emptying of the bladder as a young infant to the stage of awareness of the full bladder, usually at 12 to 18 months, when he tells the mother that he is passing urine or just about to do so. Then there is the stage of learning to inhibit the contraction of the detrusor muscle and to hold the urine through the use of the external sphincter and perineal muscles. The next stage is the control of intra-abdominal pressure through the use of the diaphragm and abdominal muscles, to the final stage when the person is able to start and stop the flow of urine at any degree of bladder filling.

Many bed-wetters have urgency and frequency of micturition by day, suggesting that bladder emptying is necessary at an earlier stage of bladder distension than usual. A factor which may be responsible is a delayed maturation of the nervous system in these patients.

There is a well-known genetic factor in enuresis.

Many observers have stressed the importance of environmental factors, including the influence of family relationships and attitudes. There is a relationship between the incidence of enuresis and insecurity in relationship to unhappiness in the home, broken homes and loss of parents. There is a higher incidence in the lower social classes.

True anatomical factors occur extremely rarely. Spina bifida occulta is not a factor. Spina bifida is closely related to enuresis only when there is a meningocele or other obvious neurological signs.

Acquired enuresis is nearly always psychological in origin, related to psychogenic factors such as emotional disturbance and insecurity.

Acquired enuresis occurs most commonly in children from the age of 5 to 8 years, and the onset is usually related to normal stresses of childhood, e.g. after an illness, an operation, the birth of a sibling, temporary or permanent loss of a loved person, etc.

Children who suffer from nocturnal enuresis not infrequently are deep sleepers.

Treatment

Methods of treatment include:
1 Psychotherapy
2 Bladder training
3 Drugs

Psychotherapy

This consists of parental guidance; anxiety must give place to confidence and hope. The child should be encouraged to make his own record of dry nights, such as putting a star in his diary for dry nights and no record being made for wet nights. A system of other rewards of dry nights is also a useful measure.

Bladder Training

Restriction of fluid intake has no therapeutic value. The child should be thoroughly wakened at the parents' bedtime and made to pass water and he should be fully conscious of the act. Older childer may be given an alarm clock to waken them at some time between 10.30 pm and rising.

Daytime training should be instituted in the school holidays. The child should be sent to the lavatory at fixed but gradually increasing intervals, beginning at one hour and increasing the interval by a quarter of an hour every second day. If the child can hold its water for three-hour periods in the day, dryness at night is facilitated. This method is most successful in children with irritable bladders and daytime frequency.

Drug Treatment

Anticholinergic drugs such as belladonna are useful, if given in adequate doses—10 minims of the tincture twice a day and 20 minims at night, increasing until signs of intolerance appear.

Probanthine bromide is slightly more successful than belladonna.

In children who sleep very deeply, amphetamine may be given; this serves the purpose of lightening sleep and also acts as a sympathomimetic agent which is similar in action on the bladder to the anticholinergic drugs.

When enuresis occurs early in the morning, the slow-acting preparations such as dexamphetamine spansules are indicated.

Tricyclic antidepressants, such as imipramine, are also used in the treatment of nocturnal enuresis. Their action appears to be partly due to their anticholinergic actions and also possibly to the fact that sleep may be somewhat lighter thus enabling the patient to wake up to micturate.

Treatment of Nocturnal Enuresis by the Electric Alarm

This apparatus consists of a pad which lies on the mattress under a draw sheet and is connected by a flex to a bedside bell activated by a $4\frac{1}{2}$ volt dry battery. Contact of the urine with the pad closes the electric circuit and rings the bell. In this method response is almost instantaneous; inhibition occurs before the patient is fully awake.

Constipation

Toilet training establishes control of bowel activity and this is one of the earliest experiences where the person has to conform to the needs of the outside world.

Constipation in children is usually due to faulty parental attitudes to bowel evacuation. Excessive concern may be a factor; at other times evacuation of the bowel may be the scene of a battle between the mother and the child and it may be only one manifestation of a general attitude of resistance. Other factors are fears of being alone or the utilization of bowel activity to get attention.

The less fuss and anxiety paid to bowel evacuation the better.

Encopresis

This is the passage of stools at inappropriate times and places after the age of 2. It is more common in boys and its maximum occurrence is between the ages of 6 and 12. The following are the usual reasons:

1 An effort to withhold bowel action in school and then soiling occurs on the way home from school, due to anxiety and the inability to hang on any longer. This explains the isolated case.
2 Continuous soiling from infancy is found sometimes with low social standards in the family.
3 Soiling after improvement may occur with emotional upsets.
4 Encopresis may occur after constipation at any time with emotional upsets.

Behaviour Problems Concerning Eating

Loss of Appetite

Loss of appetite not due to physical illness is usually due to psychological causes and is usually attributable to the attitude and management of meals by the parents. Loss of appetite or refusal of food may be the result of:

1 *An effort on the part of the child to get attention* In

other words, he may use this as a means of controlling other people.
2 *Negativism* Refusal of food may be a manifestation of negativistic behaviour. This is a common cause between the ages of 2 and 3 years. This age period is often called the period of resistance.
3 *Daydreaming* The child may be engaged in fantasy and too preoccupied to eat.
4 *Anxiety or unhappiness in the child* These emotional states can impair appetite.
5 *Parental influences* Such as (a) nagging, (b) over-solicitude, (c) threat or coercion. The child reacts to these influences by refusing food or by a loss of appetite and frequently minor battles occur between the child and the parent over the meal table. Usually the more tense and emotional the adult, the more resistant becomes the child's refusal of food.

In advising the parents on the management of these common forms of behaviour difficulty, it is important to emphasize to them that the child's health is not likely to be endangered in any way if he misses some meals. The child should come to the table at the proper times and be given the first course without fuss and no attention or threat. If the child does not want the food it should be taken away without scolding or blame. It is usually undesirable to praise children for eating, as this gives them the wrong impression and attitude with regard to taking food.

It is better to put too little food on the plate and let the child ask for more than to overload the plate to such an extent as would destroy anyone's appetite. In negativistic children, again, small quantities will result in demands for more food.

The remedy is to avoid undue tension and fuss of any kind. If this approach is consistently applied, feeding difficulties usually disappear. The child may continue to refuse food for the first few days but the parents must be prepared to persist in the new method and natural hunger usually wins in the end.

Over-eating

Over-eating may occasionally be due to psychological causes and children who for some reason or other lack adequate affection may resort to overeating as a compensation. Food is connected with love and the taking of food in some people has potent effects in relieving emotional tension. A number of cases of obesity due to psychogenically determined over-eating have been described.

Sleep Disturbances

Sleep is an essential biological need. The young infant will spend most of its time sleeping between feeds. During childhood the amount of sleep required is less but, in children, the amount of sleep required is greater than in adults.

The common problems of sleeping are:

1. Insomnia
2. Sleep-walking
3 Night terrors

Insomnia

Insomnia is frequently due to anxiety or emotional tension. The child may feel insecure, may be afraid to be on its own, or may have fears of the dark, fear of ghosts or other terrifying objects.

The process of going to sleep should be made as happy as possible and should be accompanied by giving of affection and attention to the children. The form of punishment of sending children to bed after some misdemeanour has certain specific disadvantages in so far that, if it is repeated frequently the going to bed may become associated with punishment and this, again, may go to form an unfavourable attitude to sleeping on the part of the child.

The child should be encouraged to sleep on its own as young as possible. It should be soothed and comforted by the parent before going to sleep and night lights should be avoided as far as possible. They have the effect, if anything, of confirming their fears that the darkness is something to be afraid of and postpones the successful overcoming of this fear by children.

Sleep-walking (Somnambulism)

This is a state of dissociated sleep in which the child walks about in a state of bodily activity with consciousness considerably dimmed.

Sleep-walking may be due to a number of causes. The most common causes are an over-anxious and highly strung child; occasionally the individual sleep-walking may be reliving some past experience or acting out some hidden wish.

Night Terrors

These are to be distinguished from nightmares, in so far that in night terrors the child wakes up in a state of great fear and is still, at the same time, asleep. This, again, may be regarded as a dissociated sleep.

A nightmare, on the other hand, is a terrifying dream which may wake the child. Although distinct phenomenologically, it is doubtful whether the distinction has any practical significance, although night terror is usually regarded as being a more severe symptom than nightmare.

Unhealthy Behavioural and Emotional Responses

Aggressive Behaviour Problems

Anger is an emotion we all experience when frustrated. In children it shows itself in temper tantrums such as screaming, kicking, throwing themselves about on the floor. This type of reaction most commonly occurs in the second year. Temper tantrums do not do any harm but, if they persist, they indicate that there is something wrong with the child's emotional adjustment, that the child cannot stand postponement of his demands.

The cause of temper tantrums lies often in the family's background. Parents, sometimes, may be anxious and highly strung and the family atmosphere is one of continual tension; the temper tantrum, in this instance, serves as a release mechanism for pent up emotional tensions.

Other tantrums may be a manifestation of jealousy. The best way to deal with these tantrums is to try to soothe the child; do not increase its frustration but restore a state of security.

Hyperactive (Hyperkinetic) States in Children

This is a condition manifesting in more or less marked continuous activity. These children are restless, garrulous and impulsive. They are also distractible to an extent which makes it difficult or impossible for them to keep at a given task or activity for any length of time.

Some cases show evidence of brain damage which is frequently minimal but associated with evidence of impaired coordination and deficits in attention, perception, intellect and memory.

Central nervous system stimulants such as amphetamines or methylphenidate (Ritalin) often result in improvement in behaviour.

Jealousy

Jealousy is a condition which frequently occurs in children and is a condition which is brought out when there is an element of competition. Jealousy seems to be more common in girls than in boys. The most common cause is a rivalry between brother and sister and rivalry which develops with the arrival of the new baby.

Jealousy on the arrival of a new baby may show itself in various ways, depending on the child. He may react by bed-wetting, by having temper tantrums, by being anxious and depressed or by becoming more simple and childish in his behaviour. Rivalry is a common factor in many types of mal-adjustment in children.

It is important for parents to tell children in the family of the expected new arrival and that it will be necessary for mother to devote a certain amount of time to the new baby. The parents must be tolerant of these jealousies and attempts to revert to infantile behaviour to secure similar affection. The mother must continue to give adequate affection to the other children and let them realize that they have greater enjoyment in life than a young baby.

Lying

In the first two years many mis-statements are due to inability or lack of perfection in speech. They are due to the fact that words are improperly understood and the child is not sufficiently developed intel-lectually to be precise in its expression or in its description of events.

Up to the age of 4, fantasy lying tends to become more frequent; children at this age tend to live in a world of make believe. Very often children will describe the products of their fantasy as if they existed in reality. Fantasy lying is not always an attempt to deceive but is very often just an expression of a very vivid imagination. Very often the child will tell you, when asked, whether the things he described were real or whether they were 'pretending' and, if they were a product of fantasy he will usually admit that he was pretending.

Defensive lying is carried out in order to avoid punishment or in order to get out of a difficult situation. The incidence of this type of lying increases with the probability of getting punishment. Sometimes children tell lies in order to get approval or admiration; when children are talking together there is a temptation for a child to invent stories to make himself the centre of attention; this tendency will be marked in children who feel inadequate or inferior.

Pathological lying is not a common condition; it shows itself more in late adolescence. These people are usually unstable, have a great verbal facility and very often are charming in personality; they make up stories as they go along and elaborate to a fantastic degree.

A great deal can be done in the management of children to help them avoid lying, such as if one knows that a child has done something wrong, he will not be asked **if** he has done it, but **why**. Children have to be trained to speak the truth and to regard it as a virtue.

Stealing

The word stealing is not applicable in the first two years of life because it implies that the child knows he is doing wrong. He needs to be taught the law of property and what is mine and what is thine.

Stealing may be due to a variety of factors; it may be a result of severe temptation, taking something which the child wants. The feeling will be a part of an ordinary impulse.

In individual types of stealing, a variety of motives such as an unhappy home, lack of affection or insufficient material things may be present. A child with low intelligence and with difficulty in controlling his impulses may steal indiscriminately, or stealing may serve as a release of emotional tension. This is present in emotionally unstable chil-dren.

School Phobia (School Refusal)

School phobia refers to a persistent refusal to attend school, the child remaining at home with the full knowledge of his parents. School refusal is a more appropriate term.

Truants behave differently, usually absenting themselves both from school and home. School refusers are more intelligent, of a higher social class and behave better at school. They are more timid and have been less frequently separated from their mothers in early childhood than the truant. The school refusers often have over-protective mothers and there is more neurosis in the family. School phobics are afraid of separation from their mothers and homes and this separation anxiety, rather than fear of school, is probably the underlying problem.

The treatment of early cases consists of firm support and encouragement to the mother and child towards a return to school. Attempts to force the child will only create greater panic.

If this fails, psychotherapy usually for both mother and child may be required. A compromise solution such as allowing the mother to remain with the child at school may bring about an early return.

Change of school, in itself, is useless but a change sometimes provides a fresh start and can help if combined with other methods.

Gratification Habits

Habitual manipulation of the body for pleasure in children ranges from thumb sucking to picking the nose, ears, plucking eye lashes and hairs, fondling of genitalia and masturbation, head banging and grinding of teeth. The most common are nail biting and thumb sucking. All these habits were once accorded more importance than they deserved. When marked they may indicate an underlying anxiety or insecurity and the important thing is to deal with this by parental guidance.

Educational Backwardness

When a child is educationally backward the causes are often multiple.

The following sets of causes are the most common:

1 Intellectual problems
2 Emotional problems
3 Emotional immaturity and over-dependence on the family

Intellectual Problems

The usual problem is that a child of limited intelligence or poor intelligence is pushed beyond his capacity. This leads to anxiety which further increases his difficulties.

In assessing his problem, it is not only important to assess his mental age in relationship to his chronological age in giving his intelligence quotient but, also, his attainment as measured by his educational age.

Occasionally a very intelligent child may not be doing as well as he might, because he may be bullied by other children or he may be bored and therefore has not sufficient incentive to work.

Emotional Problems

These may be due to faulty parental attitudes—over-protection, rejection and perfectionism. School refusal or school phobia is one outcome of this.

Problems of Maturation

Some children mature late, both in co-ordination and concentration.

Word Blindness (Specific Developmental Dyslexia)

Word blindness describes patients who, despite adequate vision and intelligence, are unable to read words.

Early investigators considered dyslexia to be the result of a specific lesion in or near the angular gyrus of the parietal lobe. More recently, it has been regarded as a delayed or incomplete maturation in the parieto-occipital areas. It is a difficulty in gestalt functioning, gestalt seeing, gestalt recognition, object comprehension and visual association.

There may be a category of persons in whom the language processes are imperfectly lateralized in either hemisphere and who therefore lack determinate cerebral dominance.

Genetic factors are important. Halgren confirmed that, in 88% of his cases, one or more other members of the family also had a reading problem. Another study found concordance in all 9 dyslexic monozygotic twins and discordance in 20 of 30 pairs of dizygotic twins.

Backwardness in reading may be due to a number

of causes in addition to congenital dyslexia. It may be due to low intelligence, emotional difficulties with regard to reading, negativism or other emotional difficulties. Patients with congenital dyslexia are often average, superior or very bright in intelligence.

Thirdly, the child may have a severe hearing handicap. This is another cause of poor reading.

In word blindness patients, reading and spelling are not only poor but bizarre; handwriting is cramped, uneven, variable in slant and spacing. There is no demonstrable evidence of brain damage and no primary emotional disorder. They are better than average, often of high intelligence and have relatively good ability to learn mathematics. They persist in reversing and inverting letters far beyond the age at which it is usual for children to do so. They do not express themselves fluently in writing or in speech. They often give a history of being late in learning to talk, of confusing right and left, of being ambidextrous and of having others in their families who have a similar problem in learning to read and spell.

Treatment

Prevention is always better than cure. Before entry to school, enquiries should be directed into the possibility of word blindness. This is indicated by a history of being late in talking, right–left confusion, ambidexterity, difficulty in reading or spelling in other members of the family. It is then advisable to carry out simple tests of visual and auditory recall and to recommend that an alphabetic phonetic method of teaching reading and spelling should be the one chosen for this child.

Children so taught are not rendered slower or less understanding readers. Instead, because they have become thoroughly familiar with the component parts of words, they approach them with less anxiety, more confidence and greater pleasure.

Speech Difficulties

In fully developed speech there are three phases:

1 The reception of sounds by the ear and brain
2 The interpretation and regrouping of these sounds and their associated ideas
3 The final expression of these symbolic sounds in speech.

In other words, there are receptive, formative and expressive aspects of speech.

Receptive Difficulties

Delayed development of speech can arise from failure to understand speech owing to complete or partial deafness. Children with useful hearing in the lower frequencies of sound but with deafness in the higher frequencies are sometimes difficult to detect.

Formative Difficulties

One of the simplest to understand but one of the rarest of these disorders is the aphasia which may accompany severe hemiplegia, whether congenital from birth injury or acquired in the early years of life through encephalitis or vascular accident. In some of these children the defective interpretation and regrouping of sounds and their associated ideas is further complicated by clumsy articulation. In these cases it is important to rule out mental subnormality.

Expressive Difficulties

This refers to children in whom the main difficulty is with articulation, whch can occur with general spasticity of the muscles in spastic children.

Dyslalia

This is a common disorder in which there is defective articulation of one consonant or multiple substitutions and omissions with varying degrees of intelligibility. It is probable that in these cases during the early development of speech the rapid development of language is associated with a partial failure of both perception and imitation of speech sounds, leading to faulty habits of articulation which persist even when the underlying dysfunction has passed.

This type of speech difficulty improves quickly and spontaneously. Treatment between the ages of 4 and 5, however, is useful in allaying the mother's anxiety and so rescuing the child from nagging correction.

Gilles de la Tourette Syndrome

This is a disorder which usually develops between 10 and 15 years and is more frequently found in males. The symptoms are compulsive utterances, often obscene in kind, and associated with dyskinesia of respiratory movements, and complex involuntary tics affecting various parts of the body. Treatment by haloperidol with or without behaviour therapy may help.

Psychosomatic Disorders in Children

We have already discussed certain psychosomatic disorders such as asthma, peptic ulcer, ulcerative colitis, migraine, etc., which can occur in children and our attention will now be confined to disorders which are particularly related to childhood.

Recurrent pain is probably the commonest psychosomatic disorder after infancy. Recurrent abdominal pain with no organic cause is usually psychogenically determined. Children tend to be overconscientious.

Recurrent abdominal pains, recurrent febrile attacks and recurrent headaches can be a mode of stress reaction in children as well as in adults.

The Periodic Syndrome

Some authors regard recurrent abdominal, head or limb pains as part of a wide spectrum of disorder, the periodic syndrome, of which other components are vomiting and fever. The different components may occur singly, as in cyclical vomiting or recurrent pyrexia, or together in various combinations. Vomiting in infancy tends to be superseded by abdominal pain in childhood and eventually recurrent headache or migraine in adult life.

Severe Mental Disorders in Childhood

The term childhood psychosis has created a great deal of confusion because it contains a number of different diagnostic groups in addition to schizophrenia.

We will confine our attention to childhood schizophrenia and manic-depressive illness.

It should be borne in mind that severely disturbed behaviour can occur in children suffering from epilepsy, Hurler's disease, tuberous sclerosis or as a result of toxic infective conditions, phenylketonuria, cerebral lipoidoses, congenital syphilis and encephalitis lethargica and, sometimes, because of sensory deprivations such as auditory imperception and blindness.

Childhood Schizophrenia

The following criteria are helpful in diagnosing schizophrenia in childhood:

1 Impairment of emotional relationships with others.
2 Apparent unawareness of personal identity to a degree appropriate to his age.
3 Pathological preoccupation with particular objects or certain characteristics of them without regard to their accepted functions.
4 Sustained resistance to change in the environment and a striving to maintain or restore sameness.
5 Abnormal perceptual disturbances in the absence of discernible organic abnormality.
6 Acute, excessive and seemingly illogical anxiety as a frequent phenomenon.
7 Speech either lost or never acquired, showing failure to develop beyond a level appropriate to an earlier age.
8 Distortion in motility patterns.
9 A background of serious retardation in which islets of normality or near normality, or even exceptional intellectual function or skill may appear.

Early Childhood Autism

Kanner described infantile autism as a clinical entity distinct from childhood schizophrenia. He states that infantile autism differs from childhood schizophrenia in that the disorder is clinically manifested from early infancy whereas 'childhood schizophrenia' follows more or less normal behaviour during the first two years.

The autistic child is more isolated than the schizophrenic but physically more healthy.

Many authorities believe that early childhood autism is probably the earliest form of schizophrenia although the matter must still be regarded as controversial.

Diagnostic criteria for early infantile autism

The following features aid the early diagnosis of infantile autism:

1 Gross sustained *impairment of emotional relationships* with people. This includes aloofness, withdrawal, empty clinging behaviour, and abnormal behaviour towards other people as persons, e.g. using them, or parts of them impersonally. Difficulties in mixing and playing with other children are usually severe and persistent.

2 *Apparent unawareness of personal identity* to a degree inappropriate for his age. This may be observed in abnormal behaviour towards himself, such as posturing, or exploration or scrutiny of parts of the body. Repeated self-directed aggression is another aspect of lack of integration.

3 *Pathological preoccupation with particular objects* or certain of their attributes without regard to their accepted functions.

4 *Sustained resistance to changes in the environment* and a striving to maintain or restore sameness. Sometimes this aims at producing a state of perpetual monotony.

5 *Abnormal perceptions* implied by excessive, decreased, or unpredictable response to sensory stimuli, e.g., visual and auditory avoidance or insensitivity to pain and temperature.

6 *Acute severe and apparently illogical anxiety* which is often precipitated by a change in the environment, a change in routine, or a temporary interruption of a symbiotic attachment to persons or things. Sometimes ordinary objects seem to become invested with terrifying qualities. On the other hand, an appropriate sense of fear in the face of real danger may be lacking.

7 *Speech* may be lost or not acquired, or may have failed to develop beyond a level appropriate to an earlier stage. There may be confusion of personal pronouns, echolalia and other mannerisms of diction. Words and phrases convey no sense of ordinary communication.

8 *Distortion of motility patterns*, e.g. hyperkinesis, immobility as in catatonia, bizarre postures or stereotyped mannerisms, such as rocking and spinning.

9 *A background of serious retardation* in which islets of normal, or near normal, or exceptional intellectual function or skill may appear.

Principles of management

These features indicate the need for certain prerequisites in management, for instance:

1 A regular routine is necessary with as little change as possible from day to day.

2 Operant conditioning, to help train the child towards self-help, and purposeful behaviour whose meaning he can learn to understand.

3 Overstimulation should be avoided.

4 A well-planned routine, with very gently graduated progression towards the acquirement of skills, meaningful handling of materials and the establishment of relationships with others, provide a regime which allays anxiety and greatly helps the child to realize his potentials.

Follow up studies have shown that when there is failure to achieve useful language by the age of years there is little prospect of achieving improvement in social adjustment. The main factor in ultimate prognosis is the severity of the disease.

About 70% of autistic children function in the educational subnormal range of intelligence or lower. One view is that childhood autism is primarily communication disorder, biologically determined and associated with brain dysfunction. The high rate of epilepsy in 10 to 15%, tends to confirm this view. Pharmacological treatment is not effective. Educational measures can be applied, particularly those using operant conditioning methods involving suitable rewards for appropriate behaviour. Parental guidance and advice is also very important in management.

Further Reading

Kanner, L. (1957) *Child Psychiatry*. Thomas, Springfield.

Howells, J. G. (1965) (ed) *Modern Perspective in Child Psychiatry*. Oliver & Boyd, Edinburgh.

Rutter, M. (1966) *Children of Sick Parents. Maudsley Monograph No. 16.* Oxford University Press/Institute of Psychiatry, Oxford.

Rutter, M., Graham, P. J. and Yule, E. (eds) (1970) *Neuropsychiatric Study in Childhood Clinics in Developmental Medicine No. 43*. Heinemann, London.

Rutter, M. (ed) (1971) *Infantile Autism: Concepts, Characteristics and Treatment*. Churchill Livingstone, Edinburgh.

Wolff, S. (1973) *Children under Stress.* Revised edn. Penguin Books, Harmondsworth.

Wing, L. (ed) (1975) *Early Child Autism: Clinical, Educational and Social Aspects,* 3rd edn. Pergamon Press, Oxford.

Rutter, M. and Hersov, L. (eds) (1977) *Child Psychiatry: Modern Approaches.* Blackwell Scientific, Oxford.

Last, J. and Lask, B. (1981) *Child Psychiatry and Social Work.* Methuen, London.

34

Psychiatric Emergencies

An emergency may be defined as any sudden and unexpected action which calls for immediate attention. A psychiatric emergency is a psychiatric illness which has affected the patient's behaviour and his close environment to such a degree as to demand immediate action. What constitutes an emergency not only depends on the clinical features of the patient presenting as an emergency, but on other factors such as the patient's personality and the social and environmental circumstances. Therefore, a psychiatric emergency is a composite of the clinical features, the contribution made by the patient's personality and also social and environmental factors. It is the totality of these which determines whether the particular clinical event is an emergency or not.

Suicidal Attempts and Threats

Suicide and attempted suicide have been discussed in detail in Chapter 26. Suicidal attempts or threats are nowadays one of the most common forms of psychiatric emergency. It is unwise to ignore a suicidal threat. We have already noted that between 70 and 80% of successful suicides had communicated the suicidal intent which had been ignored. The degree of risk of suicide associated with a threat has to be assessed in the light of the patient's clinical state and his social circumstances. A suicidal threat in an elderly person living alone and suffering from severe depression associated with delusions of guilt would constitute a serious risk.

It is important to inquire if a patient has left a note or a message as this often indicates that the attempt has been serious. Note should also be made of the efforts which the person may have made to avoid observation and therefore to minimize the risk of discovery and resuscitation, and whether all the available tablets were taken or only a relatively small quantity. It is desirable that patients who make a suicidal attempt should be admitted to hospital for further observation and assessment of their psychiatric and physical state, their personality and social circumstances, and that appropriate arrangements can be made for follow up treatment whether medical, psychiatric or social according to the needs of the case.

Aggressive Behaviour

The majority of psychiatric patients are not hostile dangerous or aggressive, but occasionally psychiatric illnesses present themselves in the form of gross aggressive behaviour. The following are some examples:

1 *Psychopathic personality* Some psychopaths are characterized by episodes of aggressive behaviour, sometimes coming on spontaneously or triggered by minimal provocation.

2 *Alcohol and drugs* Excessive alcohol consumption, whether in alcoholics or in normal people, can result in aggressive and violent behaviour due to diminution of self control. There are rare instances of patients with pathological intoxication who may become violent with minimal doses of alcohol (see Chapter 31).

People taking large doses of the central nervous system stimulants such as amphetamines or methylphenidate may become aggressive as a part of their overactivity and overstimulation. Heroin addicts are not usually aggressive but during the withdrawal phase if they are unable to get further supplies of the drug they become aggressive as a part of their withdrawal syndrome and desire to get further supplies.

3 *Schizophrenia* The majority of schizophrenics are not aggressive but they may exhibit hostile or aggressive behaviour as a result of their delusional beliefs. For example, if he believes that he is going to be attacked or killed a patient may get angry or hostile and may retaliate on his imaginary persecutor. Or these patients may be aggressive in response to the commands of their auditory hallucinations. Occasionally, particularly in catatonic schizophrenics, there may be outbursts of meaningless over-active, and sometimes aggressive behaviour, without necessarily provocation by an environmental stimulus.

4 *Hypomania and mania* These are not usually aggressive patients, but they may become angry and hostile if they are thwarted or obstructed.

5 *Acute toxic confusional states* These may be associated with aggressive behaviour. This is because of clouding of consciousness and diminished comprehension and sometimes because of anxiety, perplexity and delusions of persecution.

6 *Dementia* Aggressive behaviour may become manifest in dementia because of the decreased control due to cerebral damage. Sometimes when persons with dementia are faced with a very difficult task they get what is referred to as a catastrophic reaction; they get very angry, throw things round or attack people. Very often people with dementia are restless, and sometimes disturbed and aggressive, mostly at night.

7 *Epilepsy* Epileptic equivalents may take the form of aggressive behaviour, or aggression may occur in a post-epileptic confusional state.

Management of aggressive behaviour

In dealing with patients presenting with aggressive behaviour as an emergency, it is very important that doctors, nurses and relatives should treat the patient with understanding and with as much gentleness as possible.

If medication is considered to be desirable, phenothiazines, such as intramuscular injections of chlorpromazine 50–100 mg are useful in the majority of emergencies, and other useful medication is intravenous diazepam. This is the drug of choice when the disturbed behaviour is associated with epilepsy, or in disturbed behaviour in withdrawal states associated with alcoholism and barbiturate addiction.

Acute Attacks of Anxiety or Panic

The patient in an attack of acute anxiety or panic not only experiences intense terror but all the bodily concomitants of anxiety, such as sweating, dryness of mouth, feelings of distress in the chest and precordial pains which are sometimes misdiagnosed as angina. Acute anxiety is very easily transmitted to members of the family, who become extremely alarmed and very often acute anxiety attacks become emergencies at weekends or in the middle of the night even though the attack may have been present for some time.

The drugs of choice are the benzodiazepines, and intravenous diazepam will alleviate the emergency situation quickly and effectively.

Severe Depression

Severe depression may present as an emergency not only because of a suicidal threat or attempt but for other reasons as well. These patients may be unable to eat, because of lack of appetite, or may refuse food or drink because they feel they do not deserve it.

The depressed patient presenting with the above indications of such severity as to become an emergency situation will need admission to hospital, even if it has to be achieved by compulsory measures.

Acute Toxic Confusional States

These are characterized by clouding of consciousness, disorientation and sometimes by perceptual abnormalities and disturbed behaviour.

They are due to some underlying infective or toxic condition or disturbance or homeostasis, or may occur as a manifestation of the withdrawal syndromes of alcohol, barbiturates or allied hypnotics. Admission to hospital for the treatment of the underlying condition is necessary. Drugs like chlorpromazine, which do not increase the state of confusion, or the benzodiazepines, are the drugs of choice (barbiturates must be avoided).

States of Excitement

Excited over-active disturbed behaviour in patients may cause an emergency because of the damaging effects of their behaviour on themselves or on others or on their business and financial responsibilities.

This may occur in mania, in acute schizophrenic excitement, in certain epileptic states, personality disorders, in intoxications with alcohol and barbiturates and allied drugs, or during the withdrawal states from these drugs or from alcoholic drugs, or from the direct effect of central nervous system stimulants. This also occurs in confusion states, in toxic infective conditions and is associated with dementia.

For manic and hypomanic or schizophrenic excitement sedative phenothiazines or haloperidol by injection are helpful.

For excitement associated with epilepsy or alcohol or drug withdrawal intravenous diazepam is the measure of choice.

35

Forensic Psychiatry and Legal Aspects

Forensic psychiatry deals with the mentally disordered offender, and is the application of general psychiatry to those who are involved in the legal process.

Mental illness and even psychiatric abnormality is a biological concept, whereas criminal behaviour is a social concept which is arbitrarily determined by legislation.

It has been shown in the United Kingdom that approximately one-third of prison inmates have a psychiatric disorder.

Statistics reveal that courts are more likely to send offenders convicted of violent sexual offences or criminal damage, including arson, to hospital than other types of offender.

The available evidence suggests that the psychiatric disorders associated with recidivism are more likely to be personality disorders, addictions, especially alcoholism, and mental handicap.

In schizophrenia the most common determinants of violent behaviour are delusions, irresistible compulsion based on an overwhelming urge to injure or kill, or responding to the command of auditory hallucinations. Sudden violent outbursts without apparent external stimulation can occur and a small number of patients have systematized paranoid delusions, and carry out the assault as a defence against harm by their 'enemies'.

Epilepsy and Criminal Behaviour

In the past epileptic automatism was considered an important possible determinant of crimes in epileptics, particularly in relationship to crimes committed during or after an epileptic attack.

Automatism is a condition in which the epileptic carries out apparently purposive behaviour without conscious control. Research investigations have revealed that automatism is a very rare cause of violent crime.

The prevalence of epilepsy in the prison population, however, is considerably higher than the general population and the relationships between epilepsy and crime may be due to an organic brain disorder, responsible for both epilepsy and the criminal behaviour, or epilepsy causing social rejection and a sense of inferiority leading to antisocial behaviour.

Violence

Violence can be an ordinary non-pathological phenomenon, and it should not be assumed that there is a special relationship between psychiatric illness and violence. There is no evidence that psychiatric patients, as a whole, are more violent than the general population. Sometimes, violence and psychiatric illness are associated by coincidence rather than by cause and effect. However, people under stress may act destructively, attempt suicide, or carry out other forms of self-destructive behaviour and these are recognized complications of mental disorder. Violent behaviour, however, must be recognized as a possibility in psychiatrically ill patients, however low its incidence.

The evaluation of violent behaviour consists of:

1 An analysis of the behaviour, including detailed history of the episode of violence. An attempt should be made to understand the factors leading to the episode in terms of the patient's background, his stresses, his environment, his mental state and attitudes and, particularly, whether known precipitants, such as drugs, alcohol or provocation were present.
2 The identification of any pathology, such as schizophrenia, depression, alcohol abuse, brain injury, epilepsy, personality disorder or any medical abnormality.
3 The patient's responsibility for the act and an assessment of the patient's motivation.

The peak age for crimes of violence against persons is between 17 and 21 years.

Murder

When a person kills, or is a party to the killing of another, the mandatory sentence is life imprisonment. If, however, he was suffering from an abnormality of the mind, which substantially impaired his mental responsibility for his acts, the verdict is manslaughter, and not murder. Manslaughter can also be the verdict if mitigating circumstances, such as provocation, are considered to be relevant and important. In these circumstances, the crime is also manslaughter with the sentence at the judge's discretion.

The majority of murderers are male and their motives are usually emotional, and the victims are relatives or close associates. In England, victims are twice as likely to be female (wives are most vulnerable) and the common factors are quarrels, outbursts of rage, paranoid tendencies and severe depression with suicidal tendency. Fifty per cent of murderers are found to be suffering from psychiatric abnormalities, such as personality disorder, schizophrenia, and mental handicap. One-third commit suicide after murder.

The sexually sadistic murderer is usually male, solitary, uncommunicative, shy, with a precarious self-esteem, and powerful fantasy. His sex drives and abilities are low and he may be a homosexual, paedophile or transvestite. They often show an interest in black magic and sadistic pornography, and often have an extensive collection of books on such subjects.

Rape

Under the law, rape is defined as unlawful sexual intercourse with a woman without her consent. Very few rapists are suffering from any psychiatric disorder. Many are selfish, predatory, to whom rape is a part of a general cycle of aggression in which they snatch not only sex, but also property.

The remainder form a heterogeneous group including would-be rapist-murderers and sexual novitiates who misread their partner's signals.

1 Surveys have revealed that rape may be motivated by an aggressive aim, in which sexual behaviour is on the basis of anger and humiliates the victim.
2 The motivation may be a sexual aim (aggression to achieve sex gratification).
3 Sadistic men who need an element of cruelty to achieve sexual satisfaction.

Exhibitionism

An exhibitionist is a man who exposes his genitals to a woman or children as a means of sexual gratification or excitement. They are usually immature, passive individuals with an inability for appropriate expression of anger and with poor social skills, and a poor capacity for heterosexual relationships. Many exhibitionists utilize the memory of their victims' response to facilitate future masturbation, or to achieve an erection for marital intercourse. The responses most wished for are fear and disgust, and the act of exposure enables a feeling of assertion and power to be achieved in a person who is inadequate and inferior. Eighty to ninety per cent of exhibitionists who are convicted do not commit further offences. Those who continue to have the impulse or carry out acts of exhibitionism can be helped by behaviour therapy; watching the video recordings of exposure in front of a group of women who are unresponsive, followed by encouragement to participate in a normal heterosexual relationship.

Arson

The people who commit arson form a heterogeneous group with many different reasons and motives.

Broadly speaking, there are two groups.

In the first group the fire is the means of achieving something, and these arsonists set relatively few res. They may be deluded psychotic patients where ire-raising is directed by the delusion or disturbed motion. In others the motive can be revenge, anger or jealousy aimed at a specific target. In some, fire-raising may be a cry for help to draw attention to their plight. Arson may also serve to cover up evidence of a crime, or it may be an insurance fraud. Occasionally it is carried out for political motives, or it may be a gang activity for excitement, particularly in adolescents and children.

The second group involves relatively more fires. Here the motivation may be to be seen as heroes. They act bravely at the scene of the fire, feel powerful, and enjoy causing all the trouble.

The arsonist may be the victim of an irresistible impulse, or may be sexually aroused by the fire and, in others, the fire-setting serves to relieve depression or anxiety.

Shoplifting

The majority of shoplifters are women, two-thirds are usually middle-aged and suffer from a multiplicity of symptoms, such as insomnia, headaches or persistent depression. The minority (one-third) are foreign-born, usually young, and of good upbringing, regard themselves as having committed a purely technical offence, and are often well off. Male shoplifters often steal books which is very unusual in women shoplifters. Some women only commit shoplifting offences during a depressive illness, and others at the time of severe premenstrual tension or depression.

Non-accidental Injury to Children

Child abuse can range from direct physical violence (the battered child) to excessively punitive discipline, or irresponsible neglect. A child may be a subject of parental rejection, being an unwanted encumbrance, or the displaced target of parent anger.

It has been estimated that approximately 0.5% of children under three years of age are subjected to non-accidental injury per year. This amounts to 3,000 cases per annum in the United Kingdom. The death rate is 10% over a two-year period. The risk of an injured child being battered again is in the order of 60%. More than one member of a family is often subjected to physical injury.

The following injuries should arouse suspicion:

multiple bruises, burns and lacerations, bite-marks, finger-tip bruises, laceration of the inner aspects of the upper lip, multiple fractures, subdural haematoma, retinal injury, rupture of abdominal viscera, delay in reporting injury or seeking help, e.g. by more than six hours and, finally, discrepancy or vague history of the injury.

The problem, once detected, must involve both emergency action for the child and help for both the family and the child in the longer term. A 'Place of Safety' Order may be needed if the parents do not agree to hospitalization for the child's welfare.

Other important steps are: a case conference to nominate a key-worker; to achieve effective surveillance; entry into the local authority's 'At Risk' Register and, if necessary, a care order application by the Social Services.

The Mental Health Act 1983

The Mental Health Act 1983 which came into force on 30 September 1983 consolidated the Mental Health Act 1959 as amended by the Mental Health (Amendment) Act 1982. It is principally concerned with the grounds for detaining patients in hospital or placing them under guardianship and aims to improve patients' rights and the protection of staff in a variety of ways.

Most patients who need hospital care agree to be admitted informally. A minority require compulsory admission and detention in order that they may receive treatment and when no other plan of management is practicable.

Section 1—Definition of Mental Disorder

A patient must be suffering from mental disorder as defined by the Act before compulsory admission to hospital, or guardianship, can be considered.

Mental disorder means mental illness, arrested or incomplete developments of mind, psychopathic disorder and any other disorder or disability of mind.

Severe mental impairment means a state of arrested or incomplete development of mind which includes **severe** impairment of intelligence and social functioning and is associated with abnormally aggressive or seriously irresponsible conduct on the part of the person concerned.

Mental impairment means a state of arrested or

incomplete development of mind which includes **significant** impairment of intelligence and social functioning and is associated with abnormally aggressive or seriously irresponsible conduct on the part of the person concerned.

Psychopathic disorder means a persistent disorder or disability of mind (whether or not including significant impairment of intelligence) which results in abnormally aggressive or seriously irresponsible conduct on the part of the person concerned.

A person may not be regarded as suffering from mental disorder by reason only of promiscuity or other immoral conduct, sexual deviancy or dependence on alcohol or drugs.

Section 2—Admission for Assessment

This allows for admission for assessment (or for assessment followed by medical treatment) for up to 28 days. Application may be made by the nearest relative or an approved social worker. The application must be supported by two medical recommendations (one of them from an 'approved doctor'). They must agree that (a) the patient is suffering from mental disorder of a nature or degree which warrants the detention of the patient in hospital for assessment (or for assessment followed by medical treatment) for at least a limited period, and (b) that he ought to be so detained in the interests of his own health or safety or with a view to the protection of other persons. The patient has the right to apply to a Mental Health Review Tribunal within 14 days of admission. The nearest relative, the managers or the Responsible Medical Officer (RMO) can discharge the patient, although the RMO can bar discharge by the nearest relative. The patient must be discharged after 28 days unless he has been further detained for treatment.

Section 3—Admission for Treatment

This Section provides for the admission of a patient to hospital and his detention for treatment for a maximum period of six months (unless the order is renewed). The application may be made by the nearest relative or an approved social worker, founded upon the written recommendations of two doctors (one 'approved') who must indicate the grounds for their opinion and why other methods of dealing with the patient are inappropriate. The

grounds which may support an application are (a) that the patient is suffering from mental illness, severe mental impairment, psychopathic disorder or mental impairment and his mental disorder is of a nature or degree which makes it appropriate for him to receive medical treatment in a hospital; (b) in the case of psychopathic disorder or mental impairment such treatment is likely to alleviate or prevent deterioration of his condition; and (c) it is necessary for the health or safety of the patient or for the protection of other persons that he should receive such treatment and it cannot be provided unless he is detained under this Section. The patient has a right to apply to a Mental Health Review Tribunal within the first six months and once during each subsequent period for which the detention is renewed.

Section 4—Admission for Assessment in Cases of Emergency

An emergency application for admission for assessment for 72 hours may be made by the nearest relative or an approved social worker, supported by one doctor, preferably one who is acquainted with the patient. The application should state that it is of urgent necessity to admit the patient and that admission under Section 2 above would involve undesirable delay. The grounds are those defined under Section 2. The order ceases to have effect after 72 hours unless the second medical recommendation required under Section 2 is given and received by the managers within that period.

Section 5(2)—Application in Respect of a Patient Already in Hospital

This Section allows the detention of a patient already receiving any form of inpatient treatment. The application must be made by report from the doctor in charge of the case, or his nominated deputy (only one doctor may be nominated), to the managers, if it appears that an application for compulsory detention in a hospital should be made as the patient is presenting a danger to himself or others. The Section provides that the patient may be detained for up to 72 hours (including any period during which a nurse's holding power was used) after which the patient must be allowed to leave unless further powers have been taken under Sections 2 or 3.

Section 5(4)—Nurse's Holding Power

Only applicable to patients already receiving treatment for mental disorder in hospital. Allows nurses of a prescribed class, the equivalent of a registered mental nurse (including registered nurses for mental handicap), to detain a patient for up to six hours from the time that the decision is recorded on the prescribed form, while a doctor is found. It must appear to the nurse that (a) the patient is suffering from mental disorder to such a degree that it is necessary for his health or safety, or for the protection of others, for him to be immediately restrained from leaving hospital and (b) that it is not practicable to secure the immediate attendance of a practitioner for the purpose of formulating a report under Section 5(2) (above).

Section 12—Medical Recommendations

Approval for the purposes of the Act will be granted to suitable doctors by the Secretary of State (delegated to Regional Health Authorities, RHAs). Where two doctors are required to provide medical recommendations they should normally not be associated, and should preferably be the family doctor and admitting consultant, but where there may be delay involving serious risk to the health or safety of the patient in making these arrangements, two doctors from the same hospital may act as the recommending doctors. There are, however, qualifications which restrict the professional relationship of the two doctors where this arrangement is used.

Section 7—Application for Guardianship

This Section allows a patient who has attained the age of sixteen years to be placed under the supervision of a guardian. The applicant may be the nearest relative or an approved social worker (who must have seen the patient within the last fourteen days) and is made to the local Social Services authority. The application must be based upon medical recommendations from two doctors (one 'approved') who have examined the patient together or within five days of each other. The patient must be agreed to suffer from one of the forms of mental disorder (see above) and the doctor must agree that it is necessary in the interests of the welfare of the patient that he should be received into the guardianship of

an individual or of the local Social Services authority. The order is for six months unless renewed for a further six months. The patient may be discharged by a RMO (or nominated medical attendant), the authority or nearest relative. The patient may apply to a Tribunal within each six month period.

Section 8—Powers of Guardians

1 To require the patient to reside at a specified place.
2 To require the patient to attend at specified places and times for medical treatment, occupation, education or training, and
3 To require access to the patient to be given, at the patient's residence, to any doctor, approved social worker or other specified person. The guardian has no other statutory powers.

Section 20(4)—Renewal of Compulsory Powers (Hospital Treatment)

The conditions for renewing an order for compulsory hospital detention are now more detailed and renewal orders must be made more frequently. The doctor must state that the patient is (a) suffering from one of the forms of mental disorder, (b) that it is of a nature or degree which makes it appropriate for him to receive medical treatment, (c) for all forms of mental disorder, that such treatment is likely to alleviate or prevent a deterioration of his condition and (d) that it is necessary for the health or safety of the patient or for the protection of others that he should receive the treatment and that it cannot be provided in any other way. Alternatively, for patients suffering from mental illness and severe mental impairment, that the patient, if discharged, would be unlikely to be able to care for himself, to obtain the care which he needs or guard himself against serious exploitation. The doctor is required to consult other specified staff before giving his opinion. Orders must be reviewed twice as often as under the previous legislation.

Age Limits

The previous age limits for the admission of patients suffering from psychopathic disorder or mental impairment are removed but, for admission for treatment or on a hospital order, these conditions must be treatable.

Mentally Abnormal Offenders

The range of alternative provisions has been widened. There is a new provision for a court to remand a patient to hospital for a psychiatric report (Section 35) and a provision to remand to hospital to receive treatment (Section 36). A court may also make an interim hospital order (a 'trial' of a hospital order). These sections were implemented at a later date than the rest of the Act.

Section 37—Hospital and Guardianship Orders

Allows a court to order hospital admission or the reception of the patient into guardianship. It is only applicable to individuals found guilty of an imprisonable offence (except murder). Two doctors (one 'approved') must give written or oral evidence.

Section 41—Restriction Order

A Crown Court may add a restriction order, 'to protect the public from serious harm' after hearing oral evidence from one doctor (preferably the receiving doctor). The patient may not be given leave, transferred or discharged without the consent of the Home Secretary.

Consent to Treatment

A detained patient may be competent to give informed consent to treatment. The Act provides that treatment may be imposed in some circumstances even though a detained patient is incapable of consenting or refuses to consent.

With one exception, the arrangements refer to patients detained in hospital for the treatment of mental disorder. They do not apply to patients detained on emergency applications for assessment or under short-term powers, to patients remanded for a report or to conditionally discharged patients. The Sections apply to specified treatments. Other treatments do not require the formal, recorded consent of the patient or a second opinion.

Section 57—Treatment Requiring Consent and a Second Opinion

This Section applies to (a) any surgical operation for destroying brain tissue or for destroying the function of brain tissue, or (b) such other forms of treatment as may be specified by the Secretary of State in Regulations. (Regulations at the present time only specify 'the surgical implantation of hormones to reduce male sexual drive'.) No patient, detained or not detained, may be given one of these treatments (for the treatment of mental disorder) unless (a) he has given his consent, (b) an independent doctor and two other persons have certified in writing that the patient is capable of understanding the nature, purpose and likely effects of the proposed treatment and has consented to it, and (c) the independent doctor has certified in writing that, having regard to the likelihood of the treatment alleviating or preventing a deterioration of the patient's condition, that the treatment should be given. Before giving his opinion the independent doctor is required to consult two other persons who have been professionally concerned with the patient's medical treatment. One of these persons must be a nurse and the other neither a nurse nor a doctor.

Section 58—Treatment Requiring Consent or a Second Opinion

This applies to (a) such forms of treatment as may be specified by the Secretary of State in Regulations (they will include electroconvulsive therapy, ECT and (b) the administration of medicine by any means if three months have elapsed since the first occasion (during the detention for the treatment of mental disorder) that the medicine was first administered to the patient. No detained patient may be given ECT or medicine after the first three months unless (a) he has given his consent and this has been certified either by the RMO or the independent doctor or (b) the independent doctor has certified in writing that the patient is not capable of understanding the nature, purpose and likely effects of the treatment or has not given consent, but that, having regard to the likelihood of its alleviating or preventing deterioration of his condition the treatment should be given. As above (Section 57) the independent doctor must consult other staff members.

Section 59—Plans of Treatment

Consent or an independent certificate may refer to a treatment plan.

Section 60—Withdrawal of Consent

If a patient withdraws his consent, continuation of treatment will require the application of Section 57 or Section 58 as appropriate. Section 57 treatments may not be given. Section 58 treatments can only be given where a concurring second opinion is given.

Section 61—Review of Treatment

Continued treatment given as above must be reviewed when a patient's detention is renewed. This applies to all Section 57 treatments and to Section 58 treatments given after a second opinion has been obtained.

Section 62—Urgent Treatment

A treatment, otherwise restricted by Sections 57 or 58, may be given to a detained patient without the need for formal consent or a second opinion if it (a) is immediately necessary to save the patient's life, (b) (not being an irreversible treatment) is immediately necessary to prevent a serious deterioration of the patient's condition, (c) (not being irreversible or hazardous) is immediately necessary to prevent serious suffering by the patient or (d) (not being irreversible or hazardous) is immediately necessary and represents the minimum interference necessary to prevent the patient from behaving violently or being a danger to himself or others.

Irreversible treatment is a treatment which has unfavourable, irreversible physical or psychological consequences.

Hazardous treatment is a treatment which entails significant physical hazard.

Mental Health Review Tribunals

Patients have increased opportunities to apply to a Tribunal as indicated above. Restricted patients, who may apply in the second six months if on a hospital order, but in the first six months if otherwise transferred to hospital with restrictions on discharge, have a right of direct application to a Tribunal. For these patients the President of the Tribunal will be a Circuit Judge or equivalent. Further Tribunals will be able to discharge such patients directly or give them a conditional or deferred conditional discharge. Patients may apply for legal aid, to obtain advice to assist them in presenting a case and to obtain an independent medical opinion and to cover the cost of representation at a Tribunal hearing.

Mental Health Act Commission

This is a special health authority authorized by the Act with about 80 members appointed by the Secretary of State. The members are appointed from the professions of law, nursing, psychology, social work and medicine and there are lay members. They are based upon three area offices and there is a central policy committee. The Commission's medical members provide second independent opinions augmented by other doctors appointed by the Commission. All hospitals are visited regularly and the Commission is concerned with the care and welfare of individual patients. It was initially concerned only with detained patients.

Regulations and Code of Practice

Regulations are laid before Parliament as required by the Act and have the force of law. A Code of Practice, published by the Secretary of State, gives guidance on good practice, procedures on admissions and treatment.

Other Legal Aspects

The Care of Property

It is sometimes necessary for special arrangements to be made to manage the property and affairs of persons who, by reason of mental disorder, are unable to do so themselves.

This is carried out by the Court of Protection. The Court is only directly concerned with mental patients' property and not with the persons. The provision exists to protect the property of patients but not to exercise control over the patients themselves.

The normal procedure is to appoint a Receiver, who is vested by the Court of Protection with various powers of acting on behalf of the patient and who may be regarded as the statutory agent of the patient. Medical evidence is required for the Court to establish its jurisdiction. The medical evidence must satisfy the Court that the patient is incapable, by reason of mental disorder, of managing and administering his property and affairs.

Any mental illness or disorder or disability of the mind suffices to give the Court jurisdiction if, by reason thereof, the person is incapable of managing his property and affairs. The degree of mental disorder required to give the Court jurisdiction is quite distinct from and less severe than that required for compulsory detention.

The most common group of patients for whom these provisions are needed are mental disorders in elderly patients.

Testamentary Capacity

For a person to have testamentary capacity he must understand the nature of a Will, must be able to grasp the extent of his property and to form a proper judgment as to the nature of the claims to his bounty.

The doctor, when asked to advise as to testamentary capacity, should show by his report that he has considered each of these three essentials, and if he is not provided with the necessary particulars, he should refuse to advise until he is properly instructed.

Criminal Responsibility

From the legal point of view, responsibility means liability for punishment.

Defence may plead unsoundness of mind for any criminal charge but, in fact, this is usually only done in charges of murder.

In 1843 McNaughton shot and killed Sir Robert Peel's secretary. It was shown that McNaughton suffered from a number of delusions of persecution and that the killing had been inspired by these delusions, and the Judge directed the jury to find him not guilty. Public reaction was very great and culminated in a debate in the House of Lords when the now famous McNaughton Rules were formulated.

The Rules state that, in order to establish a defence on grounds of insanity, it must be proved:

1 That at the time of committing the act, the accused was labouring under such a defect of reason from disease of the mind as not to know the nature and quality of the act he was doing or, if he knew what he was doing, he did not know that it was wrong.

2 If the accused commits an act by reason of delusion, the degree of responsibility is based on the justification which the delusion would provide if it were true.

Medical men have objected to these rules ever since they were introduced, as the only thing that mattered legally was whether the accused passed the McNaughton test whilst important clinical aspects of his case might often be passed over.

From the outset, it was realized that the rule dealing with partial insanity was absurd. Attempting to evaluate insane delusions as if they were true whilst ignoring the underlying mental illness of which the delusions were themselves evidence, was recognized to be ridiculous 80 years ago.

The diagnosis of insanity was left in the hands of jurymen. The rules make no provision for the effect upon conduct of pathological emotional disturbances as opposed to disturbances of reason or knowledge.

The administration of McNaughton Rules can also be criticized on the following grounds:

1 They are inequitable as between case and case.
2 They are inequitable as between judge and witness. The judge is free to ignore the rules if he so wishes and, if he so wishes, he can always tie the medical witness down to them as strictly as he likes.
3 By applying or not applying the rules in his direction to the jury, the judge can exercise a large measure of control on the jury's decision. The judge and not the jury becomes the arbiter in what is supposedly a matter of fact. The rules are not applied candidly; if they were to be so, the judge would point out to the jury that hardly anyone is ever mad enough to be covered by the rules.

In 1957 the Homicide Act introduced the doctrine of diminished responsibility into English criminal law. The Act states that when a person kills or is a party to the killing of another, he should not be convicted of murder if he was suffering from such an abnormality of mind (whether arising from a condition of arrested or retarded development of mind or any inherent causes, or induced by disease or injury) as substantially impaired his mental responsibility for his acts and admissions in doing or being a party to the killing. If these circumstances apply the verdict is manslaughter and not murder.

The Criminal Justice Act of 1948

This deals with offences other than homicide and applies to a person charged before a Court of summary jurisdiction with an act punishable by imprisonment and, when the Court is satisfied (a) that the person did the act, (b) on the evidence of at least two doctors that he is suffering from a mental disorder, and (c) that he is a proper person to be detained, the Court may order him to be detained in a mental hospital.

The Act also empowers a Court, if satisfied by expert medical evidence that an offender shows mental abnormality not severe enough to justify compulsory detention, to place the offender on probation and to require him, for a period not exceeding twelve months, to undergo psychiatric treatment in an appropriate hospital or elsewhere as an informal resident or non-resident patient, if this is considered likely to be beneficial to the offender and providing the arrangements can be made.

Fitness to Plead

An accused person should be mentally capable of instructing counsel, appreciating the significance of pleading guilty or not guilty, challenging a juror, examining witnesses and understanding and following the evidence and Court procedure.

If the prisoner is found to be not guilty by reason of insanity or other disability, the Court will order the accused's admission to a hospital to be specified by the Secretary of State.

A Mentally Ill Person Serving as a Witness

It is admissible for a psychiatric patient to serve as a witness, but his mental state must always be taken into account in assessing his reliability. He is also to make an affidavit if his evidence is likely to be reliable.

Civil Law

Contract

A contract made by a person before the onset of mental disorder is binding. A person suffering from a mental disorder may make contracts for the necessities of life and such contracts are binding. He may also make contracts for articles other than necessities, but such contracts are not binding if it is clear that they would not have been made but for the mental disorder at the time of making the contract.

Marriage and Divorce

A marriage is not valid if, at the time of the marriage, either party was so mentally disordered as not to appreciate the nature of the contract.

Nullification of the marriage may also take place if the petitioner did not know at the time of the marriage that the other party was suffering from a mental illness or handicap or was subject to recurrent bouts of mental illness or epilepsy. The petition has to be filed within a year of the date of marriage.

A petition for divorce may be presented on the grounds that the respondent is 'incurably of unsound mind' and has been continuously under care and treatment for a period of at least five years immediately preceding the presentation of the petition.

Legislation for Scotland

The Mental Health (Scotland) Act 1960 has been amended by the Mental Health (Scotland) (Amendment) Act 1983 along broadly similar lines to the above.

Further Reading

Mowatt, R. R. (1966) *Morbid Jealousy and Murder: a Psychiatric Study of Morbidly Jealous Murderers at Broadmoor.* Tavistock Publications and Institute for the Study and Treatment of Delinquency, London.

Rolin, H. R. (1969) *The Mentally Abnormal Offender and the Law.* Pergamon Press, Oxford.

Hamilton, J. R. and Freeman, H. (eds) (1982) *Dangerousness: Psychiatric Assessment and Management.* Gaskell Books, Ashford, Kent.

Bluglass, R. (1983) *A Guide to the Mental Health Act 1983.* Churchill Livingstone, Edinburgh.

Hamilton, J. R. (1983) The Mental Health Act 1983. *British Medical Journal,* 28 May 1983, pp. 1720–1725.

Mental Health Act, 1983. HMSO, London.

36

Miscellaneous Disorders

Hypochondriasis

Hypochondriasis is a term which is vague and which over the years has been both over-used and ill-used.

A useful definition is that hypochondriasis is a preoccupation with a real or supposed physical or mental disorder with a marked discrepancy between the degree of preoccupation and the grounds for it. The interest, preoccupation and conviction are maintained with indifference to the opinion of others and do not respond to persuasion.

Controversy continues as to whether hypochondriasis is a primary disease entity or syndrome, or whether invariably it is secondary to some other disorders, such as a depressive illness or anxiety state. Comparisons of groups of patients with the diagnosis of primary hypochondriasis and those with secondary hypochondriasis showed differences in a variety of social and clinical variables which support the view that primary hypochondriasis is a true entity.

Some authorities propose the view that hypochondriasis is best seen as learned abnormal illness behaviour. An advantage of this approach is that such learned abnormal illness behaviour can be therapeutically unlearned by behaviour therapy.

Secondary hypochondriasis is associated with:

1 Depressive states
2 Anxiety states
3 Schizophrenia
4 Hysterical personality

In anxiety states the bodily concomitants of anxiety become the focus of hypochondriacal preoccupation, for example, palpitations and precordial pains give rise to fears of heart disease.

In depressive states there is a preoccupation with a variety of minor physical symptoms, such as bodily pains, dyspepsia and constipation. In severe depression a continuum of hypochondriacal symptoms may be observed. For example, the patient may believe that various organ functions are slowing down, followed by the belief that organs are abnormal and finally that serious disease is present.

These may culminate in nihilistic delusions with a belief that various organs have, in fact, disappeared.

In some grief reactions, the bereft person may develop the symptoms of the terminal illness by a process of identification and preoccupation with them.

In schizophrenia, there may be hypochondriacal symptoms of delusional intensity, often bizarre in nature.

Another category is the person with a hypochondriacal personality who is preoccupied with patent medicines, food-fads, diets, bowel function and trivial somatic phenomena. These can be very frustrating to the doctor because of incessant demands for help and their failure to respond to treatment. In these people the fear is of developing disease rather than a conviction of having already developed disease.

Hypochondriacal patients most commonly complain of pain, bodily appearance, smell, eye symptoms, sexual difficulties, gastrointestinal, cardiorespiratory and ear, nose and throat symptoms.

Monosymptomatic delusional hypochondriasis is a condition in which a single hypochondriacal delusion is held over a long period and is not secondary to any other psychiatric disorder. The person's personality, meanwhile, remains intact. Pimozide has been found to be specifically helpful in this disorder.

Treatment

The treatment and prognosis of hypochondriacal illness depend on its basis. A thorough investigation must be carried out to exclude the possibility of an underlying organic basis for the illness. In the case of secondary hypochondriasis the primary illness, depression, anxiety states and schizophrenia must receive the appropriate treatment. In the case of primary hypochondriasis, success has been reported with operant behavioural techniques.

Illness Behaviour

In the sick role the patient is excused many of his usual social responsibilities. He is not expected to cure his own illness by will-power. He should want to get well and he should seek medical help and cooperate with treatment. The way in which an individual perceives and acts as a response to his symptoms has been termed 'illness behaviour'. Various factors influence the tendency to seek medical advice for symptoms, such as degree of dependence on others, social class, religious background and interpersonal difficulties and stresses. Abnormal illness behaviour refers to the conviction of being ill rather than the presence of a physical lesion or dysfunction, and it covers any state in which the degree of invalidism is disproportionate to the degree of physical pathology.

Abnormal illness behaviour resists reassurance despite negative physical findings and laboratory investigations.

The concept of abnormal illness behaviour serves a useful purpose because it draws attention to the manner in which such patients utilize illness to deal with personal problems and predicaments.

Munchausen Syndrome

This designation is applied to patients who repeatedly seek medical or hospital treatment for feigned symptoms. A synonym is 'hospital addiction' and essentially the syndrome consists of a dramatic presentation of symptoms and history suggesting an acute emergency leading to intensive medical care, admission and sometimes surgery.

Three varieties are common:

The abdominal type which leads to repeated laparotomies

2 The haemorrhagic type, for example, haemoptysis, haemotomysis, and gynaecological (bleeding pv)
3 The neurological type often presenting with convulsions

The abdominal and haemorrhagic types are the most common. Not infrequently, patients have had hundreds of admissions in different parts of the country over a number of years.

The syndrome is best seen in terms of an extreme form of abnormal illness behaviour. These patients have an intense wish to be the centre of attention, a need to be passive but controlling, and a desire for a relationship with parental authority, such as a doctor, who they can cheat and manipulate.

Briquet's Syndrome

This syndrome comprises longstanding multiple somatic symptoms and characteristically occurs in women who manipulate their doctors and generally refuse to accept psychological or psychodynamic explanations. Sexual and gynaecological symptoms are common and most patients have a history of hospitalization and surgery before the age of thirty. A synonym for this disorder is Somatoform disorder and the diagnostic criteria include a history of several years duration, beginning before the age of thirty and including complaints of at least fourteen symptoms for women and twelve for men. These include feeling generally sick or unwell, pseudo-neurological symptoms such as difficulty in swallowing, visual disturbances, fainting attacks, muscle weakness, gastrointestinal symptoms, such as pain, nausea, vomiting, diarrhoea and food intolerance. Female reproductive symptoms are common, such as menorrhagia, psychosexual difficulties, lack of sexual desire, dyspareunia, pains in the back, in the joints and the extremities, shortness of breath, palpitations, chest pains and dizziness. These patients take up a great deal of the time and resources of Health Services, of general practitioners and hospitals, and in cost of investigations.

Whether this is a distinct and separate nosological entity is still controversial and many of the features are typical of hypochondriasis and the behaviour of patients with hysterical personalities.

Depersonalization

Depersonalization is an alteration in the perception or experience of the self so that the usual awareness of one's reality is temporarily lost or changed. The feeling of unreality is associated with a sensation of self-estrangement and a feeling of detachment. The patient may have the experience of appearing to perceive himself from a distance and he may feel mechanical as though in a dream.

The associated feelings are unpleasant. Sometimes it is accompanied by disturbances in the body image, e.g. feeling that the limbs and other parts of the body have changed in size or shape. The perception of the passage of time is sometimes changed.

He may feel that he has become an automaton and incapable of feeling emotional contact or rapport with other people.

The feeling that one is not in full control of one's actions, including speech, is often present. All these symptoms are unpleasant, and the patient maintains good contact with reality. He retains insight and recognizes that the symptom is abnormal.

The onset is usually sudden and the disorder occurs mainly in young adults.

Mild depersonalization without significant impairment has been reported to occur at some time in 30% to 60% of young adults, with fatigue, after anaesthesia, after taking hallucinogenic drugs or amphetamines.

Depersonalization can be a primary condition occurring without evidence of a form of psychiatric disorder. Derealization is often present, a condition in which the person feels a strange alteration in the perception of the environment, so that a sense of the reality of the external world is lost. This is sometimes accompanied by a change in the perception of the size and shape of external objects.

Depersonalization can occur as a symptom in many psychiatric disorders, including depression and anxiety states, and it may be precipitated by hyperventilation, schizophrenia, temporal lobe epilepsy, phobic states and obsessional states. The treatment of secondary depersonalization is the treatment of the underlying condition.

The treatment of primary depersonalization is notoriously difficult. Sometimes patients may be helped by a series of mild narcosis sessions induced by the intravenous injection of thiopentone.

Morbid Jealousy

Morbid jealousy is displayed in persons who unreasonably suspect sexual infidelity by their spouse or partner, and exhibit irritability, anger, grief, or agitation too readily or intensely in response to doubts of a partner's fidelity. They have excessive zeal in seeking confession of guilt by incessant questioning and a search for evidence of infidelity by examination of underwear, bed linen, letters, diaries and even by hiring detectives.

Morbid jealousy is more common in men than in women and very rarely it may be a syndrome in its own right. More usually, however, it is a symptom of schizophrenia or other paranoid disorder, manic depressive illness, or a personality disorder of the paranoid variety. Some are alcoholics and some have organic psychosyndromes. Drug abuse, particularly with stimulants like amphetamines and cocaine are sometimes the basis of morbid jealousy. The previous personality is often very sensitive, suspicious, unassertive and insecure. The condition is frequently associated with sexual difficulties, impotence, premature ejaculation in men, and many of the female partners of these relationships have various degrees of frigidity. Morbid jealousy may carry the risk of causing serious or grievous bodily harm, homocide or suicide.

Further Reading

Mowatt, R. R. (1966) *Morbid Jealousy and Murder: a Psychiatric Study of Morbidly Jealous Murderers at Broadmoor.* Tavistock Publications and Institute for the Study and Treatment of Delinquency, London.

37

Psychotherapy

Psychotherapy may be defined as treatment involving communication between the patient and the therapist, with the aim of modifying and alleviating illness. Many authorities would add that this form of treatment deliberately establishes a professional relationship with the patient with the object of removing, modifying or retarding existing symptoms, or disturbed patterns of behaviour, or the promotion of positive personality growth and development. There are various forms and different degrees of complexity, duration and expense of psychotherapy; e.g. psychotherapy can be:

Supportive, dealing with current problems and helping the patient to overcome his symptoms and cope more satisfactorily with them in the future and with life generally. This can be very active and skilled treatment, and for many it is the treatment that they need.
Suggestion and persuasion.
Hypnosis.
Abreactive techniques.
Intensive prolonged psychotherapy, e.g. Freudian, Jungian or other forms of analysis.
Group therapy, based on psycho-analytic principles or sometimes on other guiding rules, depending on the interest of the therapist and the type of patient he has to treat.

In most forms of psychotherapy the interview is the main vehicle of treatment. Psychotherapeutic methods have in common the fact that they depend almost entirely on communication between patient and doctor, which may be spoken or implied by expression and gesture. Before embarking on treatment, it is important to decide the objective for each case. The therapist may ascertain the factors causing the patient's symptoms quite clearly after one inter-

view, but it is usually unwise to tell the patient all you know. Premature interpretation will be rejected. Unpleasant truths may take time to be accepted. It is important for the psychotherapist to keep quiet and not to be afraid of pauses and silences. More than half the battle in psychotherapy is to be a good listener.

Doctor–Patient Relationship

Patients may exhibit positive or negative feelings of great intensity towards the doctor. The reaction depends more on the patient's personality and experience than the doctor's. The doctor must learn to tolerate his patient's emotions. If he is hostile and annoyed with his patients, he cannot get their confidence and co-operation. Doctors who regard neurotic patients as weak and spineless are not likely to help them. The doctor should be sympathetically warm and accepting at the outset, which will enable him to build up a good relationship with the patient. If later the patient has to be dealt with in a more firm and positive manner, it can be done on the basis of the patient's confidence in the doctor and in a way that he can more readily accept.

Suggestion

Suggestion is probably the oldest form of psychotherapy and one used in everyday life. Whenever one person tries to influence another, suggestion usually plays a part. It is extensively employed in advertising, propaganda, religious and political activities. It plays a part in every psychotherapeutic relationship and indeed plays a prominent part in any successful doctor–patient relationship. The bedside manner of the successful physician is compounded of a large variety of different features—his general appearance, speech, the interest he shows in the patient, his general behaviour, demeanour, his impressiveness and, in short, his 'presence'. Any treatment, whether it is in the form of a tablet, a bottle of medicine or other form of therapeutic procedure, always has an element of suggestion. The colour and the taste of a medicinal mixture sometimes have more potent effects by suggestion than the active pharmacological ingredients.

Suggestion is defined as a process of communication resulting in the acceptance, with conviction, of the communicated proposition in the absence of logically adequate grounds for its acceptance. It therefore involves the active influence of one mind upon another without any necessary logical basis. Treatment by suggestion can be traced as far back as the methods of healing used by the ancient Greeks. The therapeutic methods used in those days involved the invocation of miracles, of which there were two kinds, religious and magical. Interesting examples of religious miracles took place at the Temple of Aesculapius at Epidaurus. Patients came long distances and laid valuable gifts so as to influence the gods favourably. They spent some nights in public prayers and exhortations. Then, in front of the statue of a god, they were given advice in the form of oracles and prophetic dreams.

During the Middle Ages, churches and saints were invoked to cure particular diseases, e.g. St Clare for eye disease, St Ralph for plague, St Fiacre for haemorrhoids. By the simple authority of the name and the mere influence of the words, pious personages would sometimes produce remarkable cures, which were regarded as the outcome of divine intervention. Kings used to cure scrofula. Magical remedies in which there were all kinds of curious concoctions were used for treating diseases throughout the Middle Ages. Red coral, viper broth, crab's eye and powdered stag's horn were favourite medieval remedies.

Unobtrusive suggestion, of course, takes place in all successful methods of treatment, not only in psychiatry but in medicine and surgery. The benevolent attitude of the long-experienced general practitioner, the smile of the pleasant nurse, the clean smell of antiseptics in hospital, the colour and taste of the medicine can all play an important part by suggestion in promoting the patient's recovery. Suggestion is superficial, symptomatic treatment and

alone it is not enough. It should be combined with a further attempt to deal with the causative factor and the patient should be given some insight into his condition.

Treatments such as massage, radiant heat, sun-ray treatment, mud baths and colonic lavage owe a large part of their success to suggestion. Some physicians obtain excellent results merely by their personalities and by the suggestions they unconsciously or otherwise give. Suggestion, therefore, probably has the widest use of all methods of psychiatry. It is not only used deliberately by psychiatrists but unconsciously by good nurses, physicians and surgeons all the time. It plays a great part in our ordinary lives in many processes which we tend to think are due to the activity of the intellect but which, on closer examination, are found to operate by the subtle means of suggestion, disguised as intellectual explanation. The hoardings in the street, the reiterated policies of our newspapers, the doctrines promulgated from the pulpit are all suffused with suggestion, although disguised under the category of economical, ethical and political values. Propaganda, in all its forms, relies mainly on the power of suggestion.

The history of the treatment of many disorders shows that any spontaneous improvement occurring during the administration of treatment was put down and attributed to the treatment. Another common factor in all the treatments is that they all had an influence by suggestion. Recent work on the effect of placebo tablets, to which patients developed marked reactions, indicates that inert preparations may exert marked therapeutic effects by suggestion and may also produce marked autonomic and other bodily changes by psychogenic influences.

Reassurance

Reassurance is involved in many forms of treatment and in doctor–patient relationships generally. Patients, whatever they are suffering from, often have anxieties regarding the possibility of more serious diseases or regarding their mental stability. Many patients with mild neurotic symptoms have a severe dread of becoming insane. Patients with various bodily manifestations of emotional tension often harbour fears of cancer, or other serious diseases.

All too frequently, patients with psychiatric symptoms are told by their physicians that there is nothing wrong with them. This very often merely tends to make the patient more frightened because they know there is something wrong and they are suffering symptoms and varying degrees of unhappiness and disability. They feel bewildered and more anxious because they feel that their condition has not been properly diagnosed and that there is still something wrong which has not been found. It is important to realize that negative reassurances of this type are not by any means as effective as positive reassurances.

In patients suffering from psychiatric disorders, the physician should make the patient understand that he realizes that there is something wrong but that the trouble is not due to a physical disease and that his symptoms are manifestations of an emotional illness. A description of the nature and the origin of the symptoms should always be given in terms suitable to his intelligence and personality. Such positive reassurance with explanation is much more effective than a mere negative reassurance.

Although many general physicians and general practitioners think that psychotherapy begins and ends with reassurance, this is by no means so and very rarely does it prove to be adequate treatment in itself.

The relationship with the therapist gives the patient a feeling of acceptance and security, even though such feelings may not be expressed verbally. Reassurance is mainly effective for recent or superficial disturbances and is usually ineffective in deep-seated problems and personality difficulties.

Supportive therapy is the most commonly used method of dealing with problems of an emotional nature. The object is to bring the patient to an improved state as rapidly as possible with symptomatic improvement or recovery, so that he is able to resume normal life and activities. Supportive therapy includes guidance in such matters as education, employment, health and social relationships, always letting the patient make the final decision himself.

Environmental manipulation attempts to remove or modify disorganizing elements in his environment. Social work is the best example of trained, skilful, environmental manipulation.

Persuasion is a therapeutic method based on the belief that the patient has the ability to modify his abnormal emotional processes by will power or by application of common sense. Appeals are made to the patient's reason and intelligence, in order to help him to abandon neurotic aims and symptoms and to regain self-respect. Persuasion, in order to be effective, must be based on a good doctor–patient relationship. The patient must feel that the doctor is intensely interested in him and wants to help him. Persuasion involves explanation of the origin of the symptoms and encouragement to adopt more salutary reactions to his problems. It is probably fallacious to assume that the effectiveness of persuasion therapy depends on the operation of the intellect and it is probable that suggestion also plays an important role. Persuasion as a variety of psychotherapy can be helpful if it is effective in helping the patient's understanding of himself, helping him to relinquish neurotic reactions, tendencies and aims and if it achieves a better general readjustment. This will minimize the tendency for the patient to develop neurotic reactions or emotional tensions which, in turn, can precipitate attacks of psychosomatic disorders.

Supportive therapy is indicated for individuals with a reasonably stable personality who, up to the present illness, have made satisfactory adjustment but who have broken down under the impact of severe stress in the environment. Supportive therapy can also be helpful for less stable or more neurotic individuals.

Distributive Analysis and Synthesis

This type of treatment is a derivative of the psycho-biological school founded by Adolf Meyer. Psycho-biological therapy involves the systematic examination of all the factors that contribute to the individual—heredity, constitution, early childhood conditioning, later personal experiences, various phases of the person's life, educational, economic, work, marital, inter-personal, social, religious.

The therapeutic objective is the retraining of unhealthy or unsatisfactory attitudes. During interviews positive elements are stressed, success is emphasized and hopeful elements brought to the foreground. The patient's assets are utilized to facilitate his adjustment.

Group Psychotherapy

The treatment of patients by psychotherapy in groups was first introduced as a time-saving measure but subsequent experience demonstrated that the method had special therapeutic possibilities, which did not occur in individual psychotherapy.

The number of patients is usually six to eight. Some patients do poorly with group therapy; these include psychopathic personalities, acute severe psychotic conditions, patients who act out too readily and patients with low intelligence. The length of the group therapy session is customarily $1-1\frac{1}{2}$ hours and usually held once or twice weekly. Patients are seated around in a circle. In the first session the participants are introduced by their christian names and the purpose of group discussions is explained.

Group therapy may be conducted:

1 For purposes of re-education with a view to alteration of attitudes and behaviour patterns
2 For purposes of psycho-analytic therapy

The possible therapeutic aims and goals of group therapy are:

1 Guidance and practical advice
2 Education or orientation
3 Spiritual strength and fellowship
4 Socialization
5 Abreaction
6 Facilitation of associations and the production of deeper material for analysis
7 Symptomatic relief
8 Improved adjustment and adaptations to reality
9 Increased understanding and insight into emotional problems and conflicts
10 Modification of personality and character

Group Analytic Psychotherapy

This method has been well developed by Foulkes who states that its most significant features are:

1 Seven or eight members meet for $1\frac{1}{2}$ hours, sitting in a circle together with the analyst.
2 No programme or directions are given, so that all contributions arise spontaneously from the patients.
3 All communications are treated by the group as the equivalent of the free association of the individual under psycho-analytic conditions.

There is also a corresponding relaxation of censorship.
4 The therapist retains an attitude corresponding to that of the psycho-analyst during individual treatment.
5 All communications and relationships are seen as a part of the total field of interaction, namely the group matrix.
6 All group members take an active part in the total therapeutic process.

The natural history of the therapeutic group is as follows. In its early stages, there may be much anxiety and guilt in individual members. Conflicts are invariably present; these are related to conflicts of conformity, authority, dependency and change. It is the primary conflict of man as a group animal. The first conflict, therefore, is one of conformity to the group. The second is conflict to authority and authority figures. The third conflict evolves around the problem of dependency. The fourth, conflict of a change.

The natural history of the group usually goes through an initial phase which is termed the therapeutic honeymoon, in which great hopes are placed on the therapist; the patient has to orientate himself away from the doctor–patient axis towards the patient-to-patient axis of the group. Patients then usually get down to discussing individual symptoms. The intermediate phase is when the group truly becomes a group. The centre of reference is no longer the therapist alone. They address each other and respond directly to each other with general support and then analyse and interpret their own interactions and feelings. The terminal phase should always be gradual to allow the patient an opportunity to work through the many anxieties and depressions that in therapy, as in life, associate themselves with endings.

Group Psychotherapy for Children

This is classified according to the ages, namely: nursery, early childhood, late childhood, adolescence, also early adolescence and late adolescence.

The nursery group is about 4–5 children in a small room, with a flat tray divided into two compartments containing sand and water and some toy materials. In the early stages, areas are respected and each child cultivates his own plot. Later, they become interested in other people's work and begin working and playing with each other.

Early childhood, 5–9 years of age. Groups are formed here, according to Foulkes and Anthony, in conjunction with a sedentary occupation such as drawing, painting or modelling. The period is usually divided into a discussion phase followed by an activity phase. At the end of the discussion period, the group choose their activity for the day.

Adolescent groups. These are usually kept to one sex, optimal number about six.

Hypnosis

Hypnosis is a state of artificially induced increased suggestibility.

The technique of hypnosis usually aims at narrowing the patient's attention and awareness to the hypnotist alone and, although the condition may have the appearance of sleep, it is physiologically quite different from sleep. Electroencephalographic recordings, for example, are similar to those of the waking state.

A part of the patient's mind is 'en rapport' with the hypnotist and hypnosis is regarded by some authorities to be a state of induced dissociation.

There are different levels of hypnosis, ranging from a light hypnotic state to a deep trance.

Deep Hypnosis

Deep hypnosis, or a deep trance, is qualitatively different from the lighter stages of hypnosis. The patient is extremely relaxed, breathing becomes slower, post-hypnotic suggestions will be executed with amnesia. Suggestions are extremely effective; it is possible to make the subject hallucinate, e.g. to visualize scenes or to experience smells.

In a deep hypnotic trance the patient can open his eyes and remain in a trance; it was for this reason that the terms deep trance and somnambulism were applied to this state.

About 5% of the population can be hypnotized into a deep trance without difficulty; some others can be trained to develop a deep trance with intensive efforts over a period of time.

There are, however, many people who are not suitable subjects for hypnosis and can never be deeply hypnotized.

Hypnotic Techniques

A variety of techniques are available for inducing hypnosis.

It is necessary to prepare the patient and to explain what hypnosis means. It is important to explain that it is not a state of sleep and, secondly, that it is not essential for amnesia to occur to obtain beneficial therapeutic results.

It can be explained to the patient as a state of relaxation in which his field of awareness becomes narrowed and that, in this state, suggestions will be much more effective.

The hypnotist's rate of inducing hypnosis must be governed by the speed with which a patient responds to hypnotic suggestions.

The following are some examples of techniques used.

First of all the patients should be seated comfortably in a chair or lying down on a couch and should be encouraged to let all muscles go loose and relax; to let the body sink down in the couch, to let all the muscles be as loose and relaxed as possible. They are then asked to pay attention to what the hypnotist is saying; they are then asked to try to pay attention to the right hand or the left hand and to try to feel the sensations of touch coming from the hand; they are asked that, as soon as they feel any movement in the thumb or fingers, to lift it up to indicate which one it is. Slight movements invariably take place and the patients lift up the appropriate finger. This is then followed by suggestions that the hand and the arm is getting lighter and will rise upwards steadily to touch the forehead and, as it rises, the patients get sleepier. When the hand touches the forehead they go off into a deep sleep. The depth of hypnosis can then be increased by further suggestions, by counting ten and, by the time one has finished counting ten, they will be in a deep state of hypnosis.

The advantage of this technique is that one is unlikely to make mistakes and the rate of hypnotic suggestions for induction are governed by the response of the patients.

Other techniques are to get the patient to fixate his vision on a key or a finger or a light and to give suggestions that the eyelids are getting more and more tired and will close, and that the tiredness is passing over the head and down various parts of the body.

Sometimes one can induce a hypnotic state rapidly

by getting the patients to hyperventilate and, in some patients this, together with suitable suggestions, puts them into a deep hypnotic state.

If the patient is a suitable subject, hypnosis can be one of the quickest ways of carrying out psychotherapy:

1 For psychological investigation, i.e. to elicit the nature of underlying conflicts and problems and to facilitate the recall of forgotten experiences which may be emotionally important.
2 To abreact past experiences.
3 To modify symptoms and attitudes.
4 In the treatment of psychosomatic manifestations such as asthma. A word of warning here, it is unwise to use hypnosis in a patient suffering from status asthmaticus, particularly if they are suffering from the effects of anoxia, because any further slowing down of the respiratory rate may further endanger the patient. However, in other forms of asthmatic attacks where anoxia has not become a problem, hypnosis in certain subjects can produce dramatic results.

In the treatment of psychosomatic disorders, it is usually necessary to induce deep hypnosis to achieve the best results.

Abreactive and Other Techniques Used as Adjuncts in Psychotherapy

The term abreaction was introduced by Freud to denote the release of emotion when buried material was brought to the surface and described.

A number of aids to psychotherapy have been introduced in order to facilitate release of buried material, to help the patient to talk if he is embarrassed and to facilitate the expression of emotion.

1 *Intravenous barbiturates* 10% sodium amytal injected intravenously at the rate of 1 cm³ per minute, whilst the patient counts backwards and until he repeats a number or starts counting a normal progression. This indicates the stage of optimum narcosis; he feels relaxed, is suggestible and is able to talk more freely. Sometimes the release of emotion is hindered by the relaxing effect of the intravenous sodium amytal despite facilitating verbal expression and communication.

Intravenous sodium amytal is also useful in the diagnosis of patients with muscular pains which might be due to emotional causes or due to physical causes. The injection of a small amount of sodium amytal, insufficient to cause analgesia, will produce relief if the symptom is due to emotional tension.

Intravenous sodium amytal is useful in resistive, mute or catatonic schizophrenics, to make them amenable, communicative and easier to feed. It is also useful in doubtful cases of schizophrenia to obtain information from the patient to establish the diagnosis.

Intravenous thiopentone or methohexitone has a shorter duration of action and is preferred by some people for facilitating psychotherapy and abreaction.

2 *Intravenous methedrine* 15–30 mg methedrine injected intravenously often has powerful stimulating effects in the verbal production by the patient and the abreaction of emotions relating to past experiences.

Whereas one might describe the action of intravenous barbiturates as analogous to taking the brake off a car when the engine is running, thus enabling it to run more quickly, the action of methedrine would be compared to pressing the accelerator.

The most dramatic effects with intravenous methedrine usually occur on the first occasion. Patients will often keep on talking with great productivity for eight hours or more.

Intravenous methedrine is contra-indicated in schizophrenia and border-line schizophrenic patients and must be used with care in severely anxious patients because of its sympathomimetic effects.

Intravenous methedrine is nowadays little used in view of the danger of dependence.

3 *Hallucinogenic drugs* These include lysergic acid and sernyl and can also be used in hospital conditions for purposes of abreaction.

4 *Inhalation anaesthesia* This has also been used for abreactive purposes—chloroform, nitrous oxide, trilene and ether.

Ether has been used to facilitate an excitatory type of abreaction. It is given on an open mask and, during the phase of excitement, the patient is encouraged to remember and re-enact, with full emotional intensity, past experiences.

Muscular Relaxation

Increased muscle tension is a common manifestation of all forms of emotional tension and is responsible or a number of the patient's symptoms, e.g. certain types of headache are due to increased muscular tension of the scalp muscles; pains in the back of the neck, the back and the limbs may be due to increased muscular tension. Tremors are also manifestations of increased muscular tension.

The symptoms arising from increased muscular tension often give rise to additional anxiety, because the patient may believe that they indicate some serious disease and thereby tend to set up a vicious circle. Treatment consisting of training the patient in muscular relaxation is a valuable therapeutic adjunct. It not only can provide symptomatic relief but, in so far as states of anxiety and tension have both emotional and somatic aspects, relief of muscular tension often provides a general alleviation of the degree of anxiety felt.

Muscular relaxation may be helpful in asthmatic subjects suffering from anxiety tension symptoms, particularly when they have neuromuscular symptoms. Also, relaxation may be helpful when combined with breathing exercises, as the latter can be more effectively introduced when combined with training in muscular relaxation.

Autogenic Training

This method was developed by Schultz for treating patients with anxiety and increased muscular tension by means of muscular relaxation and exercises. The patient learns to relax each muscle group, eventually achieving complete muscular relaxation throughout the body.

Autogenic training has the advantage of being simple and effective, and can be used for groups as well as individually.

Further Reading

Balint, M. and Balint, E. (1961) *Psychotherapeutic Techniques in Medicine.* Tavistock Publications, London.

Malan, D. H. (1963) *A Study of Brief Psychotherapy.* Tavistock Publications, London.

Foulkes, S. H. and Anthony, E. J. (1973) *Group Psychotherapy.* Penguin Books, Harmondsworth.

Parry, R. (1975) *A Guide to Counselling and Basic Psychotherapy.* Churchill Livingstone, Edinburgh.

Malan, D. H. (1976) *Toward the Validation of Dynamic Psychotherapy; A Replication.* Plenum Press, New York.

Malan, D. H. (1976) *A Study of Brief Psychotheropy.* Plenum Press, New York.

Malan, D. H. (1976) *The Frontier of Brief Psychotherapy.* Plenum Press, New York.

Saunders, C. M. (1978) *The Managements of Terminal Illness.* Edward Arnold, London.

Brown, D. and Peddar, J. (1979) *Introduction to Psychotherapy. An Outline of Psychodynamic Principles and Practice.* Tavistock Publications, London.

Malan, D. H. (1979) *Individual Psychotherapy and the Science of Psychodynamics.* Butterworth, London.

Storr, A. (1979) *The Art of Psychotherapy.* Heinemann Medical, London.

Garfield, S. E. (1980) *Psychotherapy—An Eclectic Approach.* John Wiley, Bristol.

Johnson, C. W. *et al.* (1980) *Basic Psychotherapeutics.* MTP, Lancaster.

Mahoney, M. J. (1980) *Psychotherapy Process—Current Issues and Future Directions.* Plenum Press, New York.

Rachman, S. J. (1980) *Effects of Psychological Therapy.* 2nd edn of *The Effects of Psychotherapy.* Pergamon Press, Oxford.

Mandel, H. P. (1981) *Short-Term Psychotherapy and Brief Treatment Techniques.* Plenum Press, New York.

38

Biofeedback, Behaviour Therapy, Cognitive Therapy

Biofeedback and behaviour therapy are two forms of treatment aimed at modifying symptoms or behaviour by methods based on learning theory.

Biofeedback

Biofeedback involves the use of technology to provide the patient with information on the current state of the physiological system that needs to be controlled to alleviate symptoms. It is used for those symptoms or behaviour abnormalities which are normally outside voluntary control because of poor sensory information from the systems involved. Biofeedback provides information of the physiological state, usually by electronic methods which can be used in order to learn control of the relevant organ or system. Biofeedback has been used successfully in the treatment of tension headaches, also in neuromuscular rehabilitation, including muscular spasticity or defective muscular control after cerebrovascular accidents, in varieties of cerebral palsy, and torticollis. It has also been used successfully in the treatment of severe faecal incontinence.

It has been shown that if patients are given feedback regarding the size and frequency of alpha waves in their ECGs they can learn to control the amount of alpha recorded. Enhancement of alpha activity is usually associated with a relaxed and pleasant feeling. Another frequency from the sensory motor cortex has been used with success in the treatment of some forms of epilepsy.

Migraine has been successfully treated by providing feedback on bloodflow to the temporal artery. Only limited benefits have been achieved in the control of arterial hypertension. It is possible to achieve reduction in systolic pressure of approximately 10% but this is not sufficient to be of clinical importance in practice.

Promising results have been achieved in the control of cardiac arrhythmias. Feedback from cardiac activity is given by three lights, green is a signal for the patient to try to speed his heart, a red light to slow the heart, and a yellow one to inform him that he is performing correctly. Patients are taught to speed the heart and to slow the heart rates within a narrow range. Patients are able to learn to identify premature ventricular contractions. A premature beat causes a red light to flash because it comes too fast, followed by a flash of a green light which is triggered by the ensuing compensatory pause. Patients learn to identify this sequence as a premature ventricular contraction and how to prevent it.

Behaviour Therapy

Behaviour therapy is the systematic application of principles of learning to the analysis and treatment of disorders of behaviour. The rationale adopted by practitioners of behaviour therapy is that neurotic behaviour and other types of disorder are predominantly acquired and therefore should be subject to established laws of learning. Knowledge regarding the learning process concerns not only the acquisition of new behaviour patterns but the reduction or elimination of existing behaviour patterns.

Behaviour therapy has made tremendous advances in the last two decades and has made an pact on the treatment of a variety of symptoms nd behaviour disorders which previously had been sistant to treatment. A large variety of new techques are available.

eciprocal Inhibition

Many forms of neurotic behaviour are acquired in anxiety-generating situation.

Treatment can be used in the suppression of nxiety responses by responses which are phyologically antagonistic to anxiety.

The techniques of systematic desensitization onsist of enquiring first of all into the stimulus tuations which provoke anxiety in the patient, and rank these stimuli in order from the most to the ast disturbing, i.e. a hierarchy of stimulus situations.

Then the patient is asked to visualize the least isturbing stimulus when he is in a state of relaxation roduced by hypnosis or intravenous anaesthetic ich as methohexitone (Brietal).

Whenever marked disturbance occurs the theraist withdraws the stimulus and calms the patient.

Each stimulus is visualized for 5–10 seconds and –4 items are presented in each session, each item sually being presented twice.

As soon as the patient is able to visualize the ems without disturbance, the therapist moves on the next item in the next session.

Eventually the patient is able to visualize all the ormerly provoking stimuli without anxiety and this oility to imagine the provoking stimuli with tranuillity is transferred to the real life situation.

nplosion Therapy, or Flooding

 this method, in contrast to systematic desentization, the patient is confronted in imagination r reality with his most feared situation or stimulus nd then encouraged to remain in contact with that tuation until the avoidance response is extinuished.

It is a mistake to regard systematic desensitization applicable to classical phobias only. It is in fact seful in the treatment of a wide range of behavioural isorders when one is able to identify the stimuli hich elicit anxiety and which result in maladaptive r disruptive behaviour. Sometimes obsessive comulsive behaviour is stimulated by the anxiety roduced by specific objects or situations and can

be helped by systematic desensitization using a hierarchy of relevant stimuli. In stammering it can be used to decondition the anxiety associated with a range of speaking situations. Similarly, certain sexual problems such as impotence or even certain types of homosexuality may be amenable to desensitization therapy. Asthma and dysmenorrhoea have been treated by systematic desensitization.

Modelling

This is a technique used with flooding or desensitization in which the patient sees the therapist enter the phobic situation and the patient is then induced to copy him.

Operant Conditioning

Operant behaviour usually affects the environment and generates stimuli which 'feed back' to the organism. Any response or behaviour which is rewarding and therefore reinforcing increases the likelihood of further similar responses.

Shaping is based on operant conditioning principles. The patient is systematically instructed to do what he fears and is rewarded by the therapist with praise when he succeeds and with no response if he fails. This method is useful in the treatment of phobias and obsessions.

This method has been used with varying degrees of success in the treatment of behaviour disorders in children, in multiple tics, hysterical symptoms, stammering etc.

Aversion Therapy

Aversion conditioning is achieved by associating stimuli relating to the symptom to be treated with unpleasant effects following administration of apomorphine, emetine or by the administration of a painful electric shock. The latter enables a more precise timing in the presentation of the noxious stimulus and the stimuli related to the symptoms to be treated.

Aversion therapy is used when the symptom or pattern of behaviour is pleasurable to the person, e.g. alcoholism, transvestism, homosexual inclinations, etc.

Negative Learning

This has been used in the treatment of involuntary movements such as tics. It consists of getting the patient to adhere to a rigid schedule of massed practice of voluntarily carrying out the movements of the tic at intervals throughout the day. This sets up a state of inhibition which impairs or prevents the appearance of the tic movement.

It may be said that behaviour therapy achieves the best results in persons who previously were reasonably well adjusted and who have a limited number of symptoms. In many patients symptoms and unadaptive behavioural responses continue autonomously, even when the original psychodynamic factors cease to be important or active. It is extremely rare for new symptoms to develop in substitution for those treated successfully by behaviour therapy.

Cognitive Therapy

Cognitive therapy is short term, directive and structured in which the targets of treatment are symptoms, cognitions and unspoken assumptions referred to as schemata.

Cognitive therapy has been found to be particularly helpful in the treatment of depressive illness, either alone or in combination with antidepressants.

The cognitive theory of depression propounded by Beck stated that cognitions consist of thoughts and images which reflect unrealistically negative views of the self, the world and the future, and that these are based on unspoken assumptions and reinforced by current interpretation of events.

Silent assumptions (schemata) are unspoken inflexible assumptions or beliefs which form the basis for classifying, evaluating experiences and making judgements. They distort actual experience and increase the tendency to relapse. They also produce and maintain negative attitudes towards themselves, the environment and the future. Events are interpreted in negative terms of loss and/or deprivation.

Cognitive therapy teaches the patient to become aware of the views he takes of events, life changes and stresses. He is encouraged to examine himself and his environment and to test in reality his views and to correct them. In other words, the patient learns to evaluate particular meanings attributed to events by objective reality.

The behavioural techniques used are action orientated which focus on how to act and cope rather than on how to interpret events.

The methods most frequently used are:

1 Keeping a record of daily activities.
2 The patient is encouraged to relate his activities in terms of accomplishments and pleasure.
3 Assignments are given which are graded by means of a step by step approach to goals which the patient believes are impossible or very difficult.

The patient is encouraged to record his automatic thoughts both during therapeutic sessions and also daily in a diary.

The patient is helped by the therapist to recognize that personal perception of reality differs from reality itself, to examine alternative ways of interpreting events and to consider new solutions to problems.

The technique of cognitive rehearsal is helpful when patients are unable to attempt particular tasks or problems because of fear of failure. Cognitive rehearsal involves imagining performing the task in great detail in order to identify any barriers to success and then the therapist can formulate coping strategies in advance.

Treatment is further strengthened by homework in order to test old assumptions and homework to test new assumptions.

Additional techniques which are complementary and therapeutically useful are assertiveness training and anxiety management.

The course of treatment usually lasts from 12 to 20 weeks. Early sessions are given twice weekly and then the intervals are gradually increased. Further sessions may be held six to twelve months after completion of the course to review the patient's progress and to reinforce the therapeutic methods and techniques learnt during treatment.

Evidence from follow up studies indicates that cognitive therapy has substantial benefit in relieving the distress and disability of depressive illnesses and also significantly lessens the risk of relapse and recurrence.

Further Reading

Eysenck, H. J. (ed) (1960) *Behaviour Therapy and the Neuroses*. Pergamon Press, Oxford.

ates, A. J. (1970) *Behaviour Therapy*. John Wiley, New York.

Volpe, J. (1973) *Practice of Behaviour Therapy*. Pergamon Press, Oxford.

loane, R. B., Cristol, A. H., Staples, F. R., Yorkston, N. J. and Whipple, K. (1975) *Psychotherapy versus Behaviour Therapy*. Harvard University Press, Cambridge, Massachusetts.

eech, H. R. and Vaughan, M. (1978) *Behavioural Treatment of Obsessional States*. John Wiley, Chichester.

Stern, R. (1978) *Behavioural Techniques*. Academic Press, London.

Basmajian, J. V. (1979) *Biofeedback*. Williams and Wilkins, Baltimore.

Wolters, W. H. (1979) *Psychosomatics and Biofeedback*. Nijhoff, Holland.

Yates, A. J. (1980) *Biofeedback and the Modification of Behaviour*. Plenum Press, New York.

Sheldon, B. (1981) *Behaviour Modification*. Tavistock Publications, London.

39

Psychopharmacology

During the past three decades the introduction of new psychotropic drugs has transformed psychiatric treatment and provided a potent stimulus for research into mental illness.

Psychotropic drugs are pharmacological agents which exert powerful effects on the higher functions of the central nervous system. Psychopharmacology is the study of the pharmacological, biochemical, physiological, neurophysiological, psychological, clinical, therapeutic, social and epidemiological aspects of psychotropic drugs.

Psychotropic drugs can be classified according to their pharmacological and clinical effects into:

1 Hypnosedatives
2 Tranquillosedatives
3 Tranquillizers, subdivided into (a) major tranquillizers or neuroleptics and (b) minor tranquillizers
4 Central nervous system stimulants
5 Antidepression drugs
6 Psychotomimetic or hallucinogenic drugs

They may also be classified as follows:

1 Antianxiety drugs; these include some of the hypnosedatives, tranquillosedatives and minor tranquillizers
2 Antidepression drugs
3 Antipsychotic drugs— the major tranquillizers or neuroleptics

Hypnosedatives

Hypnosedative drugs are used to induce sleep and sometimes, in smaller divided doses during the day, to relieve anxiety and to produce sedation. They include the barbiturates, and others such as chloral glutethimide and paraldehyde.

Hypnosedatives have a marked action on the cerebral cortex, and patients under their influence show manifestations similar to those of alcoholic intoxication, including slurring of speech, incoordination and a slowing in reaction time. If these drugs are used at a high dosage for a sufficiently long time, physical dependence can occur, with the result that when the blood level of the drug falls, a state of anxiety is induced as a manifestation of the withdrawal syndrome. The patient feels impelled to take further doses to relieve distress.

In cases of marked physical dependence, sudden withdrawal can result in delirium, epileptic fits and sometimes cardiovascular collapse. In recent years young people, having tried drugs such as amphetamines, marihuana and heroin, have resorted to the intravenous use of barbiturates, often with disastrous and even fatal results.

Tranquillosedatives

These are used mainly for the relief of anxiety and sometimes for the alleviation of associated increased muscle tension. One of the first of these drugs to be recognized was meprobamate, derived from the muscle relaxant myanesin, which achieved widespread use in the US and other parts of the world. It is now known to be a drug of addiction causing both psychological and physical dependence with marked withdrawal symptoms.

Benzodiazapines

The benzodiazepine drugs occupy pride of place in the treatment of anxiety. There are over two thou and benzodiazepine compounds in existence but only a relatively small number have been marketed. The marketed benzodiazepine drugs constitute the most frequently prescribed drugs in medicine.

Some of the available benzodiazepine drugs are given in the following table.

Benzodiazepines	
Approved name	*Proprietary name*
Chlordiazepoxide	Librium
Diazepam	Valium
Oxazepam	Serenid
Flurazepam	Dalmane
Clorazepate	Tranxene
Lorazepam	Ativan
Prazepam	Centrax
Nitrazepam	Mogadon
Medazepam	Nobrium
Temazepam	Normison, Euhypnos
Bromazepam	Lexotan
Flunitrazepam	Rohypnol
Pinazepam	Domar
Clobazam	Frisium
Triazolam	Halcion
Alprazolam	Xanax

As a group the benzodiazepines have anxiolytic, muscle relaxant and anticonvulsant properties. They are extensively bound to plasma proteins, are lypophilic, readily passed through the placenta, and are excreted in breast milk.

They show important differences in their clinical effects which have important implications for selection of a particular benzodiazepine to meet the needs of the individual patient. The pharmacological actions and the clinical effects of benzodiazepines and other drugs are influenced by pharmacokinetic as well as pharmacodynamic actions.

Pharmacokinetics deals with rates of absorption, distribution, metabolism and elimination of drugs and, therefore, is concerned with the ways by which the body influences the movements of the drug, whereas pharmacodynamics concerns the effect the drug has on the body.

There are important pharmacokinetic differences among the benzodiazepine drugs which produce differences in clinical effect. Among the most important pharmacokinetic considerations are:

1 Effective duration of action
2 The presence or absence of active metabolites resulting from biotransformation of the parent compound
3 Tendency to accumulation of the parent compound or its active metabolites
4 Factors influencing rate of (a) absorption, (b) metabolism, (c) elimination of the benzodiazepine drug

Classification of Benzodiazepine Antianxiety Agents

An important and useful classification is based on the effective duration of clinical action of the parent drug and its active metabolites. Chlordiazepoxide, diazepam, chlorazepate and prazepam have a long duration of action with an elimination half life of between 5 to 30 hours for chlordiazepoxide, 20 to 30 hours for diazepam, 36 to 200 hours for chlorazepate by its active metabolite desmethyldiazepam, and also for prazepam which produces the same active metabolite. Lorazepam and oxazepam have a shorter elimination half life, lorazepam between 10 and 20 hours and oxazepam 5 to 10 hours and neither of these drugs has active metabolites. Lorazepam may be regarded as an intermediate compound with regard to effective duration of clinical action and oxazepam of short duration of action.

Diazepam

Diazepam is rapidly absorbed from the gastrointestinal tract and has a relatively long half life. Furthermore its active metabolite desmethyldiazepam has one of the longest half lives of any benzodiazepine derivative.

Lorazepam

Lorazepam differs in its pharmacokinetics from benzodiazepine derivatives already considered in two main respects. It has a relatively shorter half life and has no active metabolites. Lorazepam is conjugated to glycuronic acid yielding a water soluble glycuronide which is excreted by the kidneys. During multiple dose administration there is a much lesser tendency to accumulation than with chlordiazepoxide, diazepam, chlorazepate and prazepam. A steady state level is achieved within two or three days of starting therapy and termination of administration of lorazepam leads to complete elimination of the compound within a few days. Lorazepam is particularly suitable for dealing with episodes of anxiety in which prolonged sedation in between attacks is not needed. It is also suitable for anxiolytic treatment on a two or three times daily dose regime. Lorazepam when taken by mouth is completely absorbed from the digestive tract and reaches full concentration within two hours. Intramuscular injection of lorazepam results in a rapid complete absorption in contrast to intramuscular chlordiazepoxide and diazepam which are absorbed slowly and erratically.

Differences Between Various Benzodiazepines

The various benzodiazepine drugs differ in their duration of action. This is partly due to variations in the elimination half life of different drugs and also that in some benzodiazepines there are active metabolites many of which have quite a long duration of action. It is very important for the clinician to have some knowledge of the pharmacokinetics of benzodiazepine drugs. Pharmacokinetics deals with the rates of absorption, distribution, metabolism, and elimination of drugs in the living organism. It has been shown that contrary to usual clinical teaching, the intramuscular injection of chlordiazepoxide or diazepam is less likely to produce a rapid reliable clinical effect than oral medication.

There is evidence, however, that intramuscular lorazepam leads to rapid and reliable absorption and a more prompt onset of sedation. Clorazepate is hydrolysed in the stomach to an active metabolite desmethyldiazepam (nordiazepam). Patients with achlorhydria or those on antacids, or on anticholinergic agents may have considerably reduced clinically useful amounts of nordiazepam following clorazepate intake. With the exception of the hydrolysis of clorazepate to desmethyldiazepam in the stomach, the major site of biotransformation of benzodiazepines is the liver. Demethylation and/or hydroxylation are important processes in the biotransformation of some of the benzodiazapines and are affected by age, other drugs and liver disease. Age has important effects on the elimination

half life of some of the benzodiazepines, for example, in elderly subjects the chlordiazepoxide elimination half life is 60% longer than in younger subjects.

There are considerable variations in the duration of elimination half life; temazepam, oxazepam and lorazepam have a shorter elimination half life than chlordiazepoxide, diazepam, clorazepate, and furthermore, temazepam, lorazepam and oxazepam have a much simpler metabolic pathway prior to their elimination as glucoronide. They have, therefore, a clearly defined duration of action, whereas other benzodiazepines with active metabolites may continue exerting clinical and pharmacological effects for a considerable period after the administration. For example, chlordiazepoxide has three major active metabolites, desmethylchlordiazepoxide, demoxazepam, and desmethyldiazepam. Diazepam is metabolized through desmethyldiazepam as is clorazepate and medazepam.

On the basis of this pharmacokinetic evidence temazepam has considerable advantages as a hypnotic because its limited duration of action leaves it free from after effects. Oxazepam and lorazepam again are the benzodiazepines of choice for dealing with episodes of anxiety or situational anxiety. Benzodiazepines with a long half life and active metabolites may be suitable for patients with a high level of background persistent chronic anxiety. Benzodiazepines with a long elimination half life and those with long-acting active metabolites will tend to show an accumulation of effects, whereas temazepam, oxazepam and lorazepam will not tend to show accumulation. For hypnotic purposes temazepam has a mean elimination half life of 5.3 hours compared with 27 hours with nitrazepam, and 65 hours with the active metabolite of flurazepam. Temazepam does not show any accumulation because of the fact that the interval between administrations is three to four times the half life of the drug.

It should also be noted that benzodiazepines with a long half life and those with active metabolites will only show withdrawal symptoms after an interval of some days.

Accumulation tends to occur with multiple dose therapy, but the accumulation will be greater with a long elimination half life than those with active metabolites. Steady state levels are achieved much more quickly with lorazepam compared with

...azepam, and occur at a much lower blood level. ...erefore the clinical and pharmacological effects ...e much more predictable.

...e Abuse of the Benzodiazepines

...is can be considered as the risk of producing ...pendence and also the extent to which drugs may ... actively sought for or stolen. People can become ...pendent on any drug, including placebos. The ...pendence is psychological and they need to con- ...ue taking the drug even though there is no evi- ...nce of pharmacological or physical dependence. If ...e patient or the person actively seeks the drug ...cause it produces pleasurable sensations, relieves ...stress or prevents distress, this may be indicative of ...ysical dependence, based on the pharmacological ...ects, as well as psychological dependence. Further ...idence would be provided by the development of ...lerance and a rapid increase in the dose to produce ...e desired effects. Further evidence of physical ...pendence is provided by an abstinence syndrome ...nich is distinct from the anxiety state for which ...e drug was initially prescribed.

The development of tolerance to the benzo- ...azepines is infrequent with the normal dosage ...ed in treatment, but can occur when patients take ...cessively high doses of benzodiazepines. It was ...e discovery of the benzodiazepine receptors and ...e probability that there is an endogenous ligand ...hich is produced naturally for attachment to these ...ceptors, together with the association of benzo- ...azepine receptors with GABA (gamma-amino ...tyric acid) receptors and a chloride channel which ...imulated active research for the discovery of the ...tural occurring ligand. It is possible that functional ...lerance to benzodiazepines may be correlated with ... increased sensitivity of benzodiazepine receptors.

...ithdrawal syndrome

...hen benzodiazepines are withdrawn, particularly ...the patient has been on a high dosage and the ...rmination is abrupt, an increase in anxiety is ...mmon, but this by itself does not indicate the ...esence of withdrawal syndrome based on physical ...pendence. The important features to look for are ...ose manifestations which are not found in anxiety ...tes. Epileptic fits occur in 5%. More common, ...ough, are increased acuity of hearing, smell and vision. There may be abnormal perceptions; the person may see the wall or floor or ceiling moving towards him, or objects flashing across the field of vision, and many report feelings of movement of the body which is quite different from vertigo. Some experience muscle twitching, and occasionally myoclonic jerks may occur. Loss of appetite and loss of weight are frequent.

Withdrawal reaction will appear earlier when the patient has been receiving benzodiazepines with a short elimination half life (i.e. less than 20 hours) and is free from active metabolites such as alprazolam, lorazepam, lormetazepam, oxazepam, temazepam and triazolam. The onset of the withdrawal syn-drome is usually between three and ten days depend-ing on the halflife of the product. Duration of the withdrawal reaction is also variable and the longer the patient has been taking benzodiazepines the longer will the withdrawal reaction take place. One estimate is that for every year the benzodiazepines have been taken the withdrawal reaction will take one month.

Major Tranquillizers or Neuroleptic Drugs

Neuroleptic drugs fall chemically into the following groups:

1 Phenothiazine derivatives
2 Alkaloids from Rauwolfia serpentina and related synthetic drugs
3 Butyrophenone derivatives
4 Thioxanthines
5 Diphenylbutyl piperidines

Neuroleptic drugs are used in the treatment of severe psychiatric disorders such as schizophrenia and for controlling disturbed behaviour in patients with organic mental disorders and in mental sub-normality.

Neuroleptics have a general depressant action on the central nervous system but their main action is on subcortical structures, in contrast to barbiturates which predominantly affect the cerebral cortex.

Neuroleptics exert their main actions on:

1 The limbic system which is intimately concerned with emotional reactions
2 The hypothalamus, particularly autonomic centres

3 The reticular system which is intimately concerned in producing and maintaining a state of awareness

These phylogenetically older parts of the brain have a series of feedback mechanisms with the cerebral cortex which subserve the integration of visceral, emotional and somatic components of motivated behaviour.

The predominant action of neuroleptics on subcortical structures explains their capacity for controlling abnormal behaviour and various manifestations in severe psychiatric disorders, such as delusions and hallucinations in schizophrenia, without significantly affecting clarity of consciousness.

It is interesting that these areas contain large amount of neurohormones including noradrenaline and serotonin and are remarkably sensitive to psychotropic drugs.

The phenothiazines block the action of these neurohormones, whereas the Rauwolfia alkaloids deplete the neurohormonal depots.

Phenothiazine Derivatives

Chlorpromazine was the first phenothiazine tranquillizer and has stood the test of time and extensive trial in all parts of the world.

The phenothiazine nucleus consists of two benzene rings joined by a sulphur atom and a nitrogen atom as follows:

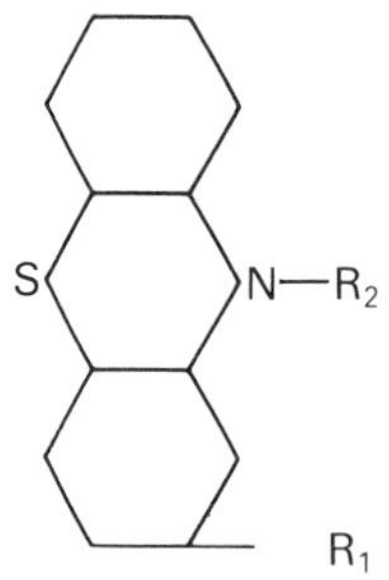

Figure 39.1

A large number of new phenothiazine tranquillizers have been derived by chemical substitution at R_1 and R_2. Differences in chemical structure are associated with differences in potency, clinical and pharmacological effects and also the production of toxic and side effects.

Potency varies according to the type of radical at R_1; for example, fluorine substituted for chlorine increases potency, whereas removal of chlorine gives rise to promazine which is one-third as potent as chlorpromazine but free from the risk of producing jaundice.

Phenothiazine drugs can be classified according to the side-chain at R_2 into:

1 Those with aliphatic side-chains
2 Those with piperidine side-chains
3 Those with piperazine side-chains (See Table 39.1).

In general, the aliphatic and piperidine derivatives are the phenothiazine drugs of choice for controlling disturbed, over-active behaviour. Piperazine derivatives are more potent, have a longer duration of action and have greater antiemetic properties, but a greater tendency to produce extrapyramidal side effects.

Chlorpromazine

Indications:

1 Psychiatry:
   (a) The treatment of schizophrenia
   (b) Controlling over-active disturbed behaviour, agitation and tension in other psychiatric disorders including organic dementia, mental subnormality and hyperkinetic states in children

2 In general medicine chlorpromazine is used:
   (a) For relieving tension and emotional distress in physical illness
   (b) For relief of pain and distress in inoperable cases of secondary carcinoma
   (c) For relief of vomiting
   (d) To help patients to regain lost weight
   (e) Management of withdrawal states in alcoholism and drug addiction

Laevopromazine is particularly effective for relieving anxiety and agitation associated with depression but does not relieve the depression itself.

Thioridazine is an almost pure psychosedative, has little antiemetic action and less potentiating effect on alcohol, barbiturates and anaesthetics.

Piperazine Derivatives

These drugs are more potent and have a longer duration of action, increase alertness, drive and

Table 39.1

Approved name	Proprietary name	Usual daily dosage range (mg)

Aliphatic series		
Chlorpromazine	Largactil	75–1000
Fluopromazine (triflupromazine)	Vespral	20–150
Methotrimeprazine (laevopromazine)	Veractil	25–700
Piperidine series		
Thioridazine	Melleril	30–600
Pericyazine	Neulactil	7.5–60/90
Piperazine series		
Prochlorperazine	Stemetil, Vertigon	15–100
Perphenazine	Fentazin	6–64
Thiopropazate	Dartalan	15–150
Fluphenazine HCl	Moditen	2.5–10
Fluphenazine enanthate	Moditen Enanthate	12.5–25 at intervals
Fluphenazine decanoate	Modecate	12.5–25 at intervals
Trifluoperazine	Stelazine	3–30

initiative and are to be preferred to chlorpromazine for schizophrenic patients who are inert, apathetic and show loss of initiative.

Trifluoperazine appears to be more effective in paranoid schizophrenia than chlorpromazine.

Piperazine drugs have a marked tendency to produce extrapyramidal side effects which include dystonic reactions of the head, neck and body, spasms and myoclonic twitches; also rigidity. These side effects are readily abolished by terminating the drug, reduction of dosage or by the administration of antiparkinsonian agents concurrently.

An innovation in the use of these drugs is the utilization of long-acting preparations such as fluphenazine enanthate and decanoate given by injection in patients who cannot be relied upon to take their medication regularly or for other reasons of convenience. Injections need only be given once every two or three weeks, and this is a major advance in the management of schizophrenics, particularly those in the community.

Alkaloids Derived from Rauwolfia Serpentina

The main alkaloid derivatives are reserpine, deserpedine and resinamine, all of which produce tranquillization and reduction of activity. In contrast to chlorpromazine, their autonomic effects are stimulation of the parasympathetic nervous system producing such side effects as slowing of the heart rate, nasal congestion, dyspepsia and diarrhoea. They also differ from the phenothiazine derivatives in taking much longer to produce their beneficial therapeutic effects; sometimes as long as six weeks administration may be necessary.

After a preliminary sedative phase lasting ten days or so, there is a stage of turbulence lasting some weeks and this is then succeeded by an integrative phase when the patient becomes more cooperative, interested, friendly and with a resolution of symptoms.

Reserpine and related alkaloids have now been

Table 39.2   Rauwolfia alkaloids used as neuroleptics

Approved name	Proprietary name	Usual daily dosage range (mg)	Principal side and toxic effects
Rauwolfia alkaloids			
Reserpine	Serpasil	0.25–5	Parasympathetic stimulation; hypotension; Parkinsonism depression
Resinamine	Moderil	0.5–1.5	Similar in type but less frequent
	Harmonyl	1–3	
Benzoquinalozone derivative			
Tetrabenazine	Nitoman	30–150	Drowsiness, sialorrhoea; Parkinsonism

superseded in the treatment of schizophrenia by the phenothiazine drugs.

A serious complication of Rauwolfia alkaloid therapy is the occurrence of severe depressive states, which may be of suicidal intensity and may need electroconvulsive therapy.

Butyrophenone Neuroleptics

The first member of this series, discovered by Janssen, was haloperidol. This drug, although differing in chemical structure from the phenothiazine drugs, has similar actions and side effects to the piperazine phenothiazines. However, it is much more potent weight-for-weight and has certain other advantages. It is particularly valuable in the management and treatment of hypomania and mania. It has a marked tendency to produce extrapyramidal side effects so that antiparkinsonian agents need to be given, usually from the beginning of treatment.

Other butyrophenones (see Table 39.3) used in psychiatry are triperidol, which is used in chronic schizophrenia when other drugs have failed; benper-

Table 39.3   Butyrophenone neuroleptics

Haloperidol	Droperidol
Triperidol	Benperidol
Methylperidol	Spiroperidol
Fluropipamide	Fluanisone

idol, used for reducing sex drives in sexual offenders and spiroperidol, which is the most potent neuroleptic known.

Thioxanthine Derivatives

These retain the sulphur atom but not the nitrogen atom in the middle ring of the phenothiazine nucleus. They provide a parallel series of psychotropic drugs to the phenothiazines (see Table 39.4).

Table 39.4   Thioxanthine neuroleptics

Approved name	Proprietary name
Chlorprothixene	Taractan
Clopenthixol	Sordinol
Flupenthixol	Depixol
Thiothixene	Narvane

Chlorprothixene is used for the treatment of anxiety and clopenthixol and thiothixene for the treatment of schizophrenia. Flupenthixol is the most potent member of the series and is used in treating schizophrenia; and a recent report indicates that it may be effective in treating depressive illnesses.

Diphenylbutyl Piperidines

This is a new series of neuroleptics introduced by Paul Janssen. The first of the series to be introduced into clinical practice in this country is pimozide which has the advantages of being effective in the treatment of schizophrenia and having few extrapyramidal or autonomic side effects. It is particularly useful in the treatment of chronic schizophrenics who are inert and apathetic. It is a specific dopamine antagonist and is used in the control of stereotyped symptoms in schizophrenia.

Fluspirilene is an injectible preparation, given once weekly for schizophrenia, and is claimed to be more activating than other depot neuroleptics.

Side Effects and Toxic Effects

It is necessary to distinguish between side effects on the one hand and toxic or hypersensitivity reactions on the other.

Side effects depend entirely on dosage and may occur in any patient if the dose is high enough. Toxic and hypersensitivity reactions occur only in some patients and are not closely correlated with dosage.

1 *Side effects* The following are common side effects: drowsiness, apathy, hypotension, dryness in mucous membranes and extrapyramidal manifestations.

2 *Toxic and hypersensitivity reactions* These include blood dyscrasias, dermatitis, which is usually light-sensitive and appearing on the exposed areas, jaundice and increased tendency to epilepsy.

Tardive Dyskinesia

Long-term treatment of antipsychotic (neuroleptic) drugs may be associated with abnormal movements described as tardive dyskinesia.

Tardive dyskinesia includes oral, lingual, buccal dyskinesia, chorea, athetosis, dystonia and tics, but not rhythmic tremor. It varies in severity from isolated dyskinesias to widespread disabling dystonias which can interfere with walking and feeding. Dyskinesias appear after many months or years of treatment with neuroleptic drugs and usually worsen during withdrawal of the drug. The differential diagnosis of tardive dyskinesia must take into account the stereotyped movements of schizophrenia, focal dystonias, Huntington's chorea, Wilson's disease and rheumatic chorea. Older people and women appear to be more at risk. Fortunately, most patients improve substantially when medication is stopped, usually within months, but sometimes up to one or two years. It is important that neuroleptic medication for schizophrenia should be evaluated at least once a year by reducing the dosage about 10% every three to seven days until the drug has been stopped

completely or the clinical condition worsens. This procedure enables the clinician to determine whether neuroleptic medication is still beneficial and would also help in detecting early withdrawal dyskinesia.

At the present time, treatment with drugs like reserpine, which deplete dopamine stores, produces only temporary benefit. Other treatments have not yet proved to be of established value.

Antidepression Drugs

There are four main groups of drugs used for elevation of mood:

1 Central nervous system stimulants including the amphetamines, pipradol and methylphenidate
2 Monoamine oxidase inhibitor drugs
3 Tricyclic antidepressants (thymoleptics) including imipramine, amitriptyline and nortriptyline
4 New generation antidepressants

Central Nervous System Stimulants

Prior to 1957, the only agents available were central nervous system stimulants which had a limited application and serious disadvantages. The disadvantages of amphetamines include tolerance, dependency and addiction. A short-lasting elevation of mood is followed by post-medication increase of fatigue, irritability and depression. They have little effect in moderately severe or severe depressions and the main indication for the amphetamine drugs is in patients with a short-lasting, early-morning depression of moderate or mild degree of severity.

Monoamine Oxidase Inhibitors

Iproniazid is similar in chemical structure to isoniazid, which for many years has been used successfully in the treatment of tuberculosis. Iproniazid was therefore first used for treating tuberculosis patients, and although it was found to be effective in promoting the healing of the tuberculous lesions, it had to be discontinued because of its side effects due to stimulation of the central nervous system. Patients became restless, over-active and sometimes frankly disturbed and abnormal in behaviour. These unwanted side effects provided a clue for the use of this drug in psychiatric treatment, and it was found to be particularly helpful in depressive illnesses, even longstanding ones which had not responded to other methods.

Iproniazid has the capacity for inhibiting the action of monoamine oxidase (MAO) as well as the actions of many other enzyme systems. There is considerable evidence that depressive illnesses are associated with a decrease in the level of biogenic amines such as noradrenaline and serotonin in certain parts of the central nervous system and it has been demonstrated both in experimental animals and in human beings that monoamine oxidase inhibiting drugs cause an increase in the levels of such amines in the central nervous system during the course of two to four weeks, corresponding with the interval of time before clinical improvement occurs in depression treated with MAO inhibiting drugs. Although iproniazid is undoubtedly efficacious in the treatment of many cases of depression, some of its adverse reactions were found to be serious, particularly its hepatotoxicity which sometimes proved fatal. It is an infrequent occurrence: approximately one in 4000 patients is affected, and the mortality rate is about 1 in 10 000.

Attempts were therefore made to discover new drugs with comparable or greater efficacy, and it was hoped, with greater safety. Some of these drugs are shown in Table 39.7. The present status regarding their clinical use may be summarized as follows. The most potent drugs in this class are iproniazid and tranylcypromine, but these also tend to have a rather high incidence of side effects. Nialamide and isocarboxazid are probably the safest, the other drugs occupying an intermediate position.

Patients treated with these drugs have to be warned to avoid eating cheese, certain wines such as red Chianti, certain beers, foodstuffs such as Marmite and Bovril, and must not take any other medication without consulting their doctor. The reason for this is that certain of these foodstuffs which contain tyramine can induce one of the most dramatic adverse reactions—the hypertensive crisis. Normally tyramine is broken down in the alimentary canal but in patients on monoamine oxidase inhibiting drugs, the enzymes responsible for breaking down tyramine are inhibited, and the latter is therefore absorbed into the blood stream causing a massive release of noradrenalin. This causes a sudden marked rise in blood pressure which is fluctuating and causes an intense headache and in some people may even cause a cerebral haemorrhage. The emerg-

ency is alleviated by administration of an alpha adrenergic blocking agent such as phentolamine to reduce blood pressure. Certain medications which contain sympathomimetic amines, such as cough mixtures containing ephedrine, may also cause elevations of blood pressure in patients on medication with MAO inhibiting drugs.

The reason that these drugs are still in use despite these practical drawbacks is that some patients will not respond to any antidepressants other than these and may be clinically unsuitable for electroconvulsive therapy. The latter is still the treatment of choice for very severe depression.

The Tricyclic Antidepressants

Imipramine, similar chemically to chlorpromazine, was first investigated for its efficacy as a tranquillizer and, as these properties were not marked, the drug was overlooked for a number of years until Kuhn (1958) tried it for the treatment of depression with good results. It has now been used for many years in all parts of the world and there is general agreement that it is an effective drug in the treatment of some forms of depression.

Experimental work has shown that it influences many brain mechanisms, stimulating some and depressing others. It is characteristic of the action of imipramine that it takes one to three weeks to produce beneficial effects, despite rapid absorption.

Table 39.5   Tricyclic antidepressants

Approved name	Proprietary name
Imipramine	Tofranil
Desipramine	Pertofran
Clomipramine	Anafranil
Amitriptyline	Tryptizol
Nortriptyline	Aventyl, Allegron
Protriptyline	Concordin
Dothiepin	Prothiaden
Dibenzepin	Noveril
Trimipramine	Surmontil
Iprindole	Prondol
Opipramol	Insidon
Doxepin	Sinequan

In practice, the tricyclic antidepressants are usually given a trial first of all because they do not demand special precautions. Those in common use are shown

Table 39.5. They vary in their clinical action; some, such as amitriptyline and trimipramine, have sedative action and these are the drugs of choice for patients suffering from depression associated with marked agitation and anxiety. The whole daily dose can be conveniently given at night-time, and this helps to promote better sleep. Sleep difficulty is one of the cardinal symptoms in depression. Some drugs are particularly indicated because of their stimulating action as well as their ability to relieve depression: these include desipramine, protriptyline and nortriptyline. Others show varying degrees of capacity for relieving depression, relieving anxiety and for stimulating drive and energy.

Current views on the mode of action of the monoamine oxidase inhibiting drugs and the tricyclic antidepressants are indicated in Fig. 39.2.

peyotl cactus from which mescaline is derived, ipomea which contains a chemical similar to lysergic acid, the psilocybe mushroom, the active principle of which is psilocybin, the plant *datura stramonium* (thorn-apple) containing scopalamine and atropine. Other plants used in South America included lianas like *banisteria caapi*, also *erythroxylon* containing cocaine, and there is at least one hallucinogenic animal, a caterpillar found in bamboo stems.

Psychotomimetic compounds including the numerous natural and synthetic drugs can be classified chemically into a number of groups: the catecholamine group, including mescaline and amphetamine derivatives; the indoleamine group, including derivatives such as lysergic acid diethylamide (LSD) and tryptamine derivatives; cannabinols, for example, tetrahydrocannabinol found in

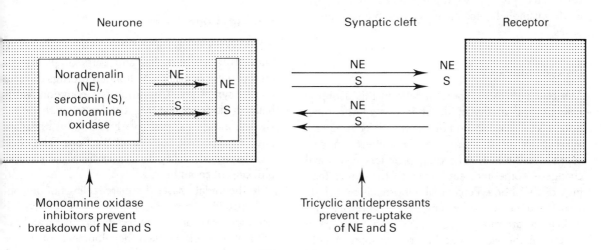

Figure 39.2

Hallucinogenic Drugs

Hallucinogenic or psychotomimetic drugs have the capacity to induce disturbances of mood, thinking, abnormalities of perception, including hallucinations. The term psychotomimetic is probably preferable as hallucinations are by no means an invariable effect of these drugs. Psychotomimetic drugs derived from various plants have been used since time immemorial. They were used for religious purposes and for festivals and orgies. The use of the poisonous toadstool *amanita mascaria* extends over thousands of years. In the Aztec and Mayan cultures of ancient Mexico a number of plants were used because of their hallucinogenic properties. They included the

Table 39.6 New generation antidepressants
(see pp. 158–9)

Approved name	Proprietary name	Recommended daily dose (mg)
Maprotiline	Ludiomil	50–150
Mianserin	Bolvidon Norval	20–60
Viloxazine	Vivalan	100–300
L tryptophan	Optimax	1000–2000
Flupenthixol	Fluanxol	1–3
Trazodone	Molipaxin	100–150

marihuana; piperidyl benzilates including anti-cholinergic drugs such as ditran and benactyzine; phencyclidine, which is chemically related to pethidine.

Catecholamines

Mescaline is not an indole but, theoretically, could undergo cyclization to form an indole. A dose of mescaline equivalent to 5 mg per kg in the average normal subject causes anxiety, sympathomimetic effects, hyper-reflexia, tremors and vivid hallucinations, which are usually brightly coloured and geometrical in form. Colour and space perception are often altered but consciousness is normal and insight is usually retained. Substituted phenyl ethylamines such as 3,4-dimethoxyphenylethylamine and substituted phenyl isopropyl amines such as trimethoxyamphetamine have psychotomimetic properties.

Indoleamines

The best known psychotomimetic in this group is lysergic acid diethylamide. It is one of the most potent known drugs and doses as low as 20–25 μg are capable of producing marked effects in susceptible individuals. The drug produces emotional changes—sometimes euphoria, at other times feelings of dysphoria. Perceptual abnormalities include visual and tactile hallucinations but auditory hallucinations are rare. Lysergic acid produces marked effects on the autonomic nervous system, mainly sympathomimetic. Some patients are enabled to remember early experiences vividly as if they were actually re-enacting the past, and this property has been used to facilitate psychotherapy, particularly as emotional release is facilitated. Certain tryptamine derivatives such as *N*-dimethyl tryptamine (DMT) have psychotomimetic properties.

Cannabis

Cannabis from marihuana, hashish and Indian hemp, has a long history, not only as a means used to produce tranquillity by Indian yogis, but for many years it has been mistakenly blamed for stimulating violent and erotic behaviour. The effects of acute intoxication of cannabis are feelings of well-being, excitement, disturbance of associations, alterations

in the appreciation of time and space, enhance auditory sensitivity with the elaborations of simpl phrases or tunes, emotional upheaval, illusior and hallucinations. Suggestibility is increased. Ver often the feeling of well-being alternates with de pression.

Some subjects experience acute anxiety as we as the initial effects. The phases of abnormality i thinking, perception and memory often come i waves, heralded by sudden violent headaches. Larg doses of the drug can produce delirium, confusioi disorientation, disturbances of mood including terrc or anger, with subsequent amnesia. This is a fairl typical toxic confusional state. Superimposed on th there may be delusions of persecution and sometime suicidal tendencies.

Piperidyl Benzilates

It has been known for many years that intoxicatic with atropine, hyoscine and parts of plants cor taining these or other anticholinergic drugs can caus mental symptoms. Confusion is a common featur hallucinations are less frequent. Some synthetic ant cholinergic drugs, particularly piperidyl benzilate have marked psychotomimetic actions. The effec are decreased ability to concentrate with marke blocking of thought.

In the initial phases there are feelings of unrealit and inability to concentrate. This is followed b fleeting visual and auditory disturbances and sul sequently more marked development of halluc nations. Occasionally paranoid delusions occur. Th general picture is much more like a toxic confusion state than that produced by the lysergic acid dieth lamide.

Phencyclidine

Unlike lysergic acid the acute effects of phencyclidir begin at once and subside in about an hour. First all there is a feeling of sleepiness, then a decrease pain and touch sensations and a decrease in auditor and visual acuity. Euphoria is usual although anxiei and depression sometimes occur, characteristical there are difficulties in thinking with feelings unreality and disturbances of body image and tim perception.

Cocaine

The plant *erythroxylon coca*, which contains cocaine, has been used for centuries in South America because it was believed to increase efficiency for work in high altitudes. Cocaine is a central nervous system stimulant, produces feelings of euphoria or even short periods of ecstasy, but it has many side effects and these are subjectively unpleasant, and this is why cocaine has not become a common drug of addiction in Great Britain.

Psychotomimetic compounds have been used as tools for research for studying the functions of the central nervous system, for producing models of schizophrenia for research investigations. They have also been used to facilitate psychotherapy in resistant patients, such as those with personality disorders, obsessional states, alcoholism and sexual deviations.

Hallucinogenic drugs are very little used in this country at the present time for therapeutic purposes. The non-therapeutic use of these drugs however, has greatly increased, particularly with regard to LSD and cannabis.

Lithium Therapy

Lithium was originally used in the treatment of mania and in hypomania, for which it was found to be efficacious. More recently lithium therapy has been found to be an effective prophylactic measure in the treatment of recurrent affective disorders, whether these are recurrent hypomania or mania, or recurrent depression (unipolar affective disorders) or recurrence of hypomania, mania and depression in the same patient (bipolar affective disorders).

The natural history of affective disorders is that they tend to be recurrent and that attacks tend to occur more frequently and sometimes with greater severity with the passage of time. Bipolar affective disorder tends to start at an earlier age and to have a shorter cycle length than unipolar affective illness. Patients who show a tendency to have attacks of affective disorder with increasing frequency as they grow older are particularly suitable for prophylactic treatment with lithium. A useful guideline for considering lithium therapy is the recurrence of an affective disorder of more than once in 2 years.

Dosage: The usual practice is to use haloperidol or chlorpromazine to treat moderate or severe mania.

When lithium is used for hypomania and mild forms of mania, the dose can be gradually built up, starting with an initial dose of 250–400 mg daily, increased gradually to produce serum lithium levels of between 0.5–1.00 mm/l within 10 to 14 days. Low levels may be necessary in the elderly because of the development of side effects. The therapeutic range for serum lithium is between 0.5–1.6 mmol. The toxic symptoms tend to occur with the levels approaching or exceeding 1.6 and, therefore, most people aim at achieving serum lithium levels between 0.5 and 1.0 mm/l. The usual dose range required is 600–1200 mg a day given in divided doses. For the elderly the dose should be between 500 and 1000 mg in divided doses, and, whereas in younger people toxic symptoms are associated with concentrations exceeding 1.5 mmol, in the elderly, toxic reactions tend to occur with serum concentration of about 1.00 mmol.

Lithium therapy should not be started unless adequate facilities for routine monitoring of serum levels are available. When therapy has started, serum levels should be measured weekly until steady states are achieved, then weekly for one month and thereafter at monthly intervals. More frequent measurements are necessary if signs of lithium toxicity occur, or when the dose is altered or when significant intercurrent disease occurs, or when signs of a relapse of mania or depression occur, or if any significant change in sodium or fluid intake occurs. As biovariability varies from product to product, particularly regarding slow release preparations, change of product should be regarded as initiation of new treatment. Blood levels should, therefore, be monitored weekly until stabilization is achieved. More frequent monitoring is required if patients are receiving diuretics. For mania, good control of symptoms is usually achieved by a serum lithium level of 1.1 mm/l. A serum lithium should be taken just before the dose after the longest interdose interval during the 24 hours, usually an interval of 12 hours is necessary after the last dose of lithium before the blood sample is taken for estimation.

Before starting treatment full physical examinations must be carried out and special investigations to include assessment of renal functions, urine analysis, assessment of thyroid function and cardiac function.

Lithium is excreted by the kidney and renal disease is a contraindication. As lithium may interfere with

Table 39.7   Monoamine oxidase inhibitors and central nervous system stimulants

Approved name	Proprietary name	Usual daily dosage range (mg)	Autonomic reactions	Hyper-flexion	Hyper-tension	Hepatic pathology	Blood dyscrasia	Peripheral oedema	Other effects
Iproniazid	Marsilid	50–150	+	+	+	+	+	+	
Phenelzine	Nardil	15–75							
Nialamide	Niamid	35–300	+	+	+	+	+	+	
Isocarboxazid	Marplan	10–30	+	+	+	+	+	+	
Tranylcypromine	Parnate	10–30	+	+	+	o	o	o	Severe headaches occasionally occur
Mebanazine	Actomol		+	+	−	−	−	+	
Amphetamines	Benzedrine Dexedrine Methedrine	5–20	+	+	+	o	o	o	Sympathomimetic side effects Addictive psychotic episodes
Phenmetrazine	Preludin	12.5–75	+	+	+	o	o	o	Sympathomimetic side effects Addictive psychotic episodes
Pipradol	Meratran	5–25							Increased anxiety
Methylphenidate	Ritalin	5–20							Anxiety symptoms, schizophrenic manifestations made worse

the electrolyte balance, circulatory failure is also a contraindication. Lithium is not effective in treating an attack of depression, but is effective in preventing the recurrences of attacks of depression in recurrent depressive disorders. It is even more effective in the prophylactic treatment of bipolar affective illness.

Unwanted Effects

Certain side effects are harmless, such as nausea, loose stools, fine tremor of the hand, polyuria and polydipsia. Other effects are serious in import and necessitate lowering of dosage. These include gross tremor of the hands, twitchings and fasciculations in the limbs, hands and face, drowsiness, unsteadiness, slurred speech, impaired concentration, disorientation, loss of memory and dizziness. Severe toxic effects include confusion, restlessness, ataxia, nystagmus, epileptiform seizures, delirium, coma and eventually death. Patients should be advised to maintain their usual salt and fluid intake. Lower doses of lithium may be needed during diuretic therapy as lithium clearance is reduced. Raised plasma levels of antidiuretic hormone may occur during treatment. Serum lithium levels may increase during concomitant therapy with indomethazine or tetracyclines.

Treatment of lithium intoxication is unsatisfactory since there is no specific antidote, but diuresis produced by intravenous urea combined with alkalinization of urine by sodium lactate helps to increase lithium excretion.

Long term treatment with lithium may result in permanent changes in the kidney and impairment of renal function. High serum concentrations of lithium including episodes of acute lithium toxicity may enhance these changes. The minimum clinically effective dose of lithium should always be used patients should be maintained on lithium therapy after 3–5 years only, if on assessment, benefit persists. Long term treatment with lithium is frequently associated with disturbances of thyroid function including raised levels of thyroid stimulating hormone, goitre and clinical hypothyroidism. Hypothyroidism is not a contraindication to the continuation of lithium treatment and can be treated with thyroid hormone.

Lithium treatment for prophylactic purposes may have to be given indefinitely and it has been noticed that sometimes its efficacy may not achieve its optimum before a year's medication. The response varies from a decrease in severity in attacks, decrease in frequency of attacks and in some, the complete prevention of recurrences.

If a patient undergoing lithium prophylactic treatment develops depression or hypomania, the appropriate pharmacotherapeutic measures for these can be given concurrently with lithium.

Prescribing for the Elderly

The reduced ability of the liver to metabolize drugs in the elderly, together with the fact that serum albumin is reduced and therefore allows a greater

uantity of the free drug to exert its phar-
nacodynamic effects, makes it imperative to give
ower doses of drugs to the elderly. This applies
articularly to tricyclic antidepressants which, if
iven in the usual adult dose, will tend to cause
oxic confusional states in the elderly. Similarly,
enzodiazepines and other drugs, unless given in
ower doses, will carry a greater risk of producing
ide effects and adverse reactions in the elderly.

Further Reading

Paykel, E. S. and Coppen, R. (eds) (1979) *Psychophar-macology of Affective Disorders.* London University Press.

Johnson, F. N. (1980) *Handbook of Lithium Therapy.* MIP.

Waxman, D. (1981) *Hypnosis.* Allen & Unwin, London.

Crammer, J., Barraclough, B. and Heine, B. (1982) *The Use of Drugs in Psychiatry,* 2nd edn. Gaskell Books, Ashford, Kent.

Silverstone, T. and Turner, P. (1982) *Drug Treatment in Psychiatry.* Routledge, London.

40

Physical Methods

Convulsive Therapy

The application of therapeutic convulsions in the treatment of mental illness was introduced in 1935 by Meduna. He induced major epileptic fits by means of intravenous cardiazol for the treatment of schizophrenic patients because of the belief held at the time that epilepsy and schizophrenia were biologically antagonistic.

Although this theory has been disproved it has continued to a restricted degree in the treatment of schizophrenia but its main field of application is in severe depressive states.

Cerletti and Bini, just before World War II, introduced the electrical method of inducing therapeutic convulsions as it was less distressing to the patient, technically easier and the effects more certain. Nowadays the treatment is given under general anaesthesia with thiopentone or methohexitone. These anaesthetics are given intravenously and then a muscle relaxant such as succinylcholine is given to modify the muscular contractions.

Therapeutic convulsions unmodified by muscular relaxants carry the risk of producing bony injury or dislocation which are definite but rare risks.

The treatment is usually given twice weekly until improvement occurs. Sometimes improvement in depression occurs after one or two treatments but, usually, after three or four or even later. The improvement, once it develops after a particular treatment, will tend to build up until complete recovery takes place. The number of treatments required varies with the individual case; some patients recover with six or seven but many require twelve or more.

When full recovery is achieved, it is wise to keep in mind that it may be necessary to give one or two more treatments after a week or longer in the event of recurrence of depression. Failure to do this has resulted in many cases not deriving as much benefit from the treatment as they otherwise could.

Classically, the electrodes are placed over each temporo-frontal area (bilateral ECT), but modern practice is tending towards administering unilateral ECT to the non-dominant cerebral hemisphere with electrodes placed over the temple and the mastoid region of the same side. This unilateral placement is followed by less unwanted side effects such as headache and memory impairment, and is claimed to be equally effective. However administered, ECT must produce a full bilateral convulsion if therapeutic benefit is to be achieved.

Electronarcosis is a more intensive and prolonged form of ECT treatment, in which there is a continued passage of the current over a period of up to seven minutes.

Electroconvulsive therapy is sometimes followed by difficulty in remembering events, but this usually passes off after varying periods of time. It is important to warn patients about this beforehand.

Indications for Electroconvulsive Therapy

1 Severe depressive states
2 Schizophrenia with an admixture of depression or, in failure to respond to phenothiazine drugs, ECT can be given concurrently

The Surgical Treatment of Mental Illness (Psychosurgery)

Moniz introduced the operation of prefrontal leucotomy for intractable psychiatric disorders.

A variety of operative procedures have been devised since, and are collectively referred to as psychosurgery.

Originally the standard prefrontal leucotomy operation consisted of severing the white matter of each frontal lobe as widely as possible. This operation had many undesirable side effects such as apathy, lethargy, inability to control aggressive impulses, high incidence of epilepsy, and the efficacy of the treatment was due to the interruption of the thalamo-frontal connections, notably between the dorsal/medial thalamic nuclei and the frontal cortex. In order to achieve the maximum therapeutic effect with the minimum undesirable effects, modified leucotomy operations have been devised since. These include bimedial leucotomy, blind rostral leucotomy, orbital undercutting, frontal undercutting.

Bimedial leucotomy involves a cut in the white matter, made under direct vision to sever the thalamo-frontal bundle, which is known to be the main pathway from the thalamus to the frontal pole and orbital frontal surface.

The variations known as bimedial leucotomy, orbital undercutting and blind rostral leucotomy are of comparable therapeutic value. Bimedial leucotomy and orbital undercutting have the advantage of being open operations and the extent of the lesion which they produce can be controlled with greater accuracy.

During recent years a number of stereotactic procedures for psychosurgery have been introduced, for example, bifrontal stereotactic tractotomy. This involves the insertion of two rows of three radioactive yttrium seeds on each side into the white matter of the posterior orbital cortex in area 13, referred to as substantia innominata,

Another new procedure is stereotactic limbic leucotomy, the object of which is to interrupt connections between the frontal cortex and the limbic system, and to make lesions in one of the main limbic circuits to the anterior cingulate gyrus.

Another method is to employ stereotactic thermal lesions by means of insulated electrodes introduced laterally to and 6–7 mm posterior to the tips of the anterior horn so as to interrupt the fronto-thalamic radiation.

In deciding on whether a leucotomy is indicated, it is usual to try all available therapeutic measures first as the operation involves causing permanent damage to the brain, but failure of therapeutic methods is not in itself an indication for leucotomy. This must be done as a result of a careful assessment of all aspects of the case, including the patient's personality, the form of his mental illness and his social circumstances.

Firstly, the main indication for leucotomy is for the relief of emotional tension and distress, whether this is in the form of an anxiety state, an agitated depression or any other form of distress, if of sufficient severity to interfere with the patient's life and well-being. Clear evidence of emotional and/or its bodily manifestations must be present before an operation is carried out. An assessment of the patient's personality is of the utmost importance because the leucotomy operation will not improve the patient's personality and, as control may be somewhat diminished, it is undesirable to carry out the operation on patients who are of ill-adjusted, unstable, anti-social, psychopathic or markedly hysterical personality. People who are in any event impulsive have difficulty in self-control; these are states of personality which are in danger of being made worse by leucotomy. The patient's personality should be reasonably well-adjusted as shown by the patient's adjustment to school, work, marriage and social relationships generally. The main point when assessing personality is that the contraindicative attributes must not be present.

The third aspect which merits careful assessment is the social circumstances of the patient. The operation of leucotomy is one stage of treatment and in order to achieve the best results, prolonged rehabilitation is usually necessary. Although immediate symptomatic improvement usually takes place, in many patients it requires careful nursing, active occupational and recreational programmes and eventually returning to suitable work with the aim of making the person an effective member of society. It is for these reasons that it is important that the patient should have relatives, friends or family who will be supporting, understanding and helpful during the process of rehabilitation.

With the careful selection of patients results of modified leucotomy are very encouraging, particularly as the operation is carried out on those patients who are of long standing and have failed to respond to the ordinary therapeutic measures.

Further Reading

Kalinowsky, L. B. and Hippus, H. (1969) *Pharmacological, Convulsive and Other Somatic Treatments in Psychiatry.* Grune & Stratton, New York.

Pippard, J. and Ellam, L. (1980) *ECT in Great Britain. A Report to the Royal College of Psychiatrists.* Gaskell Books, Ashford, Kent.

Sargant, W. and Slater, E. (1963) *An Introduction to Physical Methods of Treatment in Psychiatry.* Churchill Livingstone, Edinburgh. (6th revised edn. by P. Dally and J. Connolly, 1981.)

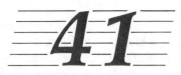

Occupational Therapy and Rehabilitation

Thomas Carlyle once wrote 'Blessed is he who has found his work, let him ask no other blessedness'. This is true for all people and is particularly true for patients who have recovered from a prolonged illness or have to spend long periods in hospital.

Rehabilitation

Rehabilitation is the process of getting a person who has been ill, or has a disability, back to as full a working capacity as is possible, commensurate with his ability to perform the tasks required, and to resume normal social activities.

Effective rehabilitation involves accurate diagnosis including assessment of physical and mental disabilities. In the diagnostic assessment it is important to note the patient's assets as well as deficits in order to plan effective rehabilitative treatment. Finally, it is essential to make a prognostic assessment so that appropriate adequate and definitive care can be planned.

A well organized rehabilitation programme includes an integrated medical and functional assessment enlisting the resources of medical, social, psychiatric, psychological and industrial expertise as necessary.

Delay in making decisions and delay in communicating them can result in increased morbidity and delayed rehabilitation. Rehabilitation in elderly patients has to take into account special problems which are especially associated with old age.

Rehabilitation in the elderly also needs to take into account various losses which tend to occur in old age. These include:

1 Loss of status following retirement
2 Decrease in income after retirement
3 Decrease in physical energy, well-being and positive good health
4 Loss of company and social contacts. The loss of contact with the circle of friends, neighbours and acquaintances which was developed during working life and which are often lost after retirement, particularly if this is also associated with moving house
5 Loss of independence
6 Loss of key persons by the death of spouse, relatives and friends

These are all major life changes constituting potentially stressful experiences and taxing a person's adaptive capacity to the full.

The quality of life in the elderly patients, as at earlier ages, depends on the ability of people to live to their full potential as human beings. This involves not only the satisfaction of the basic needs for food, rest and sleep, but also the greatest possible degree of mobility and independence in daily living and the provision of as much help as is necessary to achieve this state. In addition to the satisfaction of physical needs there are important psychological needs in the elderly, particularly when admitted to hospital. One is the importance of preserving the patient's feeling of identity and self-esteem. There is also a great need for affection and a great need to maintain as much independence as possible. In the case of those bereaved, it is important that the physiological effects of grief should be understood and that the elderly bereaved person should be given the opportunity of expressing his feelings and of working through his grief reaction. This might take time and would require understanding and tolerance on the part of those looking after him. Social needs include the maintenance of interpersonal relationships which tend to decrease with increasing age. In hospital it is very important to establish social contacts and interpersonal relationships with relatives, friends, other patients, nursing and medical staff. Interests of all kinds need to be continued and encouraged, and adequate attention given to the need for privacy.

Rehabilitation After Acute Myocardial Infarction

Following a limited period of rest in bed, depending on the severity of the infarction, walking is usually allowed about 14 days after the acute attack and thereafter an active rehabilitation calls for a gradual withdrawal of help from the patient as confidence of both the patient and his family improves. Not infrequently marked anxiety and depression in the patient may be more distressing and incapacitating than the physical damage. Appropriate reassurance and explanation are of vital importance and the patient should be given clear instructions about his activities, diet, leisure and physical training. Exercise increases cardiovascular capacity, lowers the cost of physical activity by a reduction in heart rate and blood pressure, and changes muscle metabolism and reduces serum triglycerides and free fatty acids. In addition to this, the reduction of anxiety and the knowledge that physical effort does not cause harm is of immeasurable value. The rehabilitation programme for the post-coronary patient may be summarized as follows:

1 To remove the adverse psychological effects of the illness
2 To teach the patient the prudent limits of activity and exercise
3 To remove the fear of physical activity and to improve morale
4 To increase cardiac function and to improve or relieve angina of effort

As Nichols (1946) pointed out, the major cause of persisting disability after a mild cardiac infarction is psychological. Anxiety and depression may cause the patient almost total disability even when there is no organic basis for these symptoms.

Rehabilitation should start with the treatment of the acute episode and nowadays patients are being mobilized and discharged home earlier than previously. The family doctor can play a key part in deciding and monitoring the patient's rate of progress, and liaison between the hospital and the family doctor is of the utmost importance. Rehabilitation must be planned taking into account the patient's needs and such factors as age, sex, marital status, level of physical fitness and the nature of his previous employment.

Rehabilitation After Strokes

Hemiplegia is one of the most commonly occurring physical disabilities after a cerebrovascular accident. Four common cerebrovascular lesions which may result in hemiplegia are thrombosis, intracranial haemorrhage, subarachnoid haemorrhage and cerebral embolism. Mortality is related to age, to the severity of the preceding hypertension, to the severity of the cardiac dysfunction and the duration and depth of the initial unconsciousness. With cerebral embolism, two-thirds of the patients die within three years and the average survival period is two years. With cerebral infarction only one-half die in three years and the average survival time is three or four years. The assessment of thrombosis and morbidity depends on accurate and repeated examination and an assessment of the residual disability and functional capacity in any particular patient. If complete recovery is to occur, it is accomplished usually within two months. Complete recovery does not occur in a patient who is left with a residual hemiplegia, which may be complete or incomplete, and may have, in addition to paralysis, sensory defects. If hemiplegia is the only disability, the patient with a complete residual hemiplegia can become ambulant and self-caring within four weeks. He may have to have a short or long leg brace and possibly walk with a cane in the initial stages. Assessment of the clinical condition in hemiplegia following a stroke involves the assessment of loss of motor power, loss of sensation, hemianopia, aphasia, apraxia, dementia and urinary incontinence, all of which have to be taken into account in order to plan the rehabilitation programme. Rehabilitation in the early acute stages involves physiotherapy, consisting of passive movements of all limb joints of the affected side to prevent contractures, and to prevent deformity by the use of a bed cage, foot boards, auxiliary pillow and palmar wrist splints. As soon as possible sitting and bed edge activities must be introduced, including sitting, kneeling and balancing exercises. Physiotherapy at this stage is directed towards prevention of chest complications by breathing exercises, postural drainage, continuing mobilization of joints, particularly the shoulder, prevention of contractures of hip and foot, and restoring balance and postural control. As soon as recovery starts, active rehabilitation is introduced, including standing, walking and arm mobilizing exercises, supplemented by passive movements of those joints which the patient cannot move himself. The goals of rehabilitation are set out by Hirschberg *et al* (1976) as follows:

1 The achievement of mobility and ambulation
2 The achievement of self-care
3 Psychosocial adjustment to disability
4 Prevention of secondary disability

The degree of success achieved by rehabilitation will depend as much on the patient's mental state as his physical condition. Success or failure will depend on the patient's ability to understand, to accept and to adjust himself to the level of physical disability and distress inherent in any particular stage of recovery and also upon his ability to cooperate in procedures designed to improve functions.

The deficits following a stroke may include impairment of perception, impairment of intellectual functions, changes in emotional state and changes in personality.

The ultimate prognosis will depend not only on the degree of physical disability, but on the additive effects of intellectual impairment, personality changes and psychiatric symptoms, particularly anxiety or depression. On these will depend the patient's eventual ability to undertake normal activities and to participate in social and family relationships and also individual suffering and incapacity. Persistent emotional lability tends to carry a poor prognosis.

A consistent finding is that a rehabilitation programme designed to increase sensory input and to facilitate motor output of the brain will benefit patients who have suffered from a stroke. The degree of benefit would depend on the empathy and expertise of the therapist and the cooperation and motivation which the patient is capable of mobilizing.

The psychiatrist, in liaison with the neurologist, general physician and expert on rehabilitation, can play an important role in determining the patient's mental state. He can both alleviate conditions which militate against effective rehabilitation such as depression or anxiety, and assess the patient's attitude and motivation, all of which can play as important a part in the success of rehabilitation as the physical lesion itself.

Occupational Therapy

Occupational therapy is activity and work prescribed as treatment.

Occupational therapy may be the initial, very important step towards rehabilitation.

When patients enter hospital they enter into a new life, and interests, emotions and energies taken up in their normal activities 'hang fire' as it were. Emotions do not hang fire for long and soon become attached to symptoms and magnify them.

The patient has plenty of time to think about himself and his symptoms and may become introspective. When a patient has to stay in hospital for long periods, normal habits of work tend to be lost. The ordinary motives, rewards, punishments and incentives of everyday life are missing. It is not surprising, therefore, that patients who have to stay in hospital for long periods without having any work to do may become inert, apathetic and useless, in other words 'hospitalized'.

This was found during the First World War, when large numbers of patients treated in hospitals over long periods tended to deteriorate and their morale weakened. When occupational therapy was provided, this tendency to deterioration was prevented.

Occupational therapy has the following advantages:

1 It diverts the patient's attention from himself on to other things
2 His interest and energies are directed to work
3 It maintains normal habits of work
4 It provides an incentive and a goal
5 It enables the patient to have a feeling of achievement when he completes the task
6 It stimulates interest and attention
7 It may teach the patient a new skill or hobby
8 The feeling of doing something useful and pride in achievement will help his self-esteem

9   It helps to make the patient more accessible and more cooperative with other forms of therapy

10   It aids production of positive attitudes and helps decision making

11   It aids focusing of attention and integration

Occupational therapy must arouse and sustain the patient's interest. In order to do this, the following considerations have to be borne in mind:

1   Adults must not be given childish activities

2   The initial act and the goal must not be too far removed from each other. In other words, the patient should be able to complete the work within a reasonable time so that the goal is always in sight and acting as an incentive

3   The work should be progressive in skill, difficulty and complexity so that the patient can obtain a feeling of success and continued progress

4   The standard of the expected performance must be based on the capacity of the patient and not on other people's standards

5   The work must be within the capacity of the patient but not so easy that interest is not evoked

6   Encouragement and not criticism should be used

The aims of occupational therapy are:

1   Promotion of recovery

2   Mobilization of the total assets of the patient

3   Prevention of hospitalization

4   Creation of good habits of work and leisure

5   Rehabilitation with return of self-confidence

Rehabilitation in its modern concept involves:

1   Introduction of methods of physical rehabilitation into every ward, adapted to individual disabilities and stages of recovery, commencing as early as possible after admission

2   Planning of convalescence with a view to speeding up the recovery of physical and psychological functions

3   Hospital attendance on an outpatient basis for rehabilitation after injuries which may not have necessitated inpatient treatment

The patient's daily programme should be carefully prescribed so as to fill his day with a reasonable balance of work, rest and recreation.

Passive Physiotherapy

This includes heat, massage and electrotherapy relaxation. It is only required in a minority of patients, as the main emphasis of rehabilitation is on active movements which the patients themselves carry out

This stimulates active interest and participation, inducing a feeling of responsibility for their part in the treatment.

Remedial Exercises

Two distinct but complementary aims are:

1   General bodily toning up

2   Restoration of functions to the disabled part

The exercises may be started in bed and continued, when the patient is able, in the gymnasium or out of doors.

The movements may be:

1   Assisted by the therapist

2   Free

3   Resisted by pulleys and weights or springs

Organized games such as medicine ball, volley ball, badminton etc. stimulate spontaneity and freedom of movement. The competitive spirit and excitement tends to take away the patient's anxious preoccupation with the diseased part.

Occupation Therapy

1   Diversional

2   Remedial—for particular muscle groups, e.g. basket-work, carpentry, embroidery, gardening

Lectures, Discussion Groups and Entertainments

These promote intellectual stimulation, interest and relaxation. A social worker may be required to help in home problems, so that the patient can continue with rehabilitation as free as possible from worries.

Re-employment

The Disablement Rehabilitation Officer (DRO) of the Department of Health and Social Security is specially trained to place disabled persons in suitable work.

Arrangements can be made for the DRO to see the patient in hospital before discharge, furnished with information and recommendation by the doctor in charge.

Therapeutic Community

This term is applied to a psychiatric hospital which emphasizes the importance of interpersonal influences and environmental and social factors in the treatment, management and rehabilitation of patients. Restrictions and regimentations are reduced to a minimum and the patient is helped to understand his problems in terms of interpersonal relations, and his role in relationship to other people.

Community Psychiatry

Community psychiatry is concerned with the provision of a comprehensive programme of mental health care to a defined population. In the United Kingdom the recent extensive development of psychiatric units in general hospitals which serve defined catchment areas has been coupled with support units of the psychiatric unit dealing with specific sectors of the catchment area by means of teams of psychiatrists, social workers, and nurses. This system has now become the established pattern of the psychiatric services.

A great deal still has to be done by local authorities in providing hostels, day centres, and retraining and rehabilitation services, before psychiatry achieves its maximum effectiveness.

Community psychiatry should also be committed to prevention in all its aspects. Primary prevention is the promotion of mental health and prevention of psychiatric and emotional disorders as far as this is possible. Secondary prevention is the detection of psychiatric illness in the early stages. Tertiary prevention, or rehabilitation, is the aim of returning the patient to society using his optimum potential in work and social relationships by concentrating on his assets and recoverable functions.

Further Reading

Nichols, P. J. R. and Hamilton, E. A. (1980) *Rehabilitation Medicine: Management of Physical Disabilities*, 2nd edn. Butterworth, Sevenoaks.

Wansbrough, N. and Cooper, P. (1980) *Open Employment after Mental Illness.* Tavistock Publications, London.

Wing, J. K. and Morris, B. (1981) *Handbook of Psychiatric Rehabilitation Practice.* Oxford University Press, Oxford.

Index

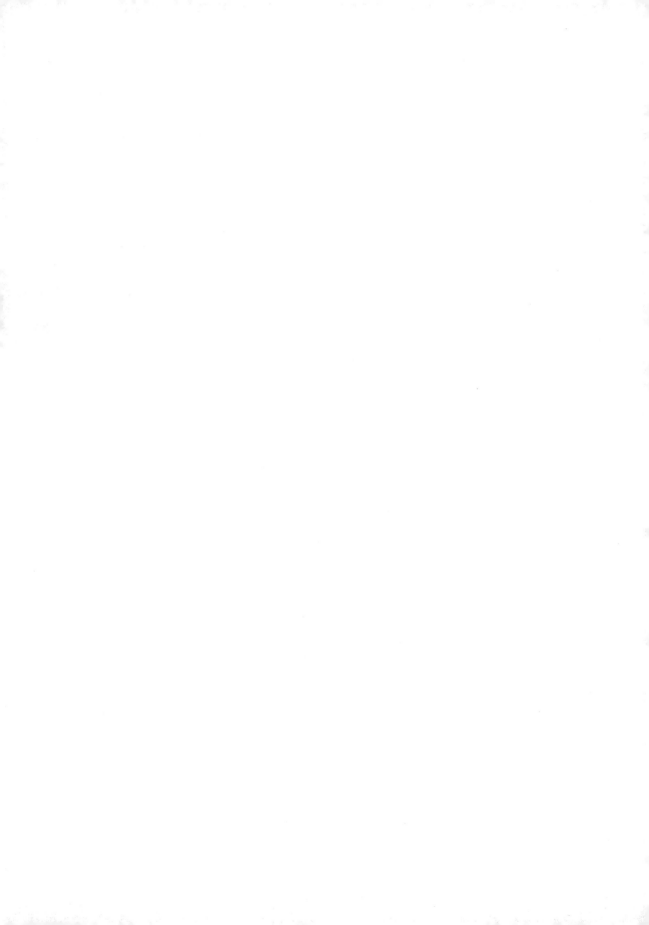